"Finally!!! After 125 years of the great divide between the mind and body, a book that gets psychoanalysis up off the couch and into everyday clinical practice. Combining his formal training as a psychoanalyst with his wealth of hands-on clinical experience and his years of practice as a psychiatrist in hospitals and outpatient clinics and as a dedicated teacher to medical learners, Dr. Steinberg illuminates the psychological factors that shape and influence patient presentations. Through a variety of eloquently described case discussions, interwoven with theoretical constructs, we are invited into the world of the unconscious, as a way of understanding that symptoms and behaviors not otherwise explained by medical models can be solutions to intrapsychic conflict. Dr. Steinberg shows us that, by integrating an understanding of the patient's psychological make-up, we as clinicians can examine and manage the frustrations we may feel, and the therapeutic nihilism we may encounter, when treating people who have complex and unsolvable problems. Moreover, this book illustrates how we can achieve more satisfactory and effective clinical practices, and how we can protect our patients from the pitfalls of overmedicalizing symptoms. This book will have a profound influence on how we think about our patients and will enrich our approaches to helping people with medical and psychiatric disorders or ill-defined symptoms. Dr. Steinberg is the consummate scholar, and most of all, he teaches us to be curious-minded and compassionate in our work with people who struggle in their lives."

David Kenneth Cochrane, MD, FRCPC, medical director General Psychiatry Services, North Bay Regional Health Centre, assistant professor University of Ottawa, assistant professor Northern Ontario School of Medicine, Canada

"Drawing on his in-depth knowledge of contemporary psychoanalytic theories and his extensive experience as a consultation-liaison psychiatrist, Dr. Steinberg provides a clear description of how early attachment experiences with caregivers become represented in children's minds as unconscious images of self and others that influence their sense of self and the quality of their relationships throughout life. Adverse childhood experiences not only affect personality functioning, but also render individuals more susceptible to medical and psychiatric disorders. Dr. Steinberg applies these concepts to patients often described as 'difficult' to manage by their family doctors or hospital specialists, making excellent use of selected case histories to illustrate the operation of defense mechanisms, as well as transference and countertransference phenomena. The book will be immensely useful to family physicians, medical and surgical specialists, and hospital-based psychiatrists."

Graeme J. Taylor, MD, FRCPC, MRCPsych, professor emeritus of Psychiatry, University of Toronto, Canada

PSYCHOANALYSIS IN MEDICINE

This book shows how contemporary psychoanalytic thinking can be applied in the everyday practice of medicine to enhance the practice of family medicine and all clinical specialties.

Dr. Steinberg analyzes his writings over the past 35 years—on psychiatry and family medicine, liaison psychiatry, and supervision and mentoring—based on developments in psychoanalytic thinking. Divided into sections based on different venues of medical practice, including family medicine clinics, inpatient medical and surgical units, and psychiatric inpatient units and outpatient programs, chapters illustrate how various concepts in psychoanalysis can enhance physicians' understanding and management of their patients. A concluding section contains applications of psychoanalytic thought in non-clinical areas pertinent to medicine, including preventing suicide among physicians, residents, and medical students, sexual abuse of patients by physicians, and oral examination anxiety in physicians.

Readers will learn to apply psychoanalytic concepts with a rational approach that enhances their understanding and management of their patients and practice of medicine generally.

Paul Ian Steinberg, MD, is clinical professor, Department of Psychiatry, University of British Columbia, member of the Western Branch – Canadian Psychoanalytic Society, and an assistant editor of the *Canadian Journal of Psychoanalysis/Revue canadienne de psychanalyse*.

PSYCHOANALYSIS IN MEDICINE

Applying Psychoanalytic Thought to Contemporary Medical Care

Paul Ian Steinberg

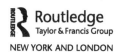
Routledge
Taylor & Francis Group

NEW YORK AND LONDON

First published 2021
by Routledge
52 Vanderbilt Avenue, New York, NY 10017

and by Routledge
2 Park Square, Milton Park, Abingdon, Oxon OX14 4RN

Routledge is an imprint of the Taylor & Francis Group, an informa business

© 2021 Taylor & Francis

Library of Congress Cataloging-in-Publication Data
Names: Steinberg, Paul Ian, author.
Title: Psychoanalysis in medicine: applying psychoanalytic thought to contemporary medical care / Paul Ian Steinberg.
Identifiers: LCCN 2020018877 (print) | LCCN 2020018878 (ebook) |
ISBN 9780367144050 (hardback) | ISBN 9780367144067 (paperback) |
ISBN 9780429031885 (ebook)
Subjects: MESH: Psychoanalytic Theory | Psychoanalytic Therapy |
Primary Health Care | Mental Disorders–diagnosis |
Mental Disorders–therapy | Psychology, Medical
Classification: LCC RC454.4 (print) | LCC RC454.4 (ebook) |
NLM WM 460.2 | DDC 616.89/14–dc23
LC record available at https://lccn.loc.gov/2020018877
LC ebook record available at https://lccn.loc.gov/2020018878

ISBN: 978-0-367-14405-0 (hbk)
ISBN: 978-0-367-14406-7 (pbk)
ISBN: 978-0-429-03188-5 (ebk)

Typeset in Baskerville
by Newgen Publishing UK

To my wife and children

With love and gratitude

CONTENTS

FOREWORD

During the past two decades, advances in psychopharmacology, molecular biology, and functional brain imaging have brought psychiatry closer to mainstream medicine. This rapprochement, however, has been accompanied by a widening of the gap between psychiatry and psychoanalysis, and by greatly reduced opportunities for psychoanalysts to be involved in the care of medically ill patients. In this scholarly and timely book, Dr. Paul Ian Steinberg restores the dialogue between psychoanalysis and medicine by describing advances in psychoanalytic thinking that have expanded understanding of the human mind and of personality characteristics that may play a role in somatic symptom formation and also influence the ways patients experience illness and interact with healthcare professionals.

Drawing on his in-depth knowledge of contemporary psychoanalytic theories and his extensive experience as a consultation-liaison psychiatrist, Dr. Steinberg provides a clear description of how early attachment experiences with caregivers become represented in children's minds as internal object relations that influence their sense of self and the quality of their relationships throughout life. Adverse childhood experiences not only affect personality functioning, but also render individuals more susceptible to medical and psychiatric disorders. Throughout the book Dr. Steinberg applies these concepts to patients who are experienced often as "difficult" to manage by their family doctors or hospital specialists. He makes excellent use of selected case histories to illustrate the operation of psychological defense mechanisms, as well as transference and countertransference phenomena. He also extends his application of psychoanalytic concepts to physicians themselves, who may experience oral examination anxiety or be at risk of suicide or of engaging in unethical behavior with a patient. The book will be immensely useful not only to family physicians and medical and surgical specialists, but also to hospital-based psychiatrists.

Graeme J. Taylor, MD, FRCPC, MRCPsych, professor emeritus of
Psychiatry, University of Toronto, Canada

PUBLICATION ACKNOWLEDGMENTS

I wish to express appreciation to the publishers of the following articles and book chapter who graciously permitted me to incorporate part or all of the latter in this book. The chapters are listed with their corresponding original versions.

Chapter 1: The psychiatry of family practice: Personality disorders. I. The problem patient. *Canadian Family Physician*, 1983, 29:1942–1947; Chapter 2: The psychiatry of family practice: Personality disorders. II. Interviewing the patient. *Canadian Family Physician*, 1983, 29:1953–1957; Chapter 3: The mis-diagnosis of depression. *Canadian Family Physician*, 1989, 35:1105–1107; Chapter 4: Psychiatric liaison to family medicine: Patient with delusional disorder (with Joseph Morrissey). *Canadian Family Physician*, 1995, 41:97–104; Chapter 5: The use of low dose neuroleptics in the treatment of patients with severe personality disorder: An adjunct to psychotherapy. *BC Medical Journal*, 2007, 49(6):306–310; Chapter 6: What psychiatry offers to medicine. *Annals of the Royal College of Physicians and Surgeons of Canada*, 1994, 27(5):283–286; Chapter 8: Broader indications for psychiatric consultation. *Canadian Family Physician*, 1987, 33:437–440; Chapter 10: Psychiatric complications of surgery in the male. *Canadian Journal of Psychiatry*, 1988, 33(1):28–33; Chapter 11: A patient with insulinoma presenting for psychiatric assessment (with Robert MacKenzie). *Canadian Journal of Psychiatry*, 1989, 34(1):58–59; Chapter 12: A case of paranoid disorder associated with hyperthyroidism. *Canadian Journal of Psychiatry*, 1994, 39(3):153–156; Chapter 13: Adrenal carcinoma and hypertension presenting with catatonic stupor. *Australia and New Zealand Journal of Psychiatry*, 1996, 30(1):146–149; Chapter 14: The inability to name a child: Depression or obsession (with Johann Aufreiter, Harold Merskey, John Mount, & Quentin Rae-Grant). *Canadian Journal of Psychiatry*, 1989, 34(3):221–226; Chapter 15: Integration of psychoanalytic concepts in the formulation and management of hospitalized psychiatric patients (with David Cochrane). *Bulletin of the Menninger Clinic*, 2013:77(1):23–40; Chapter 16: Psychodynamic approaches integrated into day treatment, and inpatient settings (William Piper, first author). Reprinted with permission from *Psychodynamic Psychotherapy for Personality Disorders: A Clinical Handbook*, John Clarkin, Peter Fonagy & Glen Gabbard, editors. (Copyright ©2010.) American Psychiatric Association. All Rights Reserved; Chapter 17: Oral examination anxiety in physicians, narcissism and object relations. *The Journal of Applied Psychoanalytic Studies*, 2002, 4(4):379–388: Chapter 18: Preventing suicide in medical students: A self and relational viewpoint. *Annals of the Royal College of Physicians and Surgeons of Canada*, 2002, 35(8):503–505; Chapter 19: Sexual abuse of adult female patients by male physicians. *Annals of the Royal College of Physicians and Surgeons of Canada*, 1993, 26(4):211–214. The excerpt in the Introduction to Consultation/Liaison section is reprinted with permission, and originally appeared in Dreams as indicators of the psychoanalytic treatment process. *Canadian Journal of Psychoanalysis*, 2018, 26(2):150–172.

ACKNOWLEDGMENTS

I have found that the term "It takes a village" applies as much to raising a psychoanalyst or writing a book as it does to raising a child. I am very grateful to many people for their help and support over the years. First I would like to acknowledge a very large group, my patients over half a century. They have been loyal, patient, tolerant of my mistakes, and active collaborators in our work. They have been my best collaborators, as Bion says, but also my best teachers.

Next, I would like to acknowledge my students, including medical students, psychiatric and family medical residents, and psychoanalytic candidates. I always found teaching to be a wonderful way of learning, because students ask questions one might not think to ask oneself. They also bring a freshness characteristic of youth and relative inexperience.

I would like to thank the following medical colleagues who generously donated their time and expertise in reviewing the chapters of this book and making constructive suggestions: Charles Chamberlaine, Lisa Gaede, Monte Glanzberg, Jerry Growe, Jean-Michel le Melledo, Stephen MacDonald, Brian Reid, Carl Rothschild, Stanley Sunshine, and Michelle Yuen. Graeme Taylor, David Salter, Theo Turpin, and David Cochrane were especially helpful in reviewing the entire book.

I wish to thank Joanne Forshaw, Nina Gutapalle, Grace McDonnell, and Liz Williams, my editors, for their consistent support, guidance, and assistance.

One has so many helpful friends and colleagues over the years that it is impossible to identify them all. I would like to thank, for their various forms of support, encouragement, and teaching, Glenn Baker, Avner Bergstein, Eva and Peter Besmer, Christopher Bollas, David Brand, Paul Cameron, Patrick Casement, Mary Gail Frawley-O'Dea, Jacques Gauthier, Irwin Hirsch, David Kligman, the late Keith Laking, Clem Loew, Nancy McWilliams (who many years ago originally encouraged me to write this book), John Mount, Thomas Ogden, Brian Shaw, Donnel Stern, the late Neville Symington, the late Bill Tillmann, Maillor Vallance, Elizabeth Wallace, and the late Bill Witchel.

I owe special thanks to the following friends and colleagues who have been especially supportive over the years: Frank Brewster, Satna Duggal, David Heilbrunn, Stephen Kline, Charles Levin, the late Roger Mesmer, Joseph Newirth, John Ogrodniczuk, Bill Piper, Elizabeth Lima da Rocha Barros, John Rosie, Angela Sheppard, Theo Turpin, Rose Vasta, et, bien sûr, Elie Debanné. I feel very fortunate to belong to the Western Branch-Canadian Psychoanalytic Society whose members collectively have maintained a very supportive atmosphere in which to practice, write, teach, and learn.

I thank my sister Heidi, my brother Joel, and my brother-in-law Brian for their ongoing support and love.

Our three sons, Reece, David, and Nicholas, continuing sources of fun, inspiration, pride, and wonder, all provided feedback on some chapters. I am enjoying getting to know their partners, Audrey and Elisha.

My wife, Carolyn Steinberg, deserves special mention. As well as becoming my closest colleague, she provided me with the time to write the articles on which this book is based, holding the fort with the children and household. She also performed a valuable function in giving me feedback about the content of the articles over the years. This book would not have been written without her.

INTRODUCTION PART 1

How could a strange treatment invented by an obscure neuropathologist-turned-clinician (only because he could not secure a research career, being Jewish) treating the "hysterical" symptoms of middle-class Viennese women at the end of the nineteenth century, have any relevance for the practice of medicine and surgery in the third decade of the twenty-first century? According to Balint (1964), at least a quarter and possibly much more of the work of family physicians is taken up with psychological issues. At a time when the practice of medicine is becoming increasingly influenced by technology, including clinical examinations by video, increasing reliance on laboratory tests at the expense of clinical data, reliance on information available on the internet rather than personally acquired knowledge, and algorithms for diagnosis and management, I propose that carefully listening to patients still has a lot to offer, especially when informed by psychoanalytic thinking.

The main theme of this book is that psychoanalytic thinking can be applied in clinically useful ways to the provision of medical/surgical care. This applies to the work of family physicians and all specialist clinicians, who inevitably need to deal with psychological aspects of their patients' conditions and management of the latter. Psychoanalytic thinking also can contribute to better understanding and practical approaches to some non-clinical areas related to healthcare. A secondary theme is that one has a capacity to keep on learning as one ages, something I have experienced between the time when the original papers on which this book is based were being written and in subsequent years, during and since my psychoanalytic training.

I can illustrate the secondary theme, that learning can be lifelong, in a couple of ways related to the primary theme of the book. I undertook psychoanalytic training relatively late in my career. When I was in psychiatric training, most psychoanalytic institutes did not accept candidates over the age of 40. Now the average psychoanalytic candidate begins training in his 40s or 50s. Similarly, when I was in psychiatric training, individuals older than 40 were generally thought to be too old to benefit from psychoanalysis. Now there is no age limit beyond which people are thought to be unable to benefit from psychoanalysis. It is not uncommon for senior citizens to undertake analysis (Segal, 1958), or even to be candidates in psychoanalytic training. Of course, not only individuals but disciplines can continue to grow and learn; this is something I have emphasized throughout this book regarding the growth of psychoanalytic theory and technique over more than 120 years.

Developments in psychoanalysis have been documented in books oriented towards mental health professionals (Symington, 1986), and in both popular (Mitchell & Black, 1995), and scholarly (Ellman, 2010) texts, which I suspect have not attracted much attention from physician readers, despite their high quality. I wish in this introduction to assume as little as possible about the reader's familiarity with psychoanalysis, and to provide an orientation for what follows. This essentially will be continued in the second introductory chapter, in which I provide some basic psychoanalytic theory.

For the sake of gender equality, I will employ both masculine and feminine personal pronouns to denote individuals such as physicians and patients, remaining consistent within any given paragraph.

WHAT IS PSYCHOANALYSIS?

Psychoanalysis is an intensive psychological "talk" therapy that explores the patient's unconscious, in particular, her unconscious motivations for how she feels, thinks, and behaves. The unconscious does not consist just of what is unbearably terrifying and painful, and is therefore repressed outside of conscious awareness. It also contains what is joyful, creative, interesting, exciting, and fantastic, which an individual may have learned early in life was too threatening to, or just neglected by, someone important to them to tolerate experiencing and developing these qualities. This can result in an individual living her life in a sterile, unsatisfying manner, not realizing her potential in relationships, work, and recreational pursuits; that is, in work, love, and play. The unconscious also includes the mechanisms of defense we employ to remain unaware of what makes us anxious, especially regarding painful truths about ourselves. There are many parts of each of us that we can profitably explore and develop. When unconscious obstacles to growth are understood, felt, experienced, and lived, this can permit renewed growth, or growth that an individual never previously has experienced.

Psychoanalysis is defined by both extrinsic and intrinsic criteria. Extrinsic criteria refer to the setting or frame of psychoanalysis. This includes the patient lying on a couch, the analyst sitting out of sight, and sessions being frequent, approximately four times a week, with duration of the analysis measured in years. Intrinsic criteria include the general technical approach being that the patient is invited to say whatever comes to her mind (the technique of free association), with the analyst's emphasis on understanding and articulating something about what the patient is communicating about which she is not consciously aware. This might include, depending on the analyst's orientation, sexual and aggressive impulses that are consciously unacceptable to the patient; mutually contradictory and disturbing unconscious images of oneself and others; terrifying experiences of the self fragmenting, falling into space, or not existing; and experiences of the analyst–patient relationship that neither partner in the analytic dyad may be prepared for. The corresponding technique in the analyst is his freely floating attention to whatever the patient says in any given session, without having preconceptions about what would be important to talk about. The analyst also needs to be open to his own thoughts, feelings, impulses, and reverie, including visual images, such as myths, songs, literature, or other aspects of culture that may occur to him, apparently "out of the blue," may represent unconscious communications from his patient. Other intrinsic factors include a technical focus on interpretations of the transference, that is, the experience the patient has of the analyst; and the analyst remaining neutral, essentially not having an agenda for the patient.

In general, the purpose of psychoanalysis is to explore the patient's mind, understanding and experiencing the patient's unconscious conflicts and unmet emotional needs that impede psychological growth and development. It is accepted that an individual's early relationships have a strong ongoing influence on the structure and content of her mind, including her characteristic ways of thinking and feeling, leaving her with specific psychological strengths and weaknesses that affect her capacity to adapt to the changes, losses, and challenges, both mundane and extraordinary, that all people experience. This involves discovering areas of both vulnerability and resilience in the patient. There is a specific focus on the analyst–patient relationship, not only because of how fruitful it is to explore that relationship in order to understand the patient's other relationships, but also because of the transformational potential of talking about an intimate relationship in a way that the patient hasn't experienced in other close relationships. Alternatively, the analytic relationship may be the first opportunity the patient has to establish a truly intimate relationship, which itself can be discussed. It is inherent in psychoanalytic work that being open to what one is thinking, and allowing oneself to experience and reflect on one's feelings before immediately acting on them, are highly valued. This involves containing one's feelings and bearing them, as opposed to evacuating them, for example, through physical violence, impulsive sexual activity, substance abuse, or other addictive behaviors, or trying to forget them. This favors the opportunity of getting acquainted with formerly unacceptable or unarticulated aspects of oneself, with the aim of integrating these split-off aspects of the self into the rest of one's personality.

Psychoanalysis is not only a method of psychological treatment, but also a theory, or, more accurately, a group of theories, to explain psychopathology, based on the positing of the existence of unconscious factors that influence one's thinking, feelings, and behavior, which can result in psychiatric symptoms. It relates psychopathology to the individual's emotional development. Psychoanalysis is also a general psychology, offering theories regarding normal human psychological development. Finally, psychoanalysis comprises a set of theories that can be applied in non-clinical disciplines such as literature (fiction, drama, and poetry), cinema, sculpture, painting, music, and academic disciplines such as sociology, anthropology, and biography.

Psychoanalysis and psychoanalytic psychotherapy, its briefer derivative, offer some benefits that time-limited, manualized, symptom-oriented treatments such as cognitive behavior therapy (CBT), which have gained much popularity and prominence in recent decades, do not. This includes an approach aimed at understanding the patient's unconscious motivations, with the richness and depth of insight that this entails, offering the opportunity for patients to undergo transformations such that they are able to cope with their unconscious conflicts and unmet emotional needs in a more constructive manner, needing to rely less on painful and unproductive symptoms and self-destructive behaviors. A symptom-oriented approach, on the other hand, does not deal with the person enduring the symptoms in exploring the meaning of his symptoms, but rather attempts to relieve him of them. When a symptom-oriented treatment is followed by symptomatic improvement, the patient remains vulnerable to having the symptoms return when he again is exposed to environmental situations that have the potential to reactivate the conflicts and the experience of unmet needs that initially led to the symptoms. Of course, symptom-oriented approaches, being quicker and cheaper, are very attractive to providers of healthcare, both government and private. They are, as well, attractive to patients who wish for quick solutions that do not involve psychological work or pain. This is not to devalue these forms of treatment. They can provide some patients with symptomatic relief, and help some patients who cannot be helped by psychoanalytic treatment. Conversely, psychoanalytic treatment can help some patients who cannot be helped meaningfully with briefer treatments.

Psychoanalysis and psychoanalytic psychotherapy also offer long-term therapeutic relationships in which the difficulties inherent in all relationships, including the patient's characteristic relationship difficulties, can be explored in the intensive here-and-now setting of the analyst–patient relationship, with the opportunity to compare the difficulties the analytic dyad experience with difficulties in the patient's previous and concurrent relationships. There also is considerable empirical evidence that longer psychotherapies have more lasting beneficial effects than shorter ones (Leichsenring et al., 2013). Psychoanalysis and psychoanalytic psychotherapy, with their focus on exploring the patient's mind, also offer patients the support of being understood in a manner much more profound than is the case with short-term symptom-oriented therapies. A psychoanalyst's very lengthy intensive training, including a personal psychoanalysis, lengthy experiences in supervision, and years of didactic teaching, provides her with the opportunity to internalize standards that have developed over 120+ years to best serve the goals of treatment and the patient's needs. Personal psychoanalysis gives psychoanalysts a perspective of being a patient that they couldn't otherwise have. No other therapeutic modality requires the therapist to undergo lengthy treatment in the therapy they are going to provide. This experience also gives the psychoanalyst familiarity with her areas of vulnerability, "blind spots," and "raw and exposed nerves," to help her manage her personal emotional reactions to her patients, that is, her countertransference. Other treatment modalities don't make this consideration an essential part of treatment. Countertransference also provides psychoanalysts with much important information about their patients that would not otherwise be available to them, such as through their reverie (Steinberg, 2017b). Therapists in non-psychoanalytic short-term therapies are not trained in this, and have very limited time to consider it.

Some authors do not make a cut-and-dried distinction between psychoanalysis and psychoanalytic psychotherapy. For many analyst–patient dyads, psychoanalysis is a richer and more profound therapeutic experience than can be achieved from once- or twice-a-week psychotherapy. Nevertheless, much valuable psychotherapeutic work can be accomplished at this frequency of sessions, depending partly on the nature and severity of the patient's difficulties, the openness of the patient to exploring her inner world, and the goodness of the therapist–patient fit. One concrete way of distinguishing psychoanalysis from psychoanalytic psychotherapy is by considering the frame mentioned above. A reliance on free association, a focus on interpretation of the transference, that is, the patient's experience of the analyst, use of the couch, and a frequency of about four sessions a week is a classic way of distinguishing psychoanalysis from psychoanalytic psychotherapy.

Psychoanalysis sometimes is characterized, usually by individuals who are not very familiar with it, as an outdated or inappropriate treatment for contemporary patients. Nothing could be further from the truth. Psychoanalysis does make great demands on patients, not only of time and money, but also of psychological work, including bearing pain that many patients would rather avoid. However, psychoanalysis continuously has changed over the decades, developing from a drive/instinct-oriented theory, to a focus on the ego, to theories of the self, internal object relations (considerations of the patient's internal world populated by unconscious images of self and others), and most recently of the analytic field. This continuous development and adaptation has enabled psychoanalysts to treat patients with an increasingly wide range of psychiatric conditions, including severe symptomatic conditions and personality disturbances that often cannot be treated effectively with other modalities.

Psychoanalysis is the original psychotherapy invented by Sigmund Freud before the turn of the twentieth century. Although one of the motivations for the reduced frequency of appointments in psychoanalytic (also called psychodynamic) psychotherapy is practical, in that it consumes less time and money, some patients who might regress too much with psychoanalysis can be treated more successfully, at least initially, with a reduced frequency of appointments. Far more people are treated with psychoanalytic psychotherapy than with psychoanalysis because of practical considerations, although psychoanalysis would be the treatment of choice in many cases. Similar techniques are used in psychoanalytic psychotherapy as in psychoanalysis, although usually in a less rigorous manner. However, there usually is considerable flexibility of technique within any given psychoanalysis, and much more variability of technique between psychoanalyses than was acknowledged in the past. Many patients with more severe symptomatic conditions and personality disturbance can be treated more effectively with psychoanalysis than with psychoanalytic psychotherapy. Some patients choose psychoanalysis because of their wish to go into as much depth as possible in their psychotherapeutic work.

WHICH OF MY PATIENTS CAN BENEFIT FROM PSYCHOANALYSIS OR PSYCHOANALYTIC PSYCHOTHERAPY?

An appendix at the end of this chapter provides diagnostic exclusion factors and relative positive and negative prognostic factors regarding the suitability of patients for psychoanalysis and psychoanalytic psychotherapy. In general, patients who wish to understand the basis of their symptoms and think in terms of their symptoms having some connection with their difficulties in life and relationships are more highly motivated to undertake psychoanalysis or psychoanalytic psychotherapy. Patients who see their symptoms as representing a medical problem completely unrelated to life circumstances, and consult their physician because they believe their physician has a medication or other treatment that will help them feel better, will be much less motivated to undertake these forms of treatment. Many of these patients will be disappointed with the limitations of an approach in which management is limited to brief supportive visits involving prescription of medication and a supportive relationship. Some of these patients may be open to manualized treatments such as CBT that demand little of them, and derive some benefit from it. The physician can perform a very valuable service by informing her patients of the availability not only of appropriate medication, such as antidepressants, but also of the availability of psychological treatments, including psychoanalysis, psychotherapy, and CBT, with which the patients may not be familiar. The physician who is aware that some patients with psychiatric conditions respond best to a combination of medication and psychological treatment will be more open to recommending that their patients consider undertaking a form of psychotherapy in addition to medication. A major goal of this book is to inform physicians about the utility of psychoanalytic thinking in daily patient care. Another goal is to inform physicians about psychoanalysis and psychoanalytic psychotherapy to enable them to feel competent to refer patients appropriately for these treatments.

I am an unapologetic proponent of psychoanalysis and psychoanalytic psychotherapy. Time-limited manualized symptom-oriented psychotherapies currently require no proponents. As noted above, they are attractive to patients, many therapists, and providers of healthcare, because of their being inexpensive, brief, relatively easy to learn and perform, and their focus on the patient feeling better soon. However, they do not deal with the difficulties of the person who is having the symptoms.

Psychiatric treatment in general and non-psychoanalytically informed psychological treatments attempt to reduce patients' symptoms. This is a reasonable goal. Psychoanalysis and psychoanalytic psychotherapy attempt to address the unconscious motivations underlying intrapsychic conflicts, difficulties in close relationships, and structural deficits in the individual's personality, including the patient's internal world of unconscious images of the self and the other (Truant, 1998, 1999). Psychoanalysis offers the opportunity for these areas of difficulty to be explored in depth in the context of the analyst–patient relationship, so for example, difficulties a patient has in his relationship with the analyst, which usually resemble some of the difficulties he has in other relationships, can be thought about together and understood in a different light. Focusing treatment only on the patient's symptoms leaves the patient vulnerable to relapse when the underlying problems, which psychoanalysis attempts to deal with, are left unaddressed. This is especially the case when the support of the therapist or psychiatrist is withdrawn, and the patient experiences a stress, especially when he is vulnerable to this on the basis of previous loss or traumatic experience. One goal of psychoanalysis is that the patient internalize the therapeutic process originally occurring between analyst and patient, so he can continue analytic work for the rest of his life, long after contact with the analyst is over. That is, in a successful psychoanalysis, the patient learns to think in an expanded fashion, both about the ways that he thinks, and the content of what he is able to think about. Problems that might have remained unthought of, to say nothing of satisfactorily resolved, can be reflected on, with the opportunity for the individual to find a satisfactory resolution, or to mourn what cannot be resolved, thus reducing the risk of symptomatic relapse.

The development of a human being into a person involves the development of one's mind. This includes the acquisition of increasingly more refined physical skills, the capacity to experience and gradually regulate emotions, and the capacity to think concretely according to the rules of logic, that is, rationally, which permits various tasks, for example, composing a grocery list and purchasing the groceries, acquiring the capacity to perform mathematical work such as the solving of quadratic equations, and applying sensory observations, judgment, and acquired knowledge to make decisions. This requires the acquisition of memory, and the capacity to pay attention, make observations, and carry out decisions in action in the world. Beyond this rational thinking lies another type of thinking less accessible to the conscious mind, and less under the power of volition. Various terms are used to describe it, such as intuition, reverie, unconscious thinking, inspiration, and even dreaming while awake. This does not involve consciously figuring something out, but rather allowing a space in one's mind where an unbidden thought may arise. For example, my psychotherapy patient and I were struggling with an impasse in our work. The sexually stimulating visual image of a record album from decades ago, *Whipped Cream and Other Delights*, eventually came to my mind. My discussing this reverie with my patient led to our work becoming enlivened, and transformed what felt like a dead relationship into a going concern (Steinberg, 2017a). Developing a mind also involves acquiring personal tastes, for example, interest in or even passion for an aspect of art, music, literature, sports, or other recreational pursuits, as well as in friends and a potential life partner, and vocational preferences and proclivities. The aim of psychoanalysis and psychoanalytic psychotherapy is to restore, or, in some cases, to initiate a process of growth of the mind of individuals whose mental growth has been limited or interrupted on the basis of the intersection between the individual's inherent vulnerability and the effects of untoward experiences in his life.

SOME HISTORICAL OBSERVATIONS

Psychoanalysis is not as popular and well known in the Western world to either medical practitioners or to the general public as it once was during its post-World War II "golden age" from the late 1940s to the 1970s. It was something of a fad then, and in parts of North America, at least, it was stylish to have psychoanalysis. Psychoanalysis also was very influential in psychiatric practice and education back then; many chairs of academic departments of psychiatry were psychoanalysts. It was also influential in several academic disciplines. Like all fads, psychoanalysis had its day, and its popularity experienced an eclipse. By the 1980s, psychoactive medications and standardized, symptom-oriented, short-term psychological treatments became increasingly popular. The limitations of medications and of shorter therapies were poorly recognized, as funders of healthcare embraced these treatments, which are much cheaper to provide, at least in the short term, than psychoanalysis and psychoanalytically oriented therapies. Recently, however, the limits of pharmacological treatment are more openly acknowledged.

Psychoanalysis as a discipline was marginalized by medicine, including psychiatry, and what it offered to medical practice was neglected. This was in spite of the evidence that psychotherapeutic attention to patients' personality and relationship difficulties can be cost-effective in the long term, with reduced visits to family physicians and emergency departments, and reduced use of inpatient beds (Altmann et al., 2018). Psychoanalysis was considered outdated and was devalued. Ironically, this occurred at a time when psychoanalysis was undergoing an intellectual renaissance, with the results of psychoanalytic clinical research demonstrating the promise of prominent psychoanalytic theoreticians/clinicians of the 1950s to the 1980s, resulting in a deeper understanding of patients' unmet psychological needs and unconscious psychological conflicts. This blossoming of psychoanalytic theory and practice has continued to the present day, resulting, as mentioned above, in a wider range of more serious mental disturbance being considered treatable. Seitler (2019) provides a recent compendium of empirical research into many areas of psychoanalysis, including adolescence, affect regulation, alexithymia, alliance, assessment and measurement, attachment, attention deficit hyperactivity disorders, brain changes, child analysis, consultation, countertransference, defense mechanisms, dream work, efficacy of psychoanalysis as compared with other psychotherapies, group psychotherapy, insight, mechanisms of change, memory, narcissism, neuroscience, psychoanalytic process studies, resistance, self, separation anxiety, separation-individuation, supervision, techniques, transference, and the unconscious.

Ironically, some non-psychoanalytic healthcare providers tend to criticize Freud's work, often without a very deep understanding of it, oblivious to the wealth of developments in psychoanalysis that have developed and extended his work since his death in 1939. Psychoanalysis is now considered passé and at best of historical interest by much of contemporary culture. It is not given much respect in many non-psychoanalytic mental health professional contexts, including psychiatry, to the extent that I was warned not to include Freud's name in the title of this book, having considered *Freud's Legacy to Medicine* as a potential title. I was told by both psychoanalysts and non-psychoanalysts that including his name was a non-starter, and would destroy chances for the book to be either published or read. It is striking that such use of the name of one of the outstanding geniuses of the twentieth century might be considered as destructive.

The envy by practitioners of other forms of treatment of the explanatory power of psychoanalysis to elucidate unconscious motivations and the meaning of symptoms, and of the early therapeutic effectiveness of psychoanalysis in an era (Victorian-Edwardian) when most improvement in treatment of psychiatric conditions was based on placebo, and therefore transient, sometimes may have been a motivation for the rejection of psychoanalysis in its early days. To what extent this envy persists in some contemporary clinicians is unknown. As well, Freud's openness regarding sexuality and his assigning it a central role in the etiology of neurosis, as well as his concept of childhood sexuality, did not find favor in an era still influenced by hypocritical Victorian prudery. These days, of course, sexuality is a less forbidden topic, and has been replaced by more contemporary concerns such as identity and alienation.

MY GOAL

The main thesis of this book, however, is not to promote psychoanalysis as a treatment approach for psychiatric disturbance and psychological difficulties, although some space will inevitably be devoted to the subject. Rather, I hope to demonstrate how contemporary psychoanalytic thinking can be applied to the practice of medicine in general, and can be practically helpful to family physicians and medical and surgical specialists, in addition to psychiatrists. This book is not intended to turn family physicians and specialists into mini-psychoanalysts, but rather to encourage you to apply psychoanalytic thought in your work in a way that enhances it. One challenge in writing this book has been to use language accessible to physicians. I have not avoided using psychoanalytic terms, but have attempted to explain them in the body of the text, in addition to providing a glossary at the end. I have always believed that if one cannot explain a concept in plain English, then one doesn't really understand it, or the concept itself has a deficiency. I still generally believe that, but have found that some ideas in psychoanalysis are difficult to understand, so it is difficult to convey one's understanding of them. I will try to indicate this when it comes up in this book. Sometimes "The fault … is not in the stars, but in ourselves, that we are underlings" (Shakespeare, 1599/1992: I, ii, 140–141). Some ideas, by their nature, are difficult to understand. That doesn't make the effort to understand them less worthwhile. This applies (for me, at least) especially to the work of Wilfred Bion and his successors. This book is not a comprehensive academic treatise, but rather a collection of observations and conclusions based on 40 years of psychiatric practice, and is intended to be practically useful to clinicians.

To the extent that this book is successful, it will interest some physicians in thinking psychoanalytically, and motivate them to learn more about psychoanalytic thought. They will be confronted with a truly massive amount of literature, including the original work of classical and contemporary theorists and practitioners, as well as writers who adumbrate and integrate the theories and practice of others. The website PEP-Web is an inexpensive and inexhaustible source of psychoanalytic information, containing all psychoanalytic papers written in practically all psychoanalytic journals, and some others, over about the last 120 years, in addition to many classic texts and some videos. The physician who wishes an accessible introduction to psychoanalytic/psychodynamic practice is referred to the work of Nancy McWilliams (1999, 2004, 2011), Patrick Casement (1985/2014, 1990/2014), and Glenn Gabbard (2000).

PSYCHOANALYTIC UNDERSTANDING

Psychoanalytic understanding of the taxonomy of mental disturbances differs from the traditional medical approach. Everyone employs unconscious mental mechanisms of defense in order to push or maintain out of awareness mental contents such as feelings, thoughts, impulses, wishes, and fantasies that they find too disturbing. Given this, no one is considered "normal." Depending on the psychological lengths that an individual must take in order to maintain these mental contents repressed out of conscious awareness (or even prevented from becoming articulated as thoughts, feelings, or impulses), a smaller or greater psychological or even physiological price is involved. In addition to repression of mental contents, contemporary psychoanalysis has developed an understanding of the ways an individual's thinking process, or her development of her thinking process, can be interfered with as well. I will elaborate on this subsequently. The price of the above attempts to reduce anxiety about one's mental contents or thinking process usually is experienced as psychiatric symptoms of variable degrees of severity, such as short-term or long-standing neurotic symptoms; acute or chronic psychotic symptoms; severe personality disturbance; paraphilias, conditions characterized by what are considered abnormal sexual desires, typically involving extreme, dangerous, or destructive behaviors; and addictive behaviors, not restricted to substance abuse. In addition, the physiological price of the above attempts can involve medically otherwise unexplainable somatic symptoms, as well as the precipitation or exacerbation of recognized medical disease. Criminal behavior is another potential outcome. The latter usually involves violence or other destructive behaviors, and often expresses a sense of entitlement to acquire assets or services without having to perform constructive work, and without a concern for others whom one materially deprives, possibly emotionally and/or physically injuring them in pursuing this goal.

I listed the above group of conditions because psychoanalysis has developed to be able to treat some patients with these conditions (excepting criminal behavior, which is not a medical condition), with outcomes of varying degrees of clinical improvement. As will become evident later in this book, individuals who are not considered to have overt psychotic symptoms still may experience, either transiently under stress, or as part of their ongoing adaptation, various disturbances in the forms of their thinking. Many people have disturbances of thought content, that is, quasi-delusional beliefs, and of their thought process, without being floridly psychotic or warranting a diagnosis of a major psychotic condition. Many more individuals demonstrate these disturbances under stressful circumstances. Everyone has a propensity to psychotic mental functioning when exposed to stressful enough circumstances (Bion, 1957). The paraphilias used to be called sexual perversions. The term "perversion" has a strongly pejorative connotation, which has no place in medical diagnosis. However, this term still performs a function in psychoanalytic parlance in describing disturbances in forms of thinking, experiencing emotions, expression of aggression, and capacity for destructive interpersonal relationships that may be manifest partly in the individual's sexual behavior (Ogden, 1996), but generally represents the individual's psychic organization.

When treatment of patients with psychiatric conditions is practiced (by physicians of whatever specialty) without the support of a psychoanalytically informed approach to understanding the patient, management necessarily focuses on symptoms, at the expense of an exploration of the meaning of the symptoms, and of what problems, internal and external, the patient is facing in his life that may be contributing to his symptoms. This favors clinicians and patients becoming frustrated, as when the patient improves, there is limited reason for hope that the improvement is sustainable. That is because nothing has changed *in* the patient to foster the continuation of remission, apart from the response to positive aspects of the therapeutic relationship, which eventually will be unavailable. Even if the patient's environment responds positively to changes in his behavior related to his improvement, he remains vulnerable to the inevitable disappointments and losses we all experience in life, which will favor an eventual relapse into a symptomatic state. In addition, loss of support of the treating clinician when the patient improves, usual when being treated by physicians, may remove one of the pillars of the patient's recovery, and lead to a relapse itself, or make the patient more vulnerable to respond to other losses with a relapse. The above, in my opinion, applies to the practice of medicine in general, not just to psychiatry. I acknowledge, of course, that one's relationship with one's family physician may continue for decades, but the same degree of support usually is not maintained when the patient has improved.

As well, an ongoing attempt to understand one's patient along psychoanalytic lines provides the clinician with the support of a theory, making possible the generation of hypotheses about what is wrong and what approach to take, which is necessary to deal with the patient and his suffering. This itself can be very challenging. The same, of course, is true in any branch of medicine. The ongoing work of trying to understand the patient provides the clinician with some meaning to her work. To the extent that she is motivated to undertake clinical work in an unconscious attempt to heal herself (which is not uncommon), it is very demoralizing when the patient doesn't improve, or relapses. If the clinician is consciously aware of this motivation in herself, especially if she has or has had the benefit of personal psychotherapy or psychoanalysis, she will tend to be less threatened by the vicissitudes and ups and downs of the patient's condition, more aware of the unconscious meaning of her attempts to cure her patient, and less dependent on needing her patient to improve, and therefore be more able to see the patient as he really is, however much he is suffering, and however limited the prospects for improvement.

This also relieves the pressure on the patient to improve for his physician's sake, enabling the patient to feel he can show himself more honestly to her, which can be therapeutic in itself, as opposed to the patient feeling that he has to take care of her by getting better, or at least by stopping complaining, and have no more genuine or authentic relationship with her than he has with others. The practice of medicine is taxing; it is very difficult to be confronted with human suffering day in and day out, especially because much of it cannot be cured, or sometimes even relieved. This is no less true when dealing with patients with psychological problems and psychiatric disturbance. A psychoanalytic understanding of one's patient provides the physician with a formulation (psychoanalytic understanding) to rest upon, as well as the hope that what understanding she can impart to her patient also may be helpful to him. Many psychiatrists and other physicians employ some psychoanalytic understanding of patients without acknowledging this to themselves. This is beneficial, but an awareness that one is using this approach facilitates learning more about it, and thereby becoming more consistent in applying one's understanding in one's work, with benefits to oneself and one's patients. Decades ago, there was an ad on New York City buses depicting a picture, probably politically incorrect according to today's standards, of a Native American smiling and wearing a hat with a feather sticking up. The caption was, "You don't have to be Jewish to like Levy's rye bread." My message is, "You don't have to be a psychoanalyst to apply psychoanalytic thinking in medicine, or, for that matter, to enjoy doing so."

THE INFLUENCE OF PSYCHOANALYSIS ON MEDICAL PRACTICE (AND ELSEWHERE)

Several generations of psychiatrists have become psychoanalysts since the discipline was invented in the mid-1890s, although relatively fewer psychiatrists become psychoanalysts now than in days past, when in many psychoanalytic institutes it was difficult or impossible to be admitted for training unless one were a physician. In spite of the preponderance of psychiatrists in the field for much of its history, little has been written by psychiatrists about their journey toward psychoanalysis. Inevitably, psychoanalysis has had less of an influence on the practice of medicine than in years past. With fewer psychiatrists having psychoanalytic training, that influence is not acknowledged or well disseminated. Nevertheless, the thesis of this book is that psychoanalytic thought can inform the practice of medicine to its benefit, both in terms of outcome of patient care, and in terms of providing physicians with an interesting and practically useful approach to understanding their patients, of which they otherwise might not be aware. This is particularly the case with family physicians, many of whose patients either present overtly with emotional distress, psychiatric symptoms, or psychological disturbance as the presenting complaint, or present this distress or disturbance in the form of somatic complaints. Another frequent presenting complaint to family physicians is difficulties in interpersonal relationships. As the range of clinical presentations to which family physicians must respond is so broad, they cannot be expected to develop expertise in dealing with these kinds of patients without some kind of theoretical basis from which to begin. Unfortunately, rotations in psychiatry undertaken in their residency training, often on an inpatient unit or a medically oriented outpatient clinic, are very unlikely to provide them with such a basis.

Ferro (2005) describes the growth of a container. The term "container" in this context refers to the capacity of a mother to contain and soothe her distressed infant, and that of a psychoanalyst to help her patient contain the latter's otherwise unthinkable thoughts and unbearable feelings. Physicians, especially family physicians, are similarly called upon to help contain their patients' unbearable feelings. "Containing" feelings involves bearing them without acting destructively or self-destructively by evacuating the feelings, for example, by abusing substances, becoming physically violent, or becoming engaged in compulsive activity. Mothers and physicians both accomplish this containment, to a greater or lesser extent, without the benefit of psychoanalytic training. Ferro (2005) suggests that the growth of a container, that is, the growth of an individual's capacity to contain, is mediated by repeated experience of intimate contact, and by the development of an ability to tolerate doubt without feelings of persecution. This is potentially available to mothers in their relationships with their infants, and to psychoanalysts and physicians in their relationships with their patients, as well as in the relationships all three groups may enjoy with family and friends. The point about tolerating doubt without feelings of persecution is important; one cannot be an effective mother, psychoanalyst, or physician without being able to accept the limitations of how much one knows, but nevertheless being able to carry on. This includes not knowing how, when, or to what extent we are able to contain an infant's or patient's unbearable emotions, but to do our best to be present in a way that might be helpful just the same. An example of the growth of a container from my own experience is how I became more comfortable with my own ambition, feelings of love and hate, and feelings of deadness and depression in treating three different patients who struggled respectively with these experiences (Steinberg, 2017a, 2017b, 2018). I believe that all physicians in clinical practice continuously are given similar opportunities for personal growth in their interactions with patients, especially patients who challenge them to help their patients contain their unbearable feelings, which can be an intimate experience in which one must tolerate doubt about one's capacity to contain.

One of my patients, not an overconfident individual, informed me with some authority in his voice that in spite of his continuing symptoms and difficulties, he was convinced that he was improving because of the increasingly benign environment and less threatening, more friendly figures he experienced in his dreams. The dream literature (Glucksman & Kramer, 2004; Kramer & Glucksman, 2012) supports his conclusion. Taylor (2016) states,

changes in the manifest content of [patients'] dreams during the course of therapy paralleled their progress in therapy and clinical improvement, which is consistent with findings from empirical research on the usefulness of manifest dream reports and documenting changes during treatment.

(2016: 64)

I could not help but agree with my patient, observing the very gradual improvement in his relationships, including with me. He was less frightened and paranoid, with a more appropriate assumption of personal agency, taking better care of his basic needs, with more logical and less psychotic thinking. He nevertheless remained an individual with very serious problems and painful symptoms, but was much better able to reflect on his inner experience and relationship with the world, and work towards finding the best solution available to him in any given situation. Rather than maintaining a deferential attitude towards me, fearing that I would retaliate, he was able to provide me with constructive criticism, much of it valid, about the way I worked with him, functioning as my "best colleague" (Bion, 1980; Ferro, 2008). This also is an illustration of the continuous development of psychoanalysis: psychoanalysts have discovered new ways of using dreams to understand their patients.

As mentioned above, psychoanalysis is not just a method of treatment, but also an approach to understanding people, and a method of academic research that can be applied in many academic and non-clinical areas. Psychoanalysis offers an approach to understanding disparate clinical situations, including traumatized individuals, and patients with paraphilias (sexual perversions), severe personality disturbance, including narcissistic and borderline personality disorders, as well as patients with neurotic symptoms, such as obsessions and compulsions, phobias, depression, anxiety, and conversions. Other psychotherapeutic approaches do not attempt to understand the psychological basis of these conditions in the same depth. Psychoanalysis also has undertaken understanding of the unconscious psychological basis for psychotic conditions. In addition, psychoanalysis has identified psychotic aspects of patients not suffering from psychotic conditions, and, in fact, the existence of psychotic aspects in everyone's personality (Bion, 1957). This has led to an understanding of the origins of thinking and the extent to which the thinking of individuals is disturbed, both in clinical and non-clinical settings. The latter is particularly relevant today, given the quality of much contemporary political discourse.

I hope this book stimulates all physicians engaged in clinical practice, who inevitably must deal with mental health aspects of their patients' management, to incorporate psychoanalytic concepts and techniques into their daily work. I will try to show how psychoanalytic ideas can be applied in a variety of clinical venues, as well as in some non-clinical situations. If this book contributes to an increased appreciation of what psychoanalysis has to offer clinicians in dealing with their patients' mental health in their everyday work, it will have served its purpose.

I have tried to emulate two prominent psychoanalytic writers, Wilfred Bion and Donald Winnicott, arguably the two most influential psychoanalytic authors of the last half-century. Winnicott's *Through Pediatrics to Psycho-Analysis* (1975) describes his development as a pediatrician becoming a psychoanalyst. This book describes my development as a psychiatrist, applying psychoanalytic ideas in different venues, eventually becoming a psychoanalyst. I include (in italics throughout the book) my new ideas about the subjects of the original papers (each represented in a chapter) on which this book is based, and indicate how my understanding of what I have written about has changed, following Bion's model in *Second Thoughts* (1967), a collection of papers with a commentary appended to show how his thoughts about the subject of each paper had changed. The introductory chapters, the chapter on psychosomatics, and the Envoi were written for this book.

Psychoanalysis is not a monolithic body of theory. It is a continuously burgeoning group of many interrelated theories and schools, some of which are to some extent mutually contradictory.

Moreover, it is now generally accepted that the person of the therapist/analyst and the way she interacts with her patient is more important than the particular theory she espouses.

DESCRIPTION OF CHAPTERS

This book is divided into sections based on the clinical venues in which I have learned about various aspects of medical practice. One might assume that each section is directed solely at practitioners working in that area, for example, the section on consultation/liaison of hospitalized patients is directed at hospital-based medical and surgical specialists, as opposed to, say, family physicians. This is not the case. I believe that all the chapters in the book are relevant, to a greater or lesser extent, to the work of all physicians in clinical practice, as well as, to a large extent, to non-medical clinicians, including nurses, psychologists, social workers, counselors and other psychotherapists, and occupational therapists. Summaries of the individual chapters are contained in the introduction to each section.

Part I contains six chapters illustrating how a psychoanalytically informed approach to patients can be helpful. They deal originally with situations in family medicine, but are relevant to medical practice in general.

Part II contains seven chapters dealing with psychoanalytically informed consultation/ liaison to hospital inpatients. These chapters should be relevant to all physicians who care for hospitalized patients.

Part III contains three chapters dealing with psychoanalytic contributions to management on inpatient psychiatry units and partial hospitalization programs, and should have some relevance for all physicians caring for patients on inpatient units or in clinics, although psychiatrists will find the clinical content most relevant to their work.

Part IV contains three chapters dealing with non-clinical subjects, including oral examinations, prevention of suicide in physicians, residents, and medical students, and boundary issues.

The book ends with an envoi in which I reflect on what I have been trying to communicate in this book, and in which I wish the reader farewell by making some suggestions to follow up the reading of this book.

MYTHS ABOUT PSYCHOANALYSIS

Psychoanalysts Treat the Worried Well

Many physicians, including, sadly, many psychiatrists, in addition to many psychologists and other mental health professionals, dismiss psychoanalysis, believing that psychoanalysts only treat the "worried well," that is, people who do not suffer from serious conditions. They consider it an old-fashioned, outdated, overly expensive and time-consuming treatment. These critics of psychoanalysis usually are ill informed about ongoing developments in psychoanalysis, which did not stop with Freud's death in 1939. (Joseph (2007) suggests, "If a thing is good enough, it will draw attacks … And you don't attack something that hasn't really held your attention.")

Freud himself did not treat the worried well. His fascinating and unparalleled case histories show that he treated patients with a wide range of serious psychiatric conditions, including what we would now characterize as severe personality disorders accompanied by psychotic symptoms, as well as patients with severe conversion, obsessional, and other neurotic symptoms. The claim that psychoanalysts treat the "worried well" is even less true now, because (as mentioned above), psychoanalysis has developed an understanding of psychosis and the psychotic part of the personality, psychosomatic conditions, sexual perversions, trauma, and addictions, and has developed techniques for treating patients suffering from these serious psychiatric disturbances.

Psychoanalysis is Not Evidence-based

There is a growing body of empirical research on the efficacy of psychoanalysis and psychoanalytic psychotherapy, including determining who will benefit from these treatments, and how the benefits come about, which critics of these treatment approaches either ignore or are unaware of (for example, de Maat et al., 2009; Doidge, 1997; Leichsenring et al., 2013; Leichsenring & Rabung, 2008, 2011; Levy & Ablon, 2009; Luborsky et al., 1988; Messer & Abbass, 2010; Shedler, 2010). It also is a well-recognized empirical finding that long-term psychotherapies are more effective in long-term follow-up than shorter therapies (Leichsenring et al., 2013). There is no question that empirical research is much more difficult to perform on unstructured, intensive, long-term treatments like psychoanalytic psychotherapy and psychoanalysis than on structured, short-term manualized treatments. Research is nevertheless being done on the former. As well, the short-term approaches mentioned have limited goals, such as symptom reduction, and research on them often involves relatively short follow-up periods. Symptom reduction is relatively easy to measure. Psychoanalytic psychotherapy and psychoanalysis, on the other hand, have much more ambitious goals, such as significant change in the patient's personality, major adaptations in life, and capacity to think, which are more difficult to measure. In addition to the increasing empirical research on psychoanalysis, if over 120 years of peer-reviewed psychoanalytic publications, consisting of a massive repository of clinical wisdom and experience, is not evidence, what is? Finally, Newirth (2018) has demonstrated how contemporary psychoanalytic, cognitive, developmental, and neuropsychological findings are consistent with and complement each other.

Psychoanalysis is Too Expensive and Impractical

Psychoanalysis is expensive in terms of the commitment of time and money required for it. In addition, it requires much of analyst and patient in terms of developing the capacity to undergo intense experiences, thinking previously unthinkable thoughts and feeling previously unbearable emotions. However, psychoanalytic candidates (trainees) often offer low-fee psychoanalysis to patients whom they treat under supervision. Also, some psychoanalysts and psychoanalytic psychotherapists offer a sliding scale of fees according to the patient's income. In some European countries, as well as in Canada and Australia, psychoanalytic psychotherapy, and to some extent, psychoanalysis, is provided by state-run medical insurance plans, and is either completely or largely covered by these plans in many jurisdictions. The demonstrated savings related to reduced emergency room and family medicine visits, and reduced need for medical investigations and surgical procedures, in patients who have undertaken psychotherapy and psychoanalysis obviate the cost of these treatments (Altmann et al., 2018).

Psychoanalysts are Crazy

I don't know if psychoanalysts are crazier than other people, but they are motivated to explore their craziness, so it becomes less of an impediment to them both in living a full life and undertaking their work. Perhaps this contributes to the observation that psychoanalysts have longer than average lifespans. It is the business of a psychoanalyst to know his craziness as well as possible in order to be able to identify his patient's craziness, bear experiencing it with her, and help her understand it in a manner that frees her from being dominated by it, to the extent that this is possible. Some of what psychoanalysts say or write might seem crazy to anyone unfamiliar with psychoanalytic literature and jargon. All this is not to say that there aren't disturbed individuals who become psychoanalysts, whose disturbance interferes with their work. As in other professions, among psychoanalytic practitioners there is a wide range of professional ability, skill, acumen, knowledge, and personalities.

Psychoanalysts perforce have the opportunity to personally learn and grow because patients confront them with what they still need to work on in themselves, and because their interactions with their patients force them to think about what the latter need them to think about. Inevitably, the unconscious conflicts, psychic deficiencies and limitations, and unmet emotional needs our patients struggle with resemble those of their psychoanalysts (and of their physicians, and everyone else). Sullivan, a pioneer in treating psychotic patients psychoanalytically, observed, "We are all much more simply human than otherwise" (1940: 7). We can only help our patients grow to the extent that we are able to grow ourselves, in our work with each patient (Slavin & Kriegman, 1998). This chance to learn about oneself is not always as much fun as a barrel of monkeys. Learning is inherently painful when it involves learning about what you have always tried not to think or feel about yourself. However, the opportunity of growing personally through one's work is one of the great attractions of psychoanalysis as a career. Ogden (2016) suggests that we have to invent psychoanalysis afresh with each patient. Physicians similarly can grow, especially when they take interest in who their patients are.

All Psychoanalysts are Preoccupied with Sex

Freud made sexuality a central part of his theory; there is some evidence that he had some personal conflicts about it. This is not unusual. It has been observed (Stolorow & Atwood, 1979) that psychoanalysts often generate their theories based on their own personalities and conflicts. This is not surprising if one considers that creating a theory may be an analyst's way of trying to help herself understand herself better. In this way, psychoanalysts are like novelists, screenplay writers, poets, and dramatists: they are writing about what they know (albeit unconsciously) best, themselves. The difference is that they are writing about it directly, rather than metaphorically.

Over its history, psychoanalytic theory has encompassed a wide range of issues, including attachment; love, hate, envy, and other powerful affects; conflicts about personal agency, aggression, alienation, money, and intimacy; a search for knowledge; and one's unconscious images of oneself and others. Sexuality is an important part of human life, and therefore a worthy object of study for psychoanalysis. However, contemporary psychoanalysis is not unduly preoccupied with sexuality. This was more of a preoccupation in Victorian times, and has been replaced with more contemporary concerns about alienation, personal emptiness, and the search for meaning in life.

The reader might be disconcerted by variations in the length of chapters and in the academic rigorousness between chapters. These depend on where I felt I could best highlight important points, and what I felt required more elaboration.

SOME PERSONAL OBSERVATIONS

My development as a psychoanalyst has been influenced by much of my work prior to becoming a psychoanalyst. I founded and led a hospital-based psychiatric consultation/liaison service, which helped me appreciate the suffering of patients who had both physical symptoms and/or medical conditions as well as psychiatric symptoms and/or personality disturbance. I also learned something about the interactions between these two groups of disturbances. My work as a medical consultant to a psychiatric outpatient service taught me something about what kinds of therapist–patient interactions led to therapists' requiring psychotherapy supervision, requesting medication for their patients, and requesting psychiatric consultation for their patients. Experience in inpatient, provincial hospital, and emergency psychiatry left me with some awareness of the stresses on staff in dealing with patients suffering from the most acute and severe psychiatric conditions, and of the stresses on patients themselves, related both to suffering from these conditions, and to being treated for them. These included, but are not limited to, considerations including enactments, therapeutic impasses, countertransference difficulties, and worsening of the patient's symptoms in treatment. Years after having co-led a psychodynamic group psychotherapy-based day treatment program for patients with severe personality disorders and comorbid Axis I disorders, largely attended by patients whom I would have previously been reluctant to treat in individual psychotherapy, I see some of the limits of what we accomplished in that program regarding not interpreting group dynamics as much as I would now. There was a containing function of the intensive group psychotherapy experience that helped patients face aspects of themselves that I believe could not be accomplished in one or two hours a week of individual psychotherapy, at least with the therapists available, given their training. Now I think that if analysts or therapists with adequate training were available, some of these patients could be reached in individual psychotherapy, to the extent that they were motivated to remain and participate actively in treatment. (It may have been financially advantageous to have these patients treated in this intensive group program before treating some of them in individual psychotherapy.) The day treatment program affected patients such that many who were considered unamenable to individual psychoanalytic psychotherapy before attending the program could be treated with it afterwards, or treated with good effect in our weekly follow-up psychodynamic psychotherapy group. My experiences as a leader in some of these programs also influenced my development, helping me to accept the limits of what can be done in working with patients, to learn to contain my frustration with staff, and to defer decisions rather than acting according to how I felt at the moment.

Like many authors, I have found writing this book a learning experience; this includes becoming aware of what I have learned that I did not know I had learned, in addition to learning a little more about the depths of what I still do not know. Many ideas occurred to me in writing this book that I believe would not have occurred to me had I not done so. Ogden (2005) shares his interesting ideas about the creativity of writing and of reading, suggesting that the reader rewrites the article she reads, making it her own.

APPENDIX: SELECTION OF PATIENTS FOR PSYCHOANALYSIS AND PSYCHOANALYTIC PSYCHOTHERAPY

What follows are some guidelines for clinicians to consider when referring patients. Much depends on the fit between analyst/therapist and patient; some patients will do very well with one therapist, and not so well with another. This is not based so much on the therapist's theoretical orientation as on her personality and other factors specific to therapist and patient.

Most of the selection criteria described below are *relative* prognostic indicators that need to be taken together, and not absolute indications or contraindications. There are very little in the way of absolute recommendations regarding selection of patients for psychoanalysis and psychoanalytic psychotherapy. Many of the positive qualities noted below are ones that our patients (and, to some extent, sometimes, we!) lack, which may reflect a dearth of motivation for psychotherapy, or make the work of therapy more difficult. However, with some patients, the very deficiency in these qualities is what brings them to analysis or therapy, and is what they need to work on. In the past, some of these criteria have been considered as absolute contraindications, which developments in psychoanalytic understanding and technique have rendered less so.

My suggestion to clinicians who feel unsure about whether or not a patient would benefit from psychoanalysis or psychoanalytic psychotherapy is to refer the patient for assessment, indicating one's concerns about the referral, and allow the consultant to form her own opinion regarding the suitability of the patient for treatment.

DIAGNOSTIC EXCLUSION FACTORS

- Acutely psychotic
- Acutely suicidal
- Active substance abuse (this is a somewhat relative factor; I have treated some people who used marijuana extensively with psychoanalytic psychotherapy. They invariably stopped or considerably reduced their marijuana use when it became clear that using marijuana to help modulate their painful feelings was diametrically opposed to our therapeutic work, which involves increasingly becoming able to bear painful feelings and expanding their capacity to think. Stopping using marijuana was followed by the patients thinking more clearly than while using marijuana. They found that the containment provided by the psychotherapy enabled them to think thoughts and feel feelings that were previously unbearable. Sometimes I have indicated I cannot treat a patient unless he curtails his marijuana use. In general, the practice of psychoanalysis and psychoanalytic psychotherapy involves avoiding prescribing behaviors to the patient. Nevertheless, if I think a behavior will obviate treatment, I indicate that. I would not undertake psychoanalysis or psychoanalytic psychotherapy with an individual who relies extensively on "harder" drugs to modulate his affects, and would recommend that he receive treatment for substance abuse/addiction before considering and undertaking treatment)
- Significant organic mental disorder or developmental delay
- Antisocial personality disorder
- Acute untreated major psychiatric disorder (some patients with these conditions may benefit from their symptoms being improved to some extent before being referred for

psychoanalysis or psychoanalytic psychotherapy. Some patients may be treated concurrently with medications while they are being referred for psychoanalytic treatment. Some other patients, for example, with a major depressive disorder who refuse to be treated with antidepressants, may still benefit from psychotherapy or psychoanalysis.)

POSITIVE PROGNOSTIC FACTORS

- Capacity for work: ability to sustain a job
- Capacity for a sustained relationship
- Ability to provide a coherent history
- Ability to provide dreams
- Appears interested in learning about herself
- Responds to interpretation with meaningful associations or enhanced understanding. Shows interest in psychological material such as a trial interpretation with a reflective response, or comments on his own unconscious motivation
- Symptoms and/or suffering serious enough to justify long-term treatment
- Willingness to look at his own contribution to difficulties, as opposed to externalizing the problem on to the world, seeing them as someone else's fault. (Often lack of this is a presenting symptom or at least needs to be addressed in treatment as a major difficulty)
- Psychological mindedness; capacity to think and reflect on internal experience, and openness to the existence of an unconscious part of his mind that is worth exploring. (See qualification in brackets immediately above)
- Conscious motivation to change
- The clinician finds something likable about the patient
- Patient can communicate his inner experience, trust his physician to some extent, imagine and fantasize, has a cooperative attitude, or can accept an intervention. (Trust is another quality the lack of which may be a presenting complaint or become an important issue to work on)
- Strength of initial therapeutic alliance formed with physician
- Capacity to think in terms of analogy and metaphor
- Ability to tolerate some emotional regression without completely losing a sense of reality, a capacity to reflect on himself, or an ability to carry on meeting the demands of daily living, as well as being able to reflect on his regression
- Adequate impulse control (lack of which may be a presenting complaint)
- Some capacity to feel guilt and remorse.

(RELATIVE) NEGATIVE PROGNOSTIC FACTORS

- Severe personality disorder: many patients with borderline, narcissistic, schizoid, passive-aggressive, self-defeating, and paranoid personality disorders make very difficult patients in psychoanalysis or psychotherapy. Nevertheless psychoanalytic theory and technique have developed such that many more can be treated than in the past. Most psychoanalysts likely would suggest that one can't treat a patient with antisocial personality disorder. I would not be that absolute, as some therapists can have some success with these patients, although most avoid attempting to treat them (McWilliams, 2011). Some clinicians feel that some of these patients are more treatable when they are older and become more capable of feeling depressed.

- Active untreated eating disorder, another relative negative prognostic factor. Patients with eating disorders that significantly threaten their health need to be treated for that symptom. Sometimes psychoanalytic treatment can be instituted concurrently. Sometimes it needs to be delayed until the patient's life is not at risk, especially if the physiological effects of the eating disorder compromise the patient's cognitive function.

- Psychosomatic expression of psychological disturbance. This is not a contraindication, but an indication of the potential depth of the patient's emotional disturbance. The motivation for the patient to accept psychoanalytic treatment may be low, as she may consider her problem to be medical. (See Chapter 7.) Some psychoanalysts have particular skill in dealing with "psychosomatic" patients (Taylor, 1987).

- History of brief psychotic episode. This is not an absolute contraindication, but an indication that the patient has a capacity to regress to a considerable and potentially destructive extent, and may have a significant psychotic part of his personality. Psychoanalytic treatment may be undertaken with special care.

- Psychological concreteness.

- Someone with whom the analyst is personally connected, however remotely, such as friend of a friend, relative of a friend, or friend of a relative. It is best for the therapist to have no previous acquaintance with the patient or his close associations, which is challenging in smaller communities.

- Concrete limitations: unavailable regarding time, lack of support of family (in young or very dependent patients), lack of money (unless treatment is covered by third party).

- Overwhelming practical problems, e.g. severe acute physical illness, acute realistic life crises.

- Tendency to see one's problem outside oneself.

- Tendency to respond with action, as opposed to tolerating painful and threatening feelings and impulses and reflecting on one's inner experience. (Often a presenting complaint.)

- Negative, devaluing attitude towards former caregivers.

- Patient who is motivated for treatment by pressure from third parties, such as a relative, employer, insurance company, or court order.

REFERENCES

Altmann U, Thielemann D, Zimmermann A, Steffanowski A, Bruckmeier E, Pfaffinger I, Fembacher A, Strauss B (2018). Outpatient psychotherapy improves symptoms and reduces health care costs in regularly and prematurely terminated therapies. *Frontiers in Psychology* 9:748.

Balint M (1964). *The Doctor, his Patient, and the Illness*, 2nd edition. New York: International Universities Press.

Bion WR (1957). Differentiation of the psychotic from the non-psychotic personalities. *International Journal of Psycho-Analysis* 38:266–275.

Bion WR (1980). *Bion in New York, and Sao Paulo*. F Bion (ed.) Perthshire: Clunie Press.

Casement P (1985/2014). *On Learning from the Patient*. London: Routledge.

Casement P (1990/2014). *Further Learning from the Patient*. London: Routledge.

de Maat S, de Jonghe F, Schoevers R, Dekker J (2009). The effectiveness of long-term psychoanalytic therapy: a systematic review of empirical studies. *Harvard Review of Psychiatry* 17:11–23.

Doidge N (1997) Empirical evidence for the efficacy of psychoanalytic psychotherapies and psychoanalysis: An overview. *Psychoanalytic Inquiry* 17(S1):102–150.

Ellman SJ (2010). *When Theories Touch: A Historical and Theoretical Integration of Psychoanalytic Thought*. London: Karnac.

Ferro A (2005). *Seeds of Illness, Seeds of Recovery: The Genesis of Suffering, and the Role of Psychoanalysis*. London: Routledge.

Ferro A (2008). The patient as the analyst's best colleague: Transformation into a dream and narrative transformations. *Italian Psychoanalytic Annual* 2:199–205.

Gabbard GO (2000). *Psychodynamic Psychiatry in Clinical Practice*, 3rd edition. Washington, DC: American Psychiatric Press.

Glucksman ML, Kramer M (2004). Using dreams to assess clinical change during treatment. *Journal of the American Academy of Psychoanalysis and Dynamic Psychiatry* 32:345–358.

Joseph B (2007). Video: *Meeting Betty Joseph*. From *Encounters Through Generations* series (an extract). The Institute of Psychoanalysis, PEP-Web videos.

Kramer M, Glucksman M (2012). The usefulness of the manifest dream report. *Academy Forum* 56:15–17.

Leichsenring F, Rabung S (2008). Effectiveness of long-term psychodynamic psychotherapy: A meta-analysis. *Journal of the American Medical Association* 300(13):1551–1565.

Leichsenring F, Rabung S (2011). Long-term psychodynamic psychotherapy in complex mental disorders: Update of a meta-analysis. *British Journal of Psychiatry* 199(1):15–22.

Leichsenring F, Abbass A, Luyten P, Hilsenroth P, Rabung S (2013). The emerging evidence for long-term psychodynamic therapy. *Psychodynamic Psychiatry* 41:361–384.

Levy RA, Ablon JS (2009). *Handbook of Evidence-Based Psychodynamic Psychotherapy*. New York: Humana Press.

Luborsky L, Crits-Christoph P, Mintz J, Auerbach A (1988). *Who Will Benefit from Psychotherapy: Predicting Therapeutic Outcomes*. New York: Basic Books.

McWilliams N (1999). *Psychoanalytic Case Formulation*. New York: Guilford Press.

McWilliams N (2004). *Psychoanalytic Psychotherapy: A Practitioner's Guide*. New York: Guilford Press.

McWilliams N (2011). *Psychoanalytic Diagnosis*, 2nd edition. New York: Guilford Press.

Messer SB, Abbass AA (2010). Psychodynamic therapy with personality disorders. In: Magnavita JF (ed.), *Evidence-Based Treatment of Personality Dysfunction*. Washington, DC: American Psychological Association, 79–111.

Mitchell SA, Black MJ (1995). *Freud and Beyond: A History of Modern Psychoanalytic Thought*. New York: Basic Books.

Newirth J (2018). *From Sign to Symbol: Transformational Processes in Psychoanalysis, Psychotherapy and Psychology*. New York: Lexington Books.

Ogden TH (1996). The perverse subject of analysis. *Journal of the American Psychoanalytic Association* 44:1121–1146.

Ogden TH (2005). On psychoanalytic writing. *International Journal of Psycho-Analysis* 86(1):15–29.

Ogden TH (2016). Some thoughts on practising psychoanalysis. *Fort Da* 22(1):21–36.

Segal H (1958). Fear of death – Notes on the analysis of an old man. *International Journal of Psychoanalysis* 39:178–181.

Seitler BN (2019). Who sez psychoanalysis ain't got no empirical research to back up its claims: An extensive bibliographic compendium of studies. *JASPER International: Journal for the Advancement of Scientific Psychodynamic Empirical Research: Spurring Research Forward* 2(1):63–103.

Shakespeare W (1599/1992). *Julius Caesar*. Folger Shakespeare Library, Mowat BA, Werstine P (eds.), New York: Washington Square Press.

Shedler J (2010). The efficacy of psychodynamic psychotherapy. *American Psychologist* 65(2):98–109.

Slavin MO, Kriegman D (1998). Why the analyst needs to change: Toward a theory of conflict, negotiation, and mutual influence in the psychotherapeutic process. *Psychoanalytic Dialogues* 8(2):247–284.

Steinberg PI (2017a). Whipped cream and other delights: A reverie and its aftermath. *Canadian Journal of Psychoanalysis* 25(2):88–105.

Steinberg PI (2017b). Love and Hate in the Countertransference, presented to Canadian Psychoanalytic Society Congress, Ottawa, June 2, 2017.

Steinberg PI (2018). Dreams as indicators of the psychoanalytic treatment process. *Canadian Journal of Psychoanalysis* 26(2):150–172.

Stolorow RD, Atwood GE (1979). *Faces in a Cloud: Subjectivity in Personality Theory*. New York: Jason Aaronson.

Sullivan HS (1940). *Conceptions of Modern Psychiatry*. New York: WW Norton.

Symington N (1986). *The Analytic Experience: Lectures from the Tavistock*. London: Free Association Books.

Taylor GJ (1987). *Psychosomatic Medicine and Contemporary Psychoanalysis*. Madison, CT: International Universities Press.

Taylor GJ (2016). Varieties of castration experience: relevance to contemporary psychoanalysis and psychodynamic psychotherapy. *Psychodynamic Psychiatry* 44(1):39–68.

Truant GS (1998). Assessment for suitability for psychotherapy I: Introduction and the assessment process. *American Journal of Psychotherapy* 52(4):397–411.

Truant GS (1999). Assessment for suitability for psychotherapy II: Assessment based on basic process goals. *American Journal of Psychotherapy* 53(1):17–34.

Winnicott DW (1975). *Through Pediatrics to Psycho-Analysis*. New York: Basic Books.

INTRODUCTION PART 2

A LITTLE THEORY

BRIEF DESCRIPTIONS OF ATTACHMENT AND OBJECT RELATIONS THEORY

I will briefly outline two related psychoanalytic theories helpful in understanding people and their difficulties (Steinberg, 1998). Attachment theory holds that an essential need for people is positive human attachments. The mothering figure's attunement and responsiveness to the infant in the first months of life are crucial in the early development of the infant's capacity to think. A child with a secure attachment is confident to explore the world as he grows. Children's relationships with their parents are important determinants of the quality of attachments that children eventually form as adults. Deprivation of positive attachments during childhood makes establishing them in adulthood difficult or impossible. Absence of, losing, or experiencing the threat of losing positive attachments or substitutes for them (see below) renders adults susceptible to adverse psychological and somatic reactions. Loss, disappointment, or frustration in an important relationship may lead to many reactions, including somatic symptoms, depression, withdrawal, search for a substitute, or hostility with accompanying guilt. Another reaction involves creativity, either in the arts, or finding a constructive solution to a problem in a relationship. Of course, one's parents are not one's only influences in childhood. To the extent that an individual who has been deprived of adequate positive experiences with his parents has meaningful positive contacts with other adults, such as extended family, friends, teachers, coaches, and leaders of youth organizations, his less-than-satisfactory experiences with his parents may be mitigated, and his psychological growth enhanced.

If an individual in childhood is deprived of positive human attachments, he may find a substitute. Three types of substitutes may be distinguished. The first group consists of direct somatic satisfaction, generally oral or genital. It includes substance abuse, overindulgence in food or alcohol, and compulsive, destructive, or self-destructive sexual behavior. The second involves "narcissistic" satisfactions, including the pursuit of power, admiration, fame, or wealth. The third involves intense investment of interest in an activity or object. This includes devotion to work, an institution, a social cause, or a group; involvement with a recreational activity; or an attachment to animals, plants, places, or even inanimate objects. Deprivation of these outlets also may lead to adverse psychological or somatic reactions. All psychological treatments offer the opportunity for a positive human attachment. To what extent learning specific to any particular form of therapy is therapeutic is an important question. Little psychotherapeutic progress is imaginable outside the milieu of a positive attachment to a therapist; experiments attempting to have computers function as psychotherapists have failed.

Attachment theory can be used in psychodynamic formulation (a psychoanalytic understanding of how a patient developed to be the way she is) to organize historical data into predisposing, precipitating, perpetuating, and protective factors, which are understood to affect an individual's development and life situation. Impoverished, interrupted, or disturbed early attachments predispose an individual (render her vulnerable) to loss or disappointment in later attachments. Maladaptive styles of attachment learned in early relationships influence the style of relating in adult life and the choice of individuals with whom attachments are formed. Our early relationships then are internalized as negative self- and object-images, that is, negative images of the self and others, which are associated with painful affects and a predisposition to psychiatric symptoms. Based on our early attachments, we are familiar with certain ways of relating and forming attachments to certain types of people. We tend as adults to relate in similar ways with similar types of people.

A common precipitating factor in the exacerbation of psychiatric symptoms is the loss of, threatened loss of, or disappointment in important attachments. It is important not only to identify these losses, but also to identify their importance and meaning to the patient, based on predisposing factors, such as early attachment patterns. Similarly, ongoing disturbed attachments are often identified as perpetuating factors. Thus, it is necessary to understand their significance to the patient in the context of early attachments. It is important to look for disappointment in, loss of, or threatened loss of an important attachment or a substitute for an attachment in trying to understand the onset of a psychiatric or psychosomatic symptom. Temporally associated precipitants for each symptom should be examined in terms of the impact or imagined impact the precipitating events have had on the patient's attachments.

A history of positive attachments in early life is an important protective factor. Ongoing positive attachments are protective factors, and also are important when considering a patient's suicide risk. Observations about the attachment between the clinician and the patient, beginning from the first interview, are utilized in formulation. This includes noting the patient's attitude towards the clinician, the characteristic defenses the patient uses, and one's emotional reaction (countertransference) to the patient. The latter may provide important clues to the patient's feelings and to feelings he elicits in others. For example, if the clinician is uncharacteristically angry when with a certain patient, she might wonder whether this represents a feeling the patient is experiencing but cannot express. Alternatively, this countertransference anger might be a clue to the clinician that what she is experiencing with this patient is something many people experience with him. Or it may represent a sensitivity of hers.

According to object relations theory, interpersonal experiences affect unconscious images of the self and others. The most powerful influences are parenting figures, who in the happiest circumstances are reliably available, protective, have the child's best interests in mind, and have a generally positive attitude towards the child. A child's self-image largely is based on an internalization of her parents' attitude. The child with parents who feel generally positive towards her tends to grow with a similarly positive attitude towards herself. The converse is true of the unfortunate child whose parents have a more negative attitude. There is not an absolute correlation between parents' attitude towards their child and the child's attitude towards herself; inborn temperamental factors (such as high sensitivity) and unavoidable environmental factors (such as a depressed mother) can influence the child's perception of her parents, which affects the internal images she develops of them. Frustration and loss in early important relationships lead to unfriendly internal images of other people ("bad internal objects"), which tend to promote less constructive reactions, whereas a history of satisfactory relationships results in more benign images of others. This in turn favors a more constructive adaptation in adult life, including in relationships and work.

The internal object, the unconscious image of the other, largely is based on the child's experience with her parents, seen through the child's eyes. There is controversy regarding the extent to which a child's perception of her parents may be unrealistic. The observation that an individual with a personality disorder can distort early memories may be used in an attempt to exonerate parents from responsibility for how the individual has developed. However, it is possible to give parents some responsibility for their children's development without blaming them for it, which is not productive.

Internal images of self and object are subject to modification based on new learning. We tend to project images of our self and our internal objects, our images of the other, on to other people. A sign of relative psychological health is that these projections are not so strong that they interfere significantly with our realistically evaluating others based on our experience with them. Persons functioning at low levels of psychological development tend to project alternately good or bad "part-objects," polar positive or negative unconscious internal images, on to other people, with a corresponding unrealistic idealization or devaluation of them. (More on this later.) They experience others as all good or all bad, as opposed to tolerating ambivalence, that is, positive and negative feelings concurrently about someone. In the severest range of pathology, individuals functioning at a psychotic level project their self- and object-representations so unrealistically that they are delusional about how they perceive themselves and others. Their auditory hallucinations are interpreted as unacceptable thoughts of their own that had been evacuated and can be experienced as coming from others.

Internal objects influence what we expect in relationships. This is obvious when an individual expects someone to be a certain way when she knows little about that person. Internal objects also influence the way that we perceive other people. Our transference, the way in which we perceive others based on our previous experiences, more or less distorts our perceptions of the other, depending on the extent to which we project our internal self-image or internal objects on to him. An individual may even influence the way someone else relates to her by unconsciously eliciting or provoking certain behaviors on the other person's part. This mechanism, called projective identification, often involves unconsciously inducing in the other person a feeling or impulse one cannot accept in oneself.

Two defensive tendencies in which interpersonal experiences are repeated instead of remembered involve an individual's projection of either a self- or object-image on to another person, concurrently identifying respectively with the internal object or with the self. In the former situation, an individual projects her self-image on to another person, and treats that individual as she experienced herself being treated as a child by her parents. The latter situation involves the projection of the internal object (the unconscious image of the other) on to the other person. The individual then reacts to the other person in a similar way to how she reacted to her parents, often unconsciously inviting the other person to treat her as her parents did (projective identification). The interpretation of these two forms of interaction, especially in the therapeutic relationship, is important in psychoanalytic therapy. The more primitive one's personality development or the more regressed one has become, the greater the tendency to rely on these projections, rather than realistically evaluating other people. The use of these observations is often crucial in the optimal medical management of "difficult" patients, who can expertly, if unconsciously, influence the attitudes of medical caregivers towards them, often in an adverse way. To the extent that we remain unaware of how these patients may provoke us, for example, to become enraged with them, our anger might distract us from providing our best medical care (Maltsberger & Buie, 1974).

Individuals who experience frustration in early attachments still need to preserve a positive internal object, an unconscious image of a friendly parent. This may require the defense of splitting, which defends against a realistically ambivalent attitude towards others. Positive and negative perceptions of and feelings about others are kept separate to prevent the negative feelings from overwhelming the positive. This results in polar opposite positive and negative part-objects, that is, one-dimensional unconscious images of the other, which may be projected into others in adult life. By "projected," I mean that the projecting individual experiences the other person as corresponding to his unconscious internal image of the other, in this case an unrealistically all-positive or all-negative image. Similarly, positive and negative aspects of the self may be split and kept separated in the mind. All this may distort one's perception of self and of others in relationships, and is characteristic of more severe personality disturbance. (People without such severe personality disturbance may regress to this type of experiencing of self and other when under stress; we all engage in this to some extent.) The projection of a good part-object is manifested in idealization, and that of a bad part-object in devaluation. Both involve unrealistic perceptions of others. An individual with these tendencies, Y, may initially idealize a person, Z, with whom he has begun a relationship. This is understood as Y projecting a good part-object on to Z. However, it is difficult for Z to live up to Y's unrealistic expectations. When Y inevitably becomes disappointed, he may then project a bad part-object on to Z, resulting in a devaluation as unrealistic as was the idealization. This pattern, when repeated, results in intense, chaotic, and disappointing relationships. This can occur in relationships involving romance, friendships, and work, but also can occur in physician–patient relationships. These oscillating and extreme attitudes towards others and towards oneself often are seen in therapeutic relationships with patients who have severe personality disturbance.

This helps explain many unsatisfactory physician–patient interactions. It may be transiently pleasant to be idealized by a patient, although one may be aware of how unrealistic this evaluation is. It is not so pleasant when the idealization is abruptly replaced by a devaluation, often expressed in very strong terms, and accompanied by a verbal attack. At this point, the physician may become aware that the patient's idealization was accompanied by very unrealistic expectations of the physician, which, when it became clear to the patient that the physician wouldn't meet these expectations, resulted in an abrupt shift in the patient's attitude towards the physician. Internally, the patient stopped projecting a good part-object and instead projected a bad part-object on to the physician. This describes the kind of alternation between positive and negative relationships a physician can experience, for example, with a person with borderline personality disorder. Freud described his understanding of transference, indicating that his patient's falling in love with him was not due to his irresistible charm, but rather to her love unconsciously being transferred on to him from the original object of her love.

ASPECTS OF PERSONALITY FUNCTIONING

One of the most important discoveries of psychoanalysis has been the concept of internal reality. External reality refers to the consensually agreed-upon concrete configuration of the world. For example, two people could agree that the table in a room has four legs. Internal reality refers to the unconscious inner world, populated by images of oneself and others, not necessarily corresponding to external reality, but based on the individual's emotional response to her cumulative experience, especially interpersonal experience. This internal reality also is affected by inborn temperamental factors unrelated to experience in the world. Unconscious fantasy is part of internal reality. It can influence one's reaction to experiences in the external world. For example, if a child's parents do not show interest in her developing internal world, that is, are not interested in her thoughts, wishes, and feelings, and generally just expect her to conform to their wishes, dismissing her ideas and initiatives, she may grow up believing that others have no interest in her thoughts or feelings, and no wish to permit her to assume personal agency, making choices about which directions she wishes to pursue in life. With this unconscious fantasy, she likely will be very sensitive to others' reactions to her initiatives and the expression of her thoughts and feelings, with a tendency to assume that they are not interested. This has a negative impact on her development as an individual and developing satisfying and close relationships with others. Also, children whose parents do not show interest in their developing internal world tend to identify with the parents, and have a similar lack of interest in their internal world. This detracts from development of cognitive abilities, a capacity for imagination and creativity, and interest in both the external world and their aspirations and wishes. Under these conditions, a child is disadvantaged regarding realizing her potential.

Living a satisfying active life as a human being requires attention to both one's internal and external worlds. The internal world is the source of feelings, ideas, wishes, impulses, and fantasies, which provide a richness to life, and which we need to inspire us regarding decisions we make about how we live our lives. The external world is a potential source of both opportunities and joy, and danger and pain, and must be perceived, thought and felt about, and accommodated to. One hallmark of relative emotional health is the capacity to distinguish between internal and external reality. This is significantly lost in psychosis, where an individual's feelings and thoughts, part of the internal world, may be experienced as if they were part of the external world, in hallucinations and delusions. However, no one is completely able to distinguish their internal and external worlds; there is inevitably some overlap.

Mechanisms of defense are unconscious attempts to reduce anxiety and other painful feelings. Too heavy reliance on what are called more primitive mechanisms of defense is typical in more disturbed personalities. These defenses, including projection, projective identification, splitting, and denial, interfere with an individual's capacity to test reality. For example, in projection and projective identification, an aspect of the self is not acknowledged as being part of the self, but is experienced as part of someone else. In splitting, two aspects of one's perception of another person, for example, are kept separate in the mind. The individual who is splitting may respond at some points to the other person as if the other person is entirely characterized by one part of the split, for example, a tendency towards openness and generosity. At other points, the individual who is splitting may respond to the other person as if he is entirely characterized by the other side of the split, for example, a tendency towards caution about money and relationships. The external reality of the other person, as it were, may be that under some circumstances, he is inclined to be generous and open, but when feeling threatened, he may be more cautious. Rather than perceiving the whole of the other individual, the patient who relies on splitting may only perceive part of it at a time, and react to that part.

In denial, an individual undoes his perception of some aspect of reality, often motivated by the individual experiencing reality as unbearably painful. For example, an investor who has relied too heavily on an investment succeeding may ignore clear signs that it needs to be sold at a loss, with the result that it loses further value, a loss that could have been prevented if the individual had been able to tolerate conscious awareness of the reality of the investments.

These more primitive mechanisms of defense also involve an impoverishment or loss of being in touch with the internal world. In projection and projective identification, aspects of the self, being attributed to someone else, are no longer available to the self. This may include positive attributes, such as a capacity to think, which are projected in order to be preserved or protected, as the patient may feel that he would destroy his capacity to think if he did not find a safe refuge for it outside himself. Similarly, in splitting, when the individual has disavowed a part of himself that has been split off, he cannot use it.

The personality structures of patients have been divided arbitrarily into different levels of severity: neurotic (including "normal"), borderline, and psychotic (McWilliams, 2011). Of course, no individual's personality corresponds exactly to any of these categories; rather, it is a question of to what extent an individual's personality structure most resembles the characteristics of each of these levels. The three criteria used in determining level of personality structure are reality testing, identity integration, and maturity of defense mechanisms. Reality testing involves a capacity to recognize consensually agreed-upon external reality. Individuals with an adequately integrated sense of identity demonstrate consistent behavior and an inner experience of continuity of the self through time. They are able to describe themselves in some depth, feel a sense of continuity with their past, and imagine their future directions. They are able to describe people they are close to in three-dimensional terms, considering both their positive and negative attributes together. It is important to note that patients with neurotic level of personality organization do not necessarily suffer from what used to be called neurotic symptoms, such as conversion, obsessive-compulsive, or phobic symptoms. Patients with borderline level of personality function do not necessarily have a borderline personality disorder. Patients with psychotic level of personality functioning do not necessarily exhibit florid psychotic symptoms. These different levels of personality functioning do not describe symptoms or specific personality constellations, but rather different levels of personality development.

Neurotic level of personality structure is characterized by good contact with reality, relatively intact integration of personal identity, and reliance on mature defenses, including altruism, humor, and sublimation (the direction of personally unacceptable or potentially destructive impulses into constructive activities, for example, playing physically active competitive sports as a way of coping with aggressive impulses). This structure is also characterized by reliance on "neurotic" defenses that are relatively mature, including intellectualization (concentrating on the concrete or intellectual aspects of a situation while distancing oneself from the associated uncomfortable feelings); reaction formation (turning unconscious wishes or impulses that are felt to be unacceptable into their opposites, for example, treating a person kindly when harboring unfriendly feelings towards her); and repression (the blocking out of conscious awareness of feelings, thoughts, and impulses that are unacceptable or threatening to the individual).

Borderline level of personality structure is characterized by adequate reality testing when these individuals are at their best. However, they have a tendency to regress when anxious or threatened; this is accompanied by more impaired reality testing. The identity integration of these patients is not as complete as those at the neurotic level. In that way they are similar to patients at the psychotic level; their sense of self is deficient. Their experience of themselves is likely to be inconsistent and discontinuous. They have difficulty describing themselves and others close to them in three-dimensional ways, considering both positive and negative aspects of the individuals at the same time. As opposed to individuals with psychotic personality organization, borderline individuals may have identity confusion, but they do know that they exist. As well, they are much more likely to react with hostility to questions about their and others' identities than patients at the psychotic level. Borderline patients rely on primitive defenses. In addition to the primitive defenses mentioned above, idealization and devaluation are common, as they alternately project positive and negative part-objects on to others, experiencing them transiently as all good or all bad.

Patients with psychotic level of personality organization characteristically have significantly impaired reality testing. Without necessarily being floridly psychotic, they may espouse unrealistic beliefs or think in idiosyncratic ways that interfere with their capacity to adapt to the external world around them, such as tangential thinking (in which their thoughts wander away from the subject at hand without returning to it). They have a very disturbed sense of personal identity, to the extent that they may not be sure they exist. Their descriptions of themselves and others are vague, inconsistent, unrealistic, and superficial. Patients at a psychotic level of personality organization rely on primitive mechanisms of defense in order to protect themselves from terror that they are not able to articulate.

For example, I diagnosed a highly trained and ostensibly highly regarded professional with a narcissistic personality disorder, likely with some antisocial features. The presence of dissociation, the unreliability of his memory, a difficulty in commitments, including repeated difficulty establishing regular times for us to meet when I tried to make arrangements for treatment, and never remembering any dreams, taken together suggested a significant level of disturbance of personality functioning. This patient could be located between borderline and psychotic levels of personality functioning.

The physician who is able to identify and consider his patient's level of personality functioning will be better prepared to predict how his patients may respond to interactions with him, and deal with the difficulties that patients at borderline and psychotic levels may present him with than will patients functioning at a neurotic level. For example, when a physician must cancel a patient's appointment, he may expect the neurotic patient to accept this, and any disappointment or inconvenience this may entail. He will be prepared for the borderline patient to experience this as a personal rejection, and to react with a degree of sadness or rage that seems incommensurate with the stimulus. He will be less bewildered when the psychotic patient becomes confused or acts as if she didn't even hear what the doctor said, and acts as if the appointment had not been cancelled.

REFERENCES

Maltsberger JT, Buie DH (1974). Countertransference hate in the treatment of suicidal patients. *Archives of General Psychiatry* 30(5):625–633.

McWilliams N (2011). *Psychoanalytic Diagnosis: Understanding Personality Structure in the Clinical Process*, 2nd edition. New York: Guilford Press.

Steinberg PI (1998). Attachment and object relations in formulation and psychotherapy. *Annals of the Royal College of Physicians and Surgeons of Canada* 31(1):19–22.

PART I

LEARNING FROM LIAISON WITH FAMILY MEDICINE

The opinions I express in this section are based primarily on my 12-year involvement with a university-affiliated family medicine clinic. Of course, I have also learned from the hundreds of family physicians who have referred me patients over the years in my contacts with them. I think being a competent family physician is the most difficult job in medicine. You have to tolerate each specialist knowing more than you in their area of specialty, and continue caring for patients the specialists send back to you, in various states of health and frames of mind. It is difficult but a sign of maturity to tolerate not knowing something. Of course, it is impossible to know everything in medicine; this applies to us all. It may be impossible to know what ails a patient. It largely may be an emotional disturbance expressed in somatic terms, which is hard to establish with any confidence, as diagnoses of exclusion are unreliable. It is difficult to interpret a somatic symptom or sign as representing a specific unconscious conflict or an unbearable feeling or experience that a patient cannot articulate in words.. Family physicians operate under considerable time pressure. I wish I could secondarily dedicate this book to all the family physicians who provide so much holding (unfamiliar with Winnicott's concept of holding) (Caldwell & Joyce, 2011) of their patients for so long, and containing their patients' unbearable affects (without knowledge of Bion's concept of container/contained) (Vermote, 2019). I think family medicine is one of the "impossible" professions, like government, education, and psychoanalysis (Freud, 1937/1964). Like the proverbial woman's work, it is never done.

Chapter 1 deals with patients with significant personality disturbance that adversely affects their relationships with their physicians, thus adversely affecting management of their medical conditions. I indicate that the physician's feelings can be a diagnostic tool, describe an approach with a patient who denies illness, and offer some ideas regarding the origins of personality disturbance, and how it can be managed.

Chapter 2 deals with patient interviewing, and how physicians can listen for themes in a patient's conversation that may hold clues to what is bothering him. I suggest avoiding giving a patient too much support in an attempt to make him feel better, because this may prevent him from going through his own thinking process and making mature decisions. It is important to eschew giving personal advice, which similarly may interfere with patients' thinking and taking responsibility for their own actions. The clinician can use her own feelings and reactions to the patient better to understand his personality and problems. Consultation with a psychiatrist can help clarify the family physician's role in assisting a particular patient.

In Chapter 3 diagnostic criteria are employed to distinguish between major depressive episode and other conditions involving depressive mood commonly presenting to physicians. Relative indications for antidepressant medication and for two types of psychotherapy are discussed. The potential disadvantages of routinely prescribing antidepressants to patients who complain of depressive mood are described. I describe the roles of psychoanalytic psychotherapy and cognitive behavior therapy in treating depressive conditions.

In Chapter 4, the liaison model of consultation illustrates how including a psychiatrist on a medical team can enhance patient care. I use a case history of a patient with a delusion about her eyes and her need for ophthalmologic surgery to illustrate diagnosis and management of patients who misinterpret or deny signs of disease. This patient's paranoid delusion complicated her physician's medical management of her. I outline a collaborative approach using a liaison model for psychiatric consultation. A discussion of mechanisms of defense in paranoid individuals is included.

In Chapter 5, I discuss patients with severe personality disorders who suffer from disturbances in the form or content of their thinking, in their affect regulation, or in their capacity to contain impulses, that may be severe enough to interfere with progress in various forms of psychotherapy. These patients are not floridly psychotic, and do not readily fit into our current diagnostic terminology. Small doses of atypical neuroleptics may help relieve their symptoms, so they can benefit from psychodynamic group psychotherapy in a day treatment program. This treatment may also be beneficial in other modalities of psychotherapy and in patients being supported by family physicians. Research is needed to determine whether this is the case, and whether patient improvement is due largely to the medication or the psychotherapy. In any situation where neuroleptic medications are used, it is important to review the potentially serious side effects of those medications with patients and to monitor patients for side effects. Advances in psychoanalytic understanding of more severe pathologies with corresponding changes in technique have made it possible to treat patients with a much broader range of disturbances initially thought to be beyond the range of psychoanalytic treatment, including not only patients with psychotic symptoms, but also patients with severe personality disorders and psychosomatic conditions. The psychoanalytic finding that everyone has a psychotic side to their personality, and that psychoanalysis or psychoanalytically informed psychotherapy may be helpful in treating patients whose psychotic parts are too prominent and interfering with their functioning, is not well appreciated in medical circles.

In Chapter 6, I note that communication and understanding between psychoanalysts and physicians often are suboptimal. Few physicians, including psychiatrists, really understand what psychoanalysts do, what psychoanalysis and psychoanalytic psychotherapy offer their patients, and which of their patients are likely to benefit from these treatments. Physicians sometimes expect too much from psychoanalysts or too little. Psychoanalysts have the potential to offer physicians assistance in many facets of medical care. They can provide a psychodynamic understanding of unconscious factors influencing not only the patient's behavior, but also that of medical and allied staff on psychiatric and other inpatient units. The latter may be important when a patient, "psychiatric" or otherwise, presents difficulties in management. The difficulty may include stirring up dissension among medical and non-medical staff on the inpatient unit, which, if not addressed, can perpetuate the difficulties they are having with the patient, as well as resulting in disharmony amongst staff that can become very destructive. The latter issue is covered in detail in Chapters 14 and 15.

Some medications described in this book may be "old-fashioned" because the patients were treated with them several decades ago.

REFERENCES

Caldwell L, Joyce A (eds.) (2011). *Reading Winnicott*. London: Routledge.

Freud S (1937/1964). Analysis terminable and interminable. In: *The Standard Edition of the Complete Psychological Works of Sigmund Freud*, Vol. XXIII. London: Hogarth Press.

Vermote R (2019). *Reading Bion*. London: Routledge.

CHAPTER 1

"PROBLEM PATIENTS": PATIENTS WITH SIGNIFICANT PERSONALITY DISTURBANCE

I have difficulty with the concept of "personality disorder" because of its binary implications, as if patients either have a personality disorder or do not, as opposed to spectra of severity of personality disturbance from less to more severe, and of forms of personality disturbance (McWilliams, 2011). We all have personalities characterized by certain traits. The more extreme and rigid these traits are manifest, the more likely they will interfere with our optimal functioning, and at some point may warrant a diagnosis of personality disorder. However, even if a diagnosis of personality disorder is never made, our personality traits can involve considerable suffering, and significant interference with our functioning.

One of the problems in discussing personality disorders is that there is no well-defined group of symptoms as there is for other psychiatric conditions. Instead, there are variations in behavior that, when observed as part of a pattern, can be classified as character traits or features. Personality disorders are described as ego-syntonic (its features are relatively comfortable for the patient) in that the patient does not experience ego-dystonic or ego-alien symptoms (that he is uncomfortable with), but rather experiences difficulties in his relationship with his environment. *Of course, patients with personality disorders do experience psychiatric symptoms, such as anxiety and depression, but these symptoms are not the hallmark of the diagnosis. Rather, it is the patient's experience of himself, and his manner of interacting with his environment, that are central to the diagnosis of personality disorder.*

Because the adaptations associated with personality disorders are ego-syntonic, they can be difficult to recognize. The clinician cannot rely on signs, symptoms, and laboratory investigations to make a diagnosis, but must be able to use her own feelings as a guide to understanding her patient's personality difficulties. Another problem in discussing personality disorder is that, while few of us have symptoms of major psychiatric conditions such as psychosis, severe depression, or a full-blown neurosis, we all have personalities. To what extent our personality styles are maladaptive determines whether we call ourselves "disordered." *Now I would say, "disturbance in the personality," as opposed to "personality disorder," to avoid making a black-and-white distinction between those who have personality disorders and those who do not. The question is, to what extent is the personality of an individual characterized by disturbance, and of what quality is the disturbance?*

Most readers of this book have in common the study of disease and the practice of medicine. Undoubtedly we all have altruistic intentions, but there is more to our motivation to become health professionals. The situation in which many, if not all, of us have found ourselves at times, that of temporarily acquiring the symptoms of the conditions we are studying, "medical students' disease," suggests that those who choose to know about and fight illness may have personal concerns about becoming ill that are brought to the fore by studying medicine. We try to master our fear of illness by learning about it, which ironically exposes the very fears we try to master. Our attempts to deal with illness result in the re-emergence of our hidden fear of illness.

To discuss personality difficulties among ourselves or to investigate them in our patients is a similarly uncomfortable procedure. We cannot avoid being reminded by our patients of aspects of ourselves that we have difficulty accepting. There is always the temptation not to be confronted with these aspects of ourselves, or of our patients. *One way of looking at this phenomenon is that people often deal with what they cannot bear to see in themselves by projecting it into others. In the case of physicians this may be our fear of disease, which motivates us to become physicians, so we are surrounded by ill people and identify them (and not ourselves) as the ill ones, or, by identifying personality disturbance in others, we are (consciously) unaware of similar tendencies in ourselves.*

PATIENT 1: THE DOCTOR'S FEELINGS AS A DIAGNOSTIC TOOL

This vignette illustrates how a patient's personality influences the medical care he receives, and may suggest how integrating an understanding of the patient's personality with clinical and laboratory investigations can lead to more effective and satisfying medical practice.

A patient complained of "worms" to her physician; stool examination was negative, but she said the worms had spread from her anal region to her abdomen. Eventually, she felt the worms were coming out of her nose. The patient presented the doctor with two specimens. One was diagnosed by microbiology as a hair. The doctor recognized the second as a millipede, but sent it off for classification because he was concerned that he might be sued by the patient if he made a mistake. He was also contemplating a neurological investigation, to rule out the possibility of an intracranial mass lesion. His fear of litigation was increased by a respected senior colleague who suggested that if the doctor missed some organic cause for this patient's complaints, he would risk a lawsuit because the patient may not have been competent to judge her need for treatment. Also, the patient's husband aggressively demanded that the physician "do something" for the patient.

The patient's husband had attended a mental health center several times for an unspecified illness, which involved troublesome and threatening behavior. The doctor's only contacts with him were a couple of phone calls in which he insisted that the doctor help his wife. The patient herself insisted that she only wanted help for her worms and was not crazy. At one point the doctor prescribed an antipsychotic medication, but the patient stopped taking it after two days because of dizziness. The doctor left it at that. The patient refused further investigation or consultations with consultants, and added to the doctor's anxiety by questioning his competence.

I might have wondered what the patient's fantasy, possibly delusional in form, of being infested by worms, might have meant. Dead people are one group that, at least in the public mind, may be inhabited by worms, during the process of decay after death. Another group are individuals who actually have a parasitic infestation, often after visiting tropical climates. Could this patient have been expressing a feeling that she was dead, or invaded by a parasite? Could this be related to what she described as the "long and bitter experience" of sharing her life with her husband, and what that experience had meant for her? What kind of "attack" from the outside might she have felt she was experiencing?

The doctor's concern about being attacked, physically and legally, could be described as a parallel process (Searles, 1955). This phenomenon originally was identified as occurring when patterns in the relationship between a psychoanalytic patient and a psychoanalyst were observed to be recapitulated in the relationship between the psychoanalyst and his supervisor. Of course, this type of process may occur between two groups of individuals who are related in other ways, especially involving hierarchies, not just a psychoanalyst/patient and supervisor/psychoanalyst pair of dyads, but, for example, a physician/patient and consultant/family physician pair, or a pupil/teacher dyad and a principal/teacher dyad.

What was the doctor's problem with this patient, such that he persisted in attempting to rule out a lesion for which there was scanty evidence, and to document that millipedes weren't intestinal parasites? All the while, he was also preoccupied with being sued, apparently without exploring the possibility that this woman might have been suffering from a major psychiatric disorder. The patient, having had long and bitter experience with her husband's history of mental illness, was ill disposed to accept that she herself might have emotional problems, especially as she had to "hold things together," because she couldn't count on her husband. Her unwillingness to be identified as a psychiatric patient might indicate she resented her husband's behavior; she wouldn't be "crazy" like him. This woman's condition could be described as paranoid. She believed she was suffering from an infestation, an attack from outside herself.

In his involvement with the patient and her husband, the family doctor had a similar, if milder, experience. He also feared attack, both a physical attack by the husband, and a legal attack if he missed making the correct diagnosis. This resulted in a concentrated attempt to perform neurological examinations, which paralleled the patient's insistence that her worms be found and eliminated. It is not necessary to examine this doctor's personality. All doctors are concerned to some extent about whether they have done the right thing in a given situation. The same obsessive character traits that enable us to study enough to pass our exams contribute to our doubts about whether we have acted competently. The senior colleague's warning, the patient's comments about the doctor's competence, and the husband's history of threatening behavior all contributed to this doctor's anxiety. Although the doctor, in prescribing an anti-psychotic medication, apparently recognized that the problem involved a psychiatric condition, these pressures encouraged him to abandon his usual competent approach to clinical investigation, beginning with a complete history. As a result, he colluded with his patient in avoiding the seriousness of her psychiatric disturbance, confining his efforts to ruling out a neurological disorder.

The patient's refusal to see a consultant and persistence in demanding that she be treated for worms may have been her way of expressing the feeling that no one, including the doctor, understood her problem. One possible approach to this patient would have been to attempt to discover if she felt the same way in other relationships, for example, in her relationship with her husband. Then reasonable medical investigations could have been pursued concurrently with a psychological investigation. With some knowledge of the utility of countertransference, this doctor would be able to use his personal feelings to help make the "diagnosis" in this case. When he found he was not managing his patient in his usual competent way, but was concerned with being attacked or prosecuted, he might have asked himself if this concern was being conveyed to him somehow by his patient. *That is, the doctor could have used his countertransference to understand what his patient was experiencing. Heiman (1950) introduced the notion of countertransference, like transference, being a helpful source of information about one's patient, as opposed to just an obstacle in treatment.*

The doctor could further his investigation by asking his patient what explanation she had for what was happening to her. He might suggest that the experiences she described must be very upsetting, and then try to find out what else might be disturbing her. A question about the husband's reaction to her illness could lead to a discussion about difficulties this woman had with her "aggressively demanding" husband. Arranging a joint appointment with husband and wife, in order to ask him exactly what he thought was wrong, and what he hoped the doctor would do, might elucidate problems in the marriage, and enlist the husband as an ally in the doctor's attempt to get his patient the treatment that she needed. It might also decrease the doctor's anxiety about the distant, but feared, husband, and help him see how afraid this patient might be of her husband.

Investigating a patient's physical complaints without considering the *person* making the complaints can result in diagnostic and therapeutic misadventure. Patients rarely present with symptoms as dramatic as delusions, but they will frequently complain of headaches or a sore throat that hardly seem to justify the appointment. Then the physician can ask himself and his patient why she is really there. Family physicians should also request a psychiatric opinion if they suspect a patient is psychotic, even if they intend to treat the patient during the psychotic episode without ongoing involvement from a psychiatrist. The psychiatrist may give helpful advice about appropriate medication, decisions on hospitalization, the best use of community treatment, and differential diagnosis. *Sadly, my comment regarding family physicians treating psychotic patients without the ongoing involvement of psychiatrists was unwittingly prophetic. With the dramatic decline in availability of hospital beds for psychotic patients since this chapter was originally published (in 1983), family physicians often are the only physicians available on an ongoing basis to psychotic patients, who no longer are routinely admitted to hospital, where the treatment they need is available, as they were in the past. Homeless psychotic patients, unfortunately now a relatively large group, very often have no physician at all available for their care.*

PATIENT 2: THE PATIENT WHO DENIES ILLNESS

This is another example of why it is important for physicians to understand their patient's personality. A family doctor diagnosed moderately severe pneumonia in a male patient. The doctor prescribed the appropriate medication in her usual competent, friendly way, and, because the illness was serious, requested that the patient return in three days for follow-up. The patient returned, in worse condition. He had not filled his prescription, but had gone to a naturopath, who reassured him that his condition was not serious, and could be managed without the use of "strong medication." The doctor, concerned and somewhat annoyed, sharply pointed out that the pneumonia *was* serious, and that the patient had better take his medicine. The patient quietly agreed, but never returned for a follow-up visit. The doctor, by now, was quite worried about her patient, who seemed to be refusing treatment for a potentially lethal illness, but was unable to get in touch with him.

What had happened? Why would a patient not fill a prescription that very likely would cure his serious illness? Perhaps he did not trust his doctor. The doctor had never seen this patient before, so the patient's experiences with the doctor could not justify such an attitude. One could hypothesize that this patient may have had a series of small, day-to-day experiences, beginning with his most important and earliest experiences with his parents, which led him gradually to develop an unconscious feeling that his caretakers were not people upon whom he could depend when he was in distress.

This patient's need not to have to depend on his doctor "when the chips were down" might be related to what he had learned in earlier relationships, that there was no one who cared when he needed caring for. Parents who are not very concerned about whether their infant is wet, or hungry, or needs to be held are also less likely to interact with and relate to their child in a satisfactory manner later in his development. The child's awareness of this relationship with his parents, and his reaction to their neglect, are painful and frightening enough that he keeps them (the awareness and emotional reaction) out of conscious awareness. However, interpersonal learning still takes place, and the experience is transferred (hence the term "transference") on to subsequent relationships (Freud, 1905/1953: 116). Perhaps this patient's unconscious belief that he could count on no one when he was in trouble led him to deny the seriousness of his illness, and made him think the prescription was unnecessary. The naturopath was attractive to this patient because he offered the only solution the patient could accept: that nothing was really wrong, and therefore he didn't have to count on anyone.

Apart from the potentially tragic practical consequences of the patient's decision, its results are interesting. The patient in effect reproduced the early situation that he presumably wanted to avoid: he became involved with an "inadequate" caregiver who he believed didn't really care what the matter was with him, and just "went through the motions" with him. By not accepting his physician's advice, the patient maintained a distressed state, similar to the hungry or wet infant's. He arranged for himself to be "abandoned" by the physician, as he may have been abandoned emotionally as a child. The doctor's insistence on the seriousness of the patient's illness only increased his need to deny the illness, and isolate himself from the doctor who "threatened" him with it.

This patient also got what he needed emotionally when the doctor worried about him. Sadly, the patient risked his life to accomplish this, and received no real benefit from the doctor's interest, because he made himself unavailable for further treatment. The patient's return to the doctor after seeing the naturopath indicates that he was somehow aware of the seriousness of the situation, and was giving the doctor another chance to come up with the right "prescription" (Balint, 1972: 5, 172, 228). However, this patient required more than just the correct medication and a sharp word from his physician. The family doctor might have benefited by looking into her patient's apparent nonchalance, which likely masked intense anxiety at the prospect of being ill. A successful investigation of this might have enabled the patient to feel confidence in his relationship with this doctor, in spite of earlier difficulties he had experienced in other relationships (Balint, 1972).

On the second visit, the doctor could have refrained from delivering a lecture on filling the prescription, but instead tried to explore *why* the patient didn't follow her advice. The patient's failure to fill the prescription should have been taken as an ominous sign. The doctor could continue exploring why her patient had difficulty following her advice. If she understood the patient's problem, he more likely would have seen that she was someone to depend on, who was interested enough to find out what was wrong in their relationship without judging him, and who acted in his best interest. The patient would then have been more inclined to follow the doctor's advice.

The doctor's expression, that the patient "had better take his medicine," has a reproachful, if not punitive, ring to my ears now. I wonder how much this patient, in not following his doctor's "orders," was inviting his physician to assume the role of a disapproving authority, which the latter conformed with, in a way that was not helpful to their relationship or to the patient's health. The physician could become aware of having a feeling different from her usual feelings when seeing an ill patient, which she could have interpreted as a communication from her own unconscious, that something she was unaware of needed to be understood and taken into account in treating this patient. Our patients, more or less, all function as directors, writers, and star actors in the dramas in which they invite us to assume supportive roles (Sandler, 1976). There is no avoiding this kind of invitation, but it is important for the physician to be aware of when the role she is being invited, or even pressured, to assume is uncomfortable, or feels unethical or just plain dangerous, either to the patient's health, for example, or to the clinician's standards of care.

My comment about the physician who was treating the patient with pneumonia needing to be interested in the patient's apparent nonchalance represents the idea that we must be interested in noticing what is missing, in this case, the expected concern about having pneumonia, as well as what is obviously present. Then we can try to ascertain what has happened to the patient's anxiety, and deal with the patient's pathological (and dangerous) defense against it.

I heard of a family physician who, at her patient's insistence, treated him for very severe depression without any conventional psychiatric medications, did not refer the patient for psychiatric consultation, and (at his request) prescribed herbs, the efficacy for which there was no evidence. The patient's condition worsened to the point where eventually a relative brought the patient to a hospital, where the patient was admitted. The attending psychiatrist ultimately reported the family physician to her licensing body for not maintaining an acceptable level of care. The only alternative the family physician appeared to have in this situation was to refuse to treat the patient with her hands tied behind her back. The patient appeared, likely for reasons related to early relational experiences, to not trust the physician's clinical judgment, and to need to feel that he was in control of the treatment. Sadly, such patients unconsciously arrange poor treatment for themselves, often recapitulating the very unsatisfactory relational experience of childhood that they unconsciously are hoping to avoid.

WHO BECOMES "PERSONALITY-DISORDERED"?

The individual who has from an early age experienced enough friendly, satisfying, loving relationships, beginning with his early attachment figures, will have an image of himself as being lovable, worthwhile, and important (Brenner, 1973: 45). In other words, his parents' attitudes towards him to a significant extent will become his own. He will likely be able to recognize other friendly people when he meets them, and become involved with them in subsequent relationships. If he happens to become involved with someone who disappoints him, he will be less likely to feel that he was rejected because he is bad or unlovable, or doesn't deserve the other person. His resistance to damage to his self-esteem is relatively high because he has internalized the image of his satisfying relationship with his parents and their attitude towards him, and feels worthwhile. The early good-enough relationships protect him from untoward reactions to present-day disappointments, and prepare him for subsequent good relationships.

On the other hand, many patients, especially the more frequent visitors to the physician's office, have had serious frustrations in their relationships with their parents. They will have been neglected, misunderstood, abused, *traumatized in other ways*, and overly controlled. *Or the parents may just not have had the qualities necessary to fulfill the child's needs, which might have been considerable.* The unconscious images of these children will correspond to their parents' attitudes towards them *(or to their experience of their parents' attitudes)*. They may feel unlovable, undeserving of friendship, or acceptable only under certain conditions, such as when they behave the way someone else wants them to. They will present with a range of personality traits, from fearful timidity to having "a chip on their shoulder." When these patients have a problem in an important relationship, they are not protected by their parents' and their own benevolent images of themselves. Rather, the present-day difficulties tend to reinforce and amplify the upsetting feelings associated with previous unsatisfactory relationships. The problem in the present relationship revives unresolved frustrations in early relationships, so the patient ends up reacting not just to the present loss or conflict, but to a series of earlier disappointments, although he usually is not aware of this. That may result in what looks like an over-reaction. The next case history describes a patient who reacted in this way.

Now I would say that individuals with adequately positive early relationships with parents are more likely to develop positive images of themselves and others, all else being equal. Other factors include the child's inherent sensitivity, the fit between parents and child, the child's temperament, and perhaps a tendency to rely on one mental mechanism, such as a defense, more than on others. In addition, factors extrinsic to the child, such as growing up in a chaotic family, growing up in a situation of environmental disturbance, such as a civil war, or an area bedeviled by climatic catastrophe, may affect the child's adaptation. There is not a simple one-to-one correlation between the child's real experience with his parents and the development of his internal world because of these factors, but there still is a strong correlation. Individuals I have assessed and treated who have quite significant character pathology do appear, in the histories I elicit from them, in their descriptions of their perception of adult relationships, in the transferences they form with me, and in my countertransference experience, to have a preponderance of negative unconscious images of themselves (self-representations) and others ("internal objects," unconscious images of others).

I referred to "trauma" because I believe we currently are much more than previously aware of and open to the varied types of trauma that people are subject to throughout the life cycle, and to the especially vulnerable nature of being a child. Traumatized patients and patients with significant personality disturbance will not be likely to have a constructive approach to the difficulties they experience in their relationships with their physicians. The latter need to have a thoughtful response to these patients' reactions to these interpersonal difficulties, which may involve, for example, withdrawal, exaggerated compliance, or overt hostility. These situations, however, are an opportunity for the physician to explore with her patient the basis for his reaction, which may involve an important experience of learning, both cognitively, in terms of having a better understanding of what "got" to the patient in his relationship with his physician, and experientially, in that the patient may learn different and more constructive ways of dealing with interpersonal conflict.

PATIENT 3: DEFINITIVE TREATMENT OF PERSONALITY DISTURBANCE AND DISORDERS

A female patient was emotionally neglected by her parents, who devoted their attention to a younger sibling. Her chief complaint was unsatisfying relationships, particularly with men, who took advantage of her. Her parents had encouraged her not to express what she wanted or to discuss her ideas, so she could not be openly angry about the frustrations in her relationships. Her reaction was to become very compliant with her parents. She never complained, but always hoped that eventually, if she were "good" enough for long enough, she would receive the love and understanding so long denied her. This day never came, and she maintained her hopefully obedient attitude towards neglectful people in her later relationships, *what we call "transference."* For instance, she chose boyfriends who clearly demonstrated their selfishness, but to whom she clung in the expectation that one day, if she complied and persisted, she would get what she needed from them.

This patient's understandable resentment was displaced on to institutions, such as the medical profession (another transference). Physicians appeared selfish, incompetent, greedy, and dangerous to her. In this way, she was able to avoid recognizing similar qualities in her boyfriends *(as her dissatisfaction with the boyfriends was displaced on to physicians, an unconscious mechanism of defense).* She also repressed *(another defense)* conscious awareness of the undesirable traits that her boyfriends shared with her parents. This enabled her to maintain the fantasy that the boyfriends would eventually love her as her parents never did, until the boyfriends' continued abuse and neglect forced her to face reality. This is an example of transference, the unconscious repetition of thoughts, feelings, and impulses that are appropriate to early relationships, and are re-experienced in current relationships. It was first described by Freud as occurring during psychoanalytic treatment. However, it actually occurs to some extent in all relationships, creating more or less distortion (depending partly on our earliest experiences) in our perceptions of others (Freud, 1910/1957: 51; Glover, 1955: 112). For example, this patient experienced similar frustrations with her boyfriends and employers as with her parents, and attempted to deal with them in the same way: by behaving "nicely" and hoping for acceptance.

This patient entered psychoanalytic psychotherapy with similar great, if unconscious, expectations. She was determined to please her therapist at whatever the cost to her integrity as an individual. It eventually emerged that she was furious with her therapist for "oppressing" her in the same way that she felt her boyfriends did. The therapist's task was to see what contribution this patient herself made to being oppressed in their relationship, and to feeling abused in other relationships. For example, she never told her therapist when an appointment was inconvenient, and then felt he was insensitive to her needs, resenting him but saying nothing. Eventually they talked about how empty, sad, and alone she felt in their relationship, and how this resembled her feelings in other relationships. When the therapist indicated that he believed this patient hoped that if she were compliant with him and allowed herself to be degraded in their relationship, he would eventually cure her, she demonstrated increasingly appropriate assertive behavior. Formerly, her passive stance was accompanied by occasional outbursts of anger that were detrimental to her. The therapist's interpretations, which helped her understand her problem, and were made in the context of an important relationship, the therapeutic relationship, were essential to the success of the treatment (Greben, 1977).

Another task of the therapist would be to consider what contributions he actually made to the difficulties in their relationship, for example, in exploiting her tendency towards compliance to his own benefit. For example, such a patient would be likely to comply with the doctor's request for a change in appointment that was not convenient for her. It would be in the interest of the therapeutic work for the physician to be sensitive to her tendency to compliance, and not take advantage of it. Inevitably, some form of re-enactment regarding this will occur, and then the physician has the opportunity to bring it up for discussion, so the therapeutic couple can think about this problem between them together, rather than merely re-enacting it. In an enactment, the therapist and patient engage in the kind of interaction that has been problematic for the patient in other relationships. The difference is that the therapist's job is to avoid when possible, or interrupt when he becomes aware of it, the enactment, so it can become a subject for the therapeutic couple to explore. It is impossible to avoid enactments completely, and they are fertile soil for planting new conceptions of how the patient can interact in relationships. However, there is a big difference between engaging in an enactment like taking advantage of a patient's compliance regarding appointments, for example, and one in which the physician takes advantage of her sexually. (See Chapter 17.) In the latter, the exploitation is too egregious; the patient has no chance to benefit by learning from the experience, but merely repeats the exploitation she has experienced at the hands of others.

This case describes psychoanalytic psychotherapy of a patient with a personality disorder, and gives an example of transference interpretation. Psychoanalysis and psychoanalytic psychotherapy are the only treatments in which the goal is changing the patient's personality by uncovering defenses and the impulses behind them, substituting more adaptive defenses, and channeling the energy of the impulses into more constructive and satisfying pursuits. By contrast, the goals of supportive, directive, or behavioral therapies, and of biological treatments, are mainly removing symptoms and altering maladaptive behavior (Stewart, 1975: 1817). *Psychoanalysis and psychoanalytic psychotherapy are different in that they do not only try to help the patient reach a* restituo ad integrum, *restoration of their previous condition, but to set in motion an ongoing process of growth, so they end up healthier than before they "fell ill," and optimally continue to grow throughout their lives, using the expanded capacity to think and experience their emotions to help them make important decisions and pursue their life goals.*

Physicians are rarely trained to do psychotherapy involving transference interpretations, but by realizing that the patient's exaggerated reaction to some aspect of his relationship with his doctor (or other healthcare provider) is based on earlier relationships, the physician knows not to react personally (for example, by behaving in an angry or defensive manner). Rather, the physician should treat the reaction as he would a physical symptom: accept it as part of the patient, and as worthy of interest. For example, if the patient expects the physician to be available to listen to him for as long as he wants, whenever he wants, the latter might enquire what the patient hopes would occur if this could happen. The main point is to try to understand what the patient is expressing, either in words or by his behavior. Both rejecting the troublesome patient and trying to make him happy by complying with him are equally futile. The real question is, what makes the patient so troublesome, and what is he searching for in his relationship with the physician? This is an important part of what is explored in psychoanalytic psychotherapy. *That is, we do not need to either refuse or agree with the patient's request of us, if it seems beyond what is reasonable. We can be interested in it, try to interest the patient in it, and explore it with him. Not all patients will cooperate with this, but some will, and we will know we have provided an opportunity for the patient to learn something in our relationship with him.*

Rather than saying that the goal of psychoanalysis and psychoanalytic psychotherapy is to change the patient's personality, I now would suggest that it is to help the patient grow and develop his personality, in particular, his mind and his capacity for thinking, for thinking previously unthinkable thoughts, and for bearing what previously have been unbearable feelings. As I suggest elsewhere, performing these treatments is an opportunity for growth for the therapist as well. I would define transference more broadly, to include the patient's entire experience of the therapist, analyst, other healthcare provider, or anyone else. I also want to refer to the contemporary notion of a transference–countertransference matrix, that is, a combined experience of patient and therapist, with each aspect indivisible from the other. I would add that the transference includes the patient's realistic perceptions, conscious or not, of the therapist, and how they affect his attitude and his behavior towards the therapist. Transference no longer is felt to be merely a repetition of past experience in present relationships, where the experiences are no longer appropriate. As suggested above, part of what the patient is reacting to in the therapist is who the therapist really is.

The above is not to deny that transference continues to be understood as a ubiquitous experience; we do perceive, interpret, and understand our present in terms of past experience. Transference occurs in all sorts of relationships, including parent–child, teacher–pupil, employer–employee, friend–friend, partner–partner, and physician–patient. The question is not whether transference occurs, but whether an individual is able to enhance his awareness of reality by reflecting on his experience, and realize that the reality of the other person may be different than his experience of her at any given time.

In this case, I described the goals of treatment in terms of instinct and ego psychology, referring to impulses and defenses. Today, I would emphasize the patient's inner world, self-representations and internal objects, changes in the patient's real relationships, and my countertransference experience, as well as the changes in the concept of transference described above. I would also describe the patient's increased capacity to mourn and his ability to bear painful affects without resorting to defensive behaviors and to modes of thinking that are destructive. I as well would comment generally on the quality of his thinking, his appreciation of reality, and any disturbances in his thinking, and what may contribute to these.

RECOGNIZING PSYCHIATRIC CONDITIONS

Psychiatric disorders can be viewed on a continuum from normality through neurotic and character (personality) disorders to psychotic disorders (Freud, 1905/1953). The use of defense mechanisms, unconscious mental devices to reduce anxiety, is universal; people vary only in the degree of their reliance on various defenses. Consider the use of the defense of projection, the attribution to others of ideas, feelings, and impulses that we cannot accept as our own. People are often reluctant to accept the responsibility for a problem, and tend to blame someone else. If this tendency is a usual reaction to difficulties, such that a person constantly imputes malicious intentions to others, is totally unwilling to accept his share of involvement in his difficulties, and has a suspicious attitude, he might have *paranoid traits* or a paranoid personality disorder. In patients with delusional and schizophrenic disorders, projection is used to such an extent that the patient is psychotic, that is, incapable of distinguishing his inner world from the external world. Two examples of excessive projection are persecutory delusions, in which the individual actually believes that an agency or other person is hostile and dangerous, and persecutory auditory hallucinations, in which a person aurally experiences a thought coming from outside himself, and thus does not accept it as his own. With both these symptoms, hostile thoughts are so unacceptable to the individual that his perception of reality is distorted, and he experiences the thought or voice as someone else's. This is a more extreme version of the unwillingness everyone experiences at times to accept personal weaknesses. The difference is the extent to which this defense is relied upon to maintain an emotional homeostasis.

Another distinction is that in the case of a hallucination or a delusion, it is not only the individual's perception of his inner psychic state that is altered, but his perception of external reality. This involves a more severe disturbance of psychic functioning, with potentially more problematic ramifications in the individual's relationship to the world.

Now, rather than making absolute distinctions between neurotic, character, and psychotic disturbances, I would refer to the extent to which a person is capable of bearing anxiety and other potentially disorganizing affects, the extent to which his thinking is dominated by more primitive defenses (like projection and denial), the extent to which he is able to distinguish his internal world from external reality, and the extent to which his wishes, fears, impulses, and fantasies take precedence over his thinking, and his awareness of consensual reality.

CHOOSING A TREATMENT

Medication

When considering the use of biological treatments in managing patients with personality disorders, it is important to realize that *no* biological agent can definitively cause personality change, because personality involves a complex system of behavior with unconscious motivations learned over a period of years. Presumably, behavior also has equally complex neuro-anatomical and biochemical substrates. It seems unlikely that such a complicated system could be changed by the administration of a drug. In medicine, medication is frequently used to relieve symptoms without the expectation of a cure; this also holds true in treating psychiatric disturbance. Antidepressants are indicated when a patient has significant depressive symptoms, and frequently are prescribed for anxiety disorders. They do not address whatever personality difficulties the patient has that made him susceptible to depression or anxiety. Antipsychotic medications are indicated when a patient has a brief psychotic episode or, sometimes, incapacitating anxiety. It is often profitable to try to understand the *source* of the anxiety, which may suggest an appropriate psychological treatment (Department of National Health and Welfare, 1981). To summarize, many patients with personality disturbance may at some time have symptoms requiring medication, but their personalities will not be improved by the medication.

Psychoanalysis or Individual Psychoanalytic Psychotherapy

The term "individual psychotherapy" covers a broad range of therapies, from supportive, directive, anxiety-suppressing therapy in which the therapist attempts to reinforce the patient's existing defenses, relieve symptoms, and enhance adaptive behavior, to psychoanalysis, in which defenses are interpreted, an attempt is made to make the unconscious conscious, anxiety is inevitably provoked, and advice, *encouragement, and reassurance* are generally not given. The long-term goal of psychoanalysis is reorganizing the personality with more adaptive defenses and understanding the patient's interpersonal difficulties. The choice of therapies is determined not so much by the patient's diagnosis as by other criteria. A psychoanalytically oriented treatment would be favored for relatively young patients who are psychologically minded or concerned with understanding the source of their problems, and who can tolerate painful feelings like anxiety and depression, which inevitably emerge in psychoanalysis (Stewart, 1975: 1812). Without these characteristics, a patient would more likely benefit from supportive therapy, which not only provides a helpful relationship, but might focus on certain specific concerns such as assertiveness or the ability to solve problems. A behavioral treatment could focus on an aspect of the patient's behavior that is a source of distress. *(See the first introductory chapter's Appendix for a more liberal contemporary approach to this.)*

With the developments in psychoanalytic theory and technique over the last half-century, psychoanalysis and the psychoanalytic psychotherapies are able to treat an increasingly broad range of patients, regarding the age, developmental level, and symptomatic severity of the patient. Older age, psychotic thinking, a history of substance abuse, and even overt psychotic symptoms are no longer factors that routinely exclude patients from these treatments. In patients with disturbances of thinking, patients who appear to lack psychological mindedness, or patients who find some affects unbearable, these limitations become important foci for psychoanalytic work, and are not necessarily contraindications for psychoanalysis or psychoanalytic psychotherapy. Psychoanalytic technique has become elastic enough to adapt to the treatment needs of many such patients, and provide beneficial therapeutic results that were not thought possible in the past.

It has been over two decades since I served as psychiatric consultant to a family medicine center. During that time, psychiatrists trained in psychoanalysis and psychoanalytic psychotherapy as a group, in my opinion, have not adequately informed their family medical colleagues about the indications, contraindications, techniques, goals, and scope of these treatments. At the same time, psychotherapists trained in psychoanalytic psychotherapy no longer practice this form of treatment in publicly funded settings in North America, including hospital outpatient psychiatric departments and mental health clinics, as was done decades previously. These treatments therefore are less available to the population in a publicly funded venue than in the past. The challenge is still there for psychiatrists practicing psychoanalytic psychotherapy and psychoanalysis better to inform family physicians and their specialist colleagues about these treatments. Family physicians can inform themselves about these treatment approaches through reading or attending educational events.

OTHER TREATMENTS

If a patient with significant personality disturbance has difficulties in his relationships with his spouse or family, couples or family therapy can be considered. Sometimes changes in relationships can be effected better in couples or family therapy than in an individual therapy. There are as many choices in family and group therapies, from more insight-oriented to more supportive, as there are in individual therapies.

Chapter 2 addresses the disadvantages of physicians providing advice, reassurance, and encouragement about personal matters, which they are not qualified by their training to give, and which on a transient basis may feel gratifying for the physician to provide and the patient to receive, but does not change anything in the long run, and certainly does not help patients expand their capacity to think and bear painful feelings.

CONCLUSION

When the physician considers the personalities of her patients, her management of them is enhanced. Treatment is likely to be more effective, and the physician's professional satisfaction will probably be greater, too.

REFERENCES

Balint M (1972). *The Doctor, his Patient, and the Illness*, revised ed. New York: International Universities Press.

Brenner C (1973). *An Elementary Textbook of Psychoanalysis*, revised ed. New York: International Universities Press.

Department of National Health and Welfare (1981). Therapeutic monograph of anxiolytic-sedative drugs. *Canadian Medical Association Journal* 124:1439–1446.

Freud S (1905/1953). Fragment of an analysis in a case of hysteria. In: *Complete Psychological Works of Sigmund Freud,* Vol. VII. London: Hogarth Press and the Institute of Psychoanalysis.

Freud S (1910/1957). Five lectures on psychoanalysis. In: *Complete Psychological Works of Sigmund Freud,* Vol. XI. London: Hogarth Press and the Institute of Psychoanalysis.

Glover E (1955). *Technique of Psychoanalysis.* New York: International Universities Press.

Greben S (1977). On being therapeutic. *Canadian Psychiatric Association Journal* 7:371–380.

Heiman P (1950). On counter-transference. *International Journal of Psychoanalysis* 31:81–84.

McWilliams N (2011). *Psychoanalytic Diagnosis: Understanding Personality Structure in the Clinical Process,* 2nd edition. New York: Guilford Press.

Sandler J (1976) Countertransference and role responsiveness. *International Review of Psycho-Analysis* 3:43–47.

Searles HF (1955). The informational value of the supervisor's emotional experience. *Psychiatry* 18:135–146.

Stewart R (1975). Psychoanalysis and psychotherapy. In: Freedman A, Kaplan H, Sadock B (eds.), *Comprehensive Textbook of Psychiatry,* 3rd edition. Baltimore, MD: Williams and Wilkins.

CHAPTER 2

INTERVIEWING THE PATIENT

This chapter is based mainly on conclusions drawn from my experience in interviewing patients I have assessed and treated personally, those interviewed by trainees while I observed, and those described by their physicians in Balint training seminars. Balint (1972) deserves credit as a pioneer in research on patient interviewing and what family physicians can accomplish. Balint met with groups of family physicians who briefly described situations with their patients that Balint and the other physician participants could think about together, focusing on what was happening between doctor and patient that unconsciously communicated something important about the patient. When assessing their patients, family physicians should be prepared to weigh the importance of their patients' personalities and current emotional states in their presentation. The physician's interested attitude will frequently uncover emotional concerns that sometimes render extended physical examinations and laboratory investigations unnecessary.

THE VALUE OF LISTENING

The physician may indicate explicitly that she is interested in hearing what the patient has to say, and encourage him to talk about what is bothering him. (Of course, the patient will tune in to non-verbal indications that the physician is interested in what the patient has to say as well, including the physician's posture, visual focus, facial expression, and encouragements to the patient to elaborate further, "mm-hmm?") This implicit invitation sometimes is more effective than asking direct questions that may inhibit the patient from bringing up something embarrassing or painful. Although it is presumptuous to suggest that one can do something about a problem the patient brings up, he experiences considerable support if he feels that his physician is willing to listen to and try to understand what he has to say. At least, then he is not alone with his troubles.

However, sometimes the physician's assumptions or convictions related to her ethnicity, religion, ethical standards, or other aspects of who she is make it difficult for her to remain objective. She must then judge whether she can tolerate the stress of trying to remain objective, or should suggest a referral on the grounds that another physician may be better prepared to deal with this particular patient.

It is often helpful to listen for a theme in the patient's conversation. This theme may appear in various ways. For instance, after the doctor changes her appointment time, a patient may make a mildly sarcastic remark that the doctor keeps him waiting too long when he does visit the office, and then express dissatisfaction with his employer, who he feels is not respectful enough. *(Or he might just make a crack about the employer, and it is up to the doctor to sense that this is about her too, and perhaps enquire about this. For example, "You mentioned your frustration about your employer, but I wonder if what you said might also apply somewhat to me, as my secretary rebooked your appointment at a time I suspect is not very convenient for you." Saying this in a non-threatening way invites the patient to be candid with the doctor about their relationship. If he sees the doctor accepting this, he may feel emboldened to tell her more about his other relationships.)* By identifying that the patient feels that people *(including the doctor)* aren't considerate of him, and asking to what extent this is the patient's experience, the physician may initiate a meaningful discussion of marital difficulties, for example, or even of lifelong distress beginning with the patient's relationship with his parents. At times discretion is necessary if the physician believes the theme is too upsetting for the patient to hear, given his circumstances or his mental state, whether in general, for example in a patient with developmental delay; on that occasion, if the patient is too upset; or because of the person's personal vulnerabilities. An example of the latter would be a traumatized patient who is not ready to face something.

PSYCHIATRIC CONSULTATION

The family physician then may feel she has ended up with more problems than she started with, but she really only has discovered more precisely where the difficulties lie. A few meetings in which the doctor works with the patient to learn what is bothering him about his relationships may provide enough support for some relief. If it does not, or if the patient indicates an interest in finding out more about his problems, even though he presently feels better, the physician could consider recommending a consultation with a psychiatrist whose work is psychoanalytically informed.

A psychiatric consultation can be helpful to investigate further the nature and background of the patient's difficulties, and advise about appropriate treatment and who can administer it. The family physician benefits most from a consultation when she specifically indicates that she is interested in the psychiatrist's opinion of the meaning of the patient's symptoms and the difficulties in his relationships. She can also ask how she can best help her patient, and how to strengthen her relationship with him. This is more beneficial than only providing a diagnosis and suggestions for symptomatic treatment that do not address the patient's psychological needs or the family physician's concerns.

GIVING PATIENTS ADVICE

My most important advice to physicians is not to give advice. I mean, it is unwise to give concrete advice regarding the patient's relationships with the external world. This kind of advice is usually based on the advisor's wishes, aspirations, fantasies, and conflicts, and cannot be expected to address the patient's needs. I am excluding from this comment medical advice such as, "You need an appendectomy," which physicians are qualified to give, and advice designed to avert a destructive situation, such as "If you don't slow down you'll hit that car," which practically everyone is qualified to give.

However, many patients will ask questions about important life decisions, such as whether they should accept a job offer or leave their spouse. The physician cannot give a correct answer, as she cannot know. An appropriate response is to enquire what difficulty the patient is having in making the decision, or what he believes the physician could say that would help. The doctor can ask the patient to describe important considerations in making the decision, and then enquire again what the difficulty is in deciding.

Giving an opinion is destructive because it infantalizes the patient, does not solve his problem, and encourages the unrealistic notion that the physician "has the answers." The physician would then tend to become burdened with demanding patients whom she attracts with her omniscient attitude. This attitude actually indicates that the physician has a problem that neatly fits in with the desires of some of her patients to depend on her for answers. It is a greater service to the patient to investigate with him why he needs the advice than to reinforce his inability or refusal to think by supplying the answer. Moreover, if the physician's advice is "wrong," the patient has a legitimate complaint against her, and someone to blame.

Psychoanalysts and psychotherapists are no better trained to give concrete advice about their patient's relations with the outside world than are physicians. We are trained to help our patients think about their destructive behaviors and plans, and try to help them to understand their unconscious motivation to engage in these behaviors. Also, physicians, psychoanalysts, and therapists usually are not the first people to attempt to give their patients concrete advice. Family and friends almost always do, often with the patient's invitation. How much do people listen to advice, even if they request it? If we think people will listen to our advice, we likely are ignoring to what extent people's motivations are governed by unconscious factors about which they have no awareness, to say nothing of control over. That is, the motivation for people's behavior is largely outside of conscious awareness, so advice is unlikely to affect it.

CONSTRUCTIVE SUPPORT

A common misconception is that supportive psychotherapy consists of the physician giving friendly encouragement and reassurance to the patient. This may mean the physician and patient are on a first-name basis, and involve the doctor's giving practical advice, or behaving in a way that will "make the patient feel better." This may calm both physician and patient, and is an essential part of a parent's relationship with a young child. It also has a place in psychoanalysis and psychoanalytic psychotherapy (Gedo, 1979: 34). *I did not mean to imply that encouragement, advice giving, and reassurance are an inherent part of psychoanalytic treatment. The forms of listening, clarification, and interpretation that are techniques of psychoanalysis, however, may have a very calming effect on the patient.* However, if applied on a wholesale basis, reassurance, advice, and encouragement prevent the physician from ever finding out much about her patients' problems, and cause her to participate in the problems because of her own need to be a soothing parental figure.

There are at least two problems with providing reassurance. Again, I am excepting reassurance that a physician is qualified to provide, for example, regarding the prognosis of an illness. First, unless we have a crystal ball, we cannot predict the future. Our patients know that, so our reassurance inevitably seems hollow, and we then are encouraging an unhealthy complacency and lack of personal agency in our patients. As well, reassuring our patients is antithetical to what we attempt to accomplish in psychoanalysis or psychotherapy, which physicians might also support; that is, to help patients feel what feels unbearable and think what has hitherto been unthinkable. Another consideration is, who do we most need to reassure, our patients or ourselves? If we need to reassure our patients, they may conclude that we cannot bear to hear what they have to say, and decide to protect us from it. A therapeutic tea party ensues, which is polite but sterile, and provides limited results.

A more constructive concept of support than providing advice, encouragement, and reassurance is the support of the patient's mature functioning. That is, the physician should help the patient to function at the most mature level he is capable of. By her behavior and attitudes, the physician can model a reasonable, thinking individual who has the patient's interest in mind and does not ignore reality. A sign that a patient is beginning to internalize the physician's attitude occurs when, rather than acting impulsively as in the past, he thinks, "My doctor wouldn't think this was the right thing to do," or even, "Doctor X would tell me not to do this." *When this happens, the physician should enquire why the patient believes she (the physician) wouldn't think so. Then she can show him how he really decided himself what to do. This last action, identifying that it is the patient who assumed the agency regarding this decision, both implicitly gives the patient permission to "use" the physician this way, and acknowledges that the patient has learned something and is applying it constructively. With patients who may be hesitant to take advantage of what they learn in their interactions with me, I feel comfortable indicating that they are free to use anything I say in a way that will be helpful to them, and what they get from our interaction does not come at the price of me losing something. In fact, I am open with my belief that it is not just the patient who can benefit from our interaction, but I as well, and that our work is an opportunity for me to learn.*

Family physicians can also support patients in other ways. At times of stress, when the patient is not functioning at his best, and is perhaps showing signs of decompensation, such as depersonalization, extreme anxiety, or exaggerated character traits that may be unhelpful or destructive, the physician can lend support as an auxiliary ego. That is, he may have to complement the patient's executive functioning, helping him avoid destructive situations, even if it means giving advice such as "Perhaps you should give yourself a little time to think before quitting your job." *In general, I do not believe that we have the training or experience to give practical advice. However, implicit in much of the work of a psychoanalyst or psychotherapist, which can be applied in the practice of medicine, is the advice that it is better to think before acting. Of course, this may not apply to the same extent in some emergency situations, where there is little time for the leisure of protracted thinking. Most of the difficult decisions our patients make, however, do not involve emergencies.* The physician can also tactfully point to hard facts that the patient may be ignoring. *For example, "I am not sure that in the heat of your feelings about the dilemma about whether to go out for dinner with your boss, you are taking into account what you told me some time ago about your concerns about his personal interest in you."* Occasionally it may be necessary to provide some relief for the most severe symptoms, such as overwhelming anxiety, with medication, which should be employed in conjunction with the supportive approach described above.

TAKING OVER PATIENTS' RESPONSIBILITIES

The physician must tread a fine line between taking over the patient's responsibility for decision making and for perceiving reality, which may encourage further regression on his part, and emotionally abandoning him. The physician may have to "take over" at some point if the patient needs to be certified, if he is dangerous to himself or to others, or is not capable of consenting to treatment or managing his financial affairs. It is especially important in these cases to take over only the area in which the patient cannot function independently, no more than necessary, and to withdraw from it as soon as he can function independently. So, for example, one might be obliged to render someone incompetent to manage his financial affairs, but otherwise be able to respect his decisions regarding consent for treatment, and not need to hospitalize him against his will. Meanwhile the physician can foster the patient's improved functioning by indicating that the situation is temporary and limited to specific areas of responsibility. The doctor can also explain in a factual way, attempting not to humiliate the patient, why she has taken over a responsibility that generally is his.

ATTEMPTING TO UNDERSTAND PATIENTS' PROBLEMS

It is best not to presume that one understands what a patient tells one. *It is painful to feel one doesn't understand.* I indicate to patients that I will try to understand, and this is a major goal of our work. It is better to enlist the patient's cooperation and learn something together. The patient is then free to use what you both have learned. Even if the patient is too impulsive or rigid, or seems not intelligent enough, to collaborate, it should still be the physician's goal to understand, just as it is good medicine to make an accurate traditional diagnosis, regardless of how limited the management options may be.

The physician's attempts to understand offer a healthy model to the patient. The patient sees a physician who is interested in learning about him, who is patient, and who can tolerate ideas and feelings that may be upsetting to her. This attitude of trying to understand discourages maladaptive coping behaviors such as ignoring reality or acting impulsively in a way that temporarily decrease anxiety but are destructive in the long run. The patient's identification with the physician's attitudes can at times be of even greater benefit than the increased understanding of his difficulties he gains from his physician.

Technically, one can ask the patient for details about problems he may generalize about, and ask whether his current situation reminds him of other experiences. The physician can ask her patient to identify how he feels in the current situation, and when else he has felt that way. Making a general comment about what the patient has told you may help the patient have an association to it. For example, a patient complained to me that his employer did not really give their clients good service, but pressed them to financially overcommit themselves to his company. I was interested in why the employer's behavior was emotionally significant to this patient, and pointed out that he seemed to think that his employer was using the clients, offering something that he wasn't delivering, and extracting all he could get from them. My patient was reminded of his mother, and went on to describe how his employer and mother behaved in a similar way.

THE PHYSICIAN'S FEELINGS AS A DIAGNOSTIC TOOL

The physician can use her emotional reactions (countertransference) while interviewing to help understand her patient. This is the proper use of emotions in a clinical setting. It usually is unproductive for physicians to openly react emotionally to a patient when they feel offended, defensive, or depressed about what their patient says. I generally advise physicians not to tell their patients what their emotional reaction to the patient is. This is an additional burden to someone who may already be emotionally weighed down. The last thing the patient needs to worry about is how the physician will take what he says; he already may be anxious about this. Rather, the physician should use her feelings in an attempt to understand what the patient is going through. This understanding can often be shared with gratifying results. My student used her feelings like this. Initially, she reacted to a patient who overtly demanded a lot of time with her by avoiding him whenever she could. She arranged appointments with him at 11:30 a.m. so she would "have" to stop at noon for lunch. This allowed her to avoid dealing with his demanding nature, and with her resultant anger, which she felt ashamed of, and tried to suppress. A more satisfactory result was obtained when we discussed the student's anger, making it acceptable for her to experience it and contain it. I encouraged her to explore with her patient what it was that he hoped to get from her, and why he felt he needed so much time with her. At that point they began a therapeutic collaboration. He stopped his hopeless pursuit for attention from someone who was fleeing, his experience in many previous relationships, and began to think about this with my student. He tolerated this collaboration because he knew that my student would see him regularly for a predictable period of time, and was willing to try to understand how much he needed and why, even if she could not fulfill all of his demands. This collaboration also removed the student's reason for being angry, as she did not have to escape from her patient after they had agreed on a predictable schedule of meetings.

A different student used his emotional response to a patient less effectively. He was usually very quiet, but became quite animated with one of his patients, a young woman who contributed little to conversations, felt empty, and had impoverished relationships. I interpreted this student's many questions of and frequent suggestions for his patient as an unconscious attempt to liven up this patient, and revive his flagging interviews with her. His lively way of interacting, which the patient evidently enjoyed, allowed her to ignore her difficulty. He tried to provide what she had been looking for: someone to "liven her up." This was more than anyone could accomplish, as she had very valid (albeit unconscious) motivations for her psychic deadness. My student's approach precluded any exploration of the patient's emotional lifelessness. Because the student attempted to provide what the patient unconsciously requested, she did not have to put her difficulty into words, which could have been the beginning of a psychotherapeutic exploration of her deadness and its antecedents. I believe my student's struggles with his own deadness made it difficult to tolerate his patient's deadness.

GOALS OF THERAPY

The physician must not expect that she will be able to solve her patient's problems. The best she can do is to help her patient to change his attitude towards the problems, think in different ways about the problems, and improve his methods of dealing with the problems. The physician needs to consider her own limitations of time, expertise and interest, and to make an assessment of the patient that allows her to make constructive decisions about treatment, and about whether or not she will suggest a psychiatric consultation or referral to a qualified therapist (Ramesar & McCall, 1983). Although few family physicians can expect to undertake psychoanalytic psychotherapy with a patient who has a personality disorder, they can perform a great service by helping – with the patient's collaboration – to explore his difficulties. Naturally, it is dangerous to force this approach on a patient who is too rigid or too disturbed to benefit from it. Otherwise, however, this can be instrumental in motivating the patient to continue investigating his difficulties, either with the family physician or with a psychoanalyst or psychotherapist.

BALINT GROUPS

Family physicians interested in further developing interviewing skills used in their frequent contacts with patients can organize Balint training seminars (Balint, 1972). This involves regular meetings between a group of family physicians and a trained Balint leader, who is usually a psychiatrist with psychoanalytic training or a special interest in psychoanalytic psychotherapy and physician–patient relationships. The aim of such groups is to help physicians better understand the difficulties they face in their relationships with patients. This often elucidates difficulties patients have in other relationships, and can suggest constructive approaches to take with patients. *In these seminars, family physicians briefly present situations that confront them in their daily experiences with patients whom they find difficult to deal with. The group thinks together about each situation, guided by the leader. Different perspectives on understanding the patient, the doctor's experience, and the doctor-patient relationship arise from the seminar. In these seminars, participants grow in terms of their capacity to think about what is happening with their patients. This gives them more freedom in responding creatively to their patients. Balint groups are an original contribution of psychoanalysis to the practice of family medicine.* They have been incorporated into some family medicine training programs, and employed with inpatient psychiatric nurses (Steinberg & Shaw, 1989).

The poet Keats used the term "negative capability" to describe the ability to tolerate not knowing. This of course is an essential quality for a physician to have, because there is so much about medicine and about our patients that we can't and don't know. If we tolerate not knowing, as opposed to assuming a position of omniscience or, more modestly, an exaggerated confidence about how well we know our patients, we have the potential to learn something about them. One needs to open a space in one's mind for an unbidden thought, which might represent one's patient unconsciously communicating something important about himself. This is very different from asking a patient direct questions in order to elicit information that will help you draw a conclusion, the opposite of the "Where is the lesion, and what is the lesion?" approach I learned in neurology. Of course, trying to understand something personal about a person is a very different venture than performing a neurological examination to locate and then establish the nature of a discrete lesion.

The family physician needs to tolerate not knowing, sometimes for long periods of time. The advantage the family physician has over specialists is that she usually has multiple exposures to her patients, and often their families, over a period of many years. At some point, a patient may openly say something very genuine about his situation when he trusts his family physician enough. He may never do this with a specialist, unless, for example, it is a psychiatrist who is his psychotherapist or psychoanalyst and sees him regularly over a lengthy period of time. Another possibility is that the family physician may notice a theme in what a patient says, or experience some intuition, or a reverie, which may be based on an unconscious communication between her and her patient. An example from my experience follows. Those wishing to learn more about the use of reverie may read the original article (Steinberg, 2018).

I had been seeing a patient in psychotherapy for a couple of years. The patient complained of the deadness and emptiness of his life. I eventually ended up experiencing this in my interactions with him, which felt lifeless. The therapy seemed to be going nowhere. One day, towards the end of a session, I thought of the LP album cover Whipped Cream and Other Delights *by the trumpeter Herb Alpert. This is a sensually exciting image from the 1960s depicting an attractive young woman with an inviting look on her face, clothed only in whipped cream. This kind of experience is called a reverie. Feeling that I had nothing else to contribute, I shared this image with my patient, who readily recalled it. He then recounted a dream involving a trumpet the previous night, which he had forgotten until then. My recollection of this album cover livened me up at the time, and my patient's recollection of his dream led to a discussion over several sessions of how he had deadened himself as a way of dealing with the premature death of his father during his childhood. His longing for his father became something we could experience together rather than just talk about. These discussions initiated liveliness in the therapy. The point of this anecdote is to suggest that there was an unconscious communication between my patient and me, with him somehow indicating that something related to a trumpet could lead to something lively and significant.*

I am suggesting that these kinds of communication often may happen between family physicians and their patients as well, and can lead to fruitful discussions when they are noticed.

The family physician is the professional her patient has come to see on the day of the consultation. It is not practicable, even if it were desirable, to refer every patient whom you may suspect of having an unconscious emotional conflict or an unarticulated feeling or fantasy that is contributing to his distress or to a physical symptom to a psychiatrist or a psychoanalyst. The family physician needs to be patient with her patient, within any given session and over a longer period of time. Something about the essence of the patient may be communicated to the family physician. The question then is what to do with what the family physician believes she has understood. The first issue is whether she should communicate to the patient what she feels she understands about him. This raises the question of what a patient is ready to hear. What the family physician has understood may be helpful to the patient to hear, or may be experienced as catastrophic. Of course, one of the factors involved is how the family physician presents what she understands to her patient. Can this be communicated in a tactful, gentle, bearable way? This depends in part on how the family physician feels about what she has learned. If it is almost unbearable for her to think about it, she may have trouble communicating it to the patient in a way he can bear. One may take a graduated and tentative approach, not blurting out what one is thinking directly, but rather saying something more general or vague, inviting the patient to think about this and elaborate on it. For example, if a physician has the impression that her patient wants to talk about being abused by her partner but is uncomfortable broaching the subject, one might say, "I have the impression that there is something you want to tell me about your relationship with your spouse, but are having some difficulty telling me," or, "It seems to me that you are hinting at feeling mistreated, but do not seem comfortable giving me the details," or, "I think you want to tell me something about your relationship with your husband, but are concerned about my reaction. Would it help to know that my approach will be to try to understand the difficulty with you? I will encourage you to think through whatever difficulty you want to discuss, as opposed to your making decisions before you are ready to." Another factor influencing what you can tell a patient, of course, is how comfortable a relationship the patient and family physician share. A mutually comfortable relationship contributes to a firmer foundation on which to say something that may be upsetting.

Alternatively, if a physician believes that her patient is thinking of something and is conflicted about discussing it, needing to discuss it, but apprehensive about the physician's reaction or ashamed of the subject, one may gently suggest that the patient seems to have a conflict about bringing something up. Rather than asking about the content of what the patient is struggling with, one can address the process, that is, the conflict, and ask the patient about what difficulty the patient is having in bringing the subject up. Once the patient has discussed this difficulty and the physician has given appropriate reassurance (as above, that you are there to think together, rather than feeling pressure to act), the content often is no longer as difficult to discuss. An example of appropriate reassurance when a patient is concerned about his physician's reaction to what he will say would be, "I am not sure how I will react to what you have to tell me, but I will do my best to contain myself, whatever my reaction is, and focus on how I can be helpful to you regarding the difficulty you want to discuss." In my opinion, that is more reassuring and will seem more realistic to a patient than a physician who claims that nothing the patient says will surprise or shock her.

REFERENCES

Balint M (1972). *The Doctor, his Patient and the Illness*, revised ed. New York: international Universities Press.

Gedo J (1979). *Beyond Interpretation*. New York: International Universities Press.

Ramesar S, McCall M (1983). Coping with the negative therapeutic response in psychosocial problems in family medicine. *Canadian Journal of Psychiatry* 28:259–262.

Steinberg PI (2018). Whipped cream and other delights: A reverie and its aftermath. *Canadian Journal of Psychoanalysis* 25(2):88–105.

Steinberg PI, Shaw BF (1989). The effectiveness of Balint training for psychiatric nurses. *Journal of the Balint Society* 17:28–32.

CHAPTER 3

"ARE ALL MY PATIENTS DEPRESSED?":
THE (MIS-)DIAGNOSIS OF DEPRESSION

"Depression" is a common presenting symptom in the family physician's office, especially including vague complaints such as fatigue, dizziness, and malaise for which no medical diagnosis is made. Overall, however, the incidence of major depressive disorder is thought to be relatively low (Weissman & Boyd, 1985: 766.) This is explained by the fact that the diagnostic criteria for depressive illness ("major depressive episode," MDE) permit physicians to make this diagnosis only in cases of relatively prolonged depression in which neurovegetative signs of depression are usually prominent (American Psychiatric Association, 2013). The restrictive nature of this diagnosis is useful as it implies the need for biological treatments such as antidepressant medication or, in more severe or refractory cases, electroconvulsive therapy. Given this management, the prognosis for symptomatic recovery from a depressive episode is relatively good. *(I am not dealing here with indications for psychotherapy in patients with major depressive disorder.)*

Conditions such as persistent depressive disorder (PDD) (formerly dysthymic disorder) and adjustment disorder with depressed mood (ADDM), which present very frequently to family physicians, are less responsive to antidepressants. Nevertheless, antidepressant medication often is prescribed for patients complaining of depressive mood, regardless of whether they have symptoms suggesting that their "depression" would be responsive to antidepressants.

Perhaps prescribing antidepressants thus has lowered the incidence of severe depressive illness in the community. However, the price that many patients pay for this result is that they are often given a treatment that offers little hope of relieving their complaints, *apart from the limited benefits of a placebo effect*; that involves potentially serious side effects; and that is dangerous in overdose. *(The original article on which this chapter is based was published when tricyclic antidepressants and monoamine oxidase inhibitors were the main antidepressant medications being prescribed. However, the purportedly less toxic antidepressants in current usage can potentiate suicide risk.)* Physicians can prescribe antidepressants that "satisfy" both themselves and their patients that something is being done for their patients, while unwittingly withholding psychological treatments that may offer a better chance of helping these patients.

MAJOR DEPRESSIVE EPISODE

MDE is usually relatively easy to diagnose. The family practitioner rarely sees a patient with a psychotic depression with mood-congruent delusions, for example of guilt or impoverishment, or hallucinations, such as accusatory auditory hallucinations (Lehmann, 1985: 786). A reliable diagnostic sign of MDE is that the depression has become "autonomous"; that is, it has become the main preoccupation of the patient, whose social and occupational functioning is impaired. The depressive mood of these patients is persistent, as distinct from patients with ADDM. Many if not most patients with MDE warrant admission to a psychiatric unit because of their increased suicide risk. Such a setting can also provide the necessary support to them that cannot be provided on an outpatient basis. *Sadly, what was routinely the standard of psychiatric care available when this originally was published no longer obtains, and patients with MDE are rarely admitted to hospital, and then very briefly, unless they present a very active suicide risk. They generally are discharged as soon as their suicide risk is felt to be acceptably reduced. The intensive psychiatric care that patients with MDE used to receive, often amounting to two or three weeks in hospital, is no longer available, except for the few who are able to afford private hospitalization.*

"NON-MAJOR" DEPRESSION

The diagnosis of adjustment disorder with depressed mood (ADDM) is appropriate when a patient experiences depressive mood following a psychosocial precipitant. Such a precipitant is often a disappointment or loss in a relationship, or some other blow to the patient's self-esteem. The patient may be acutely miserable, and may present in a "crisis" shortly after the precipitant has occurred. By definition, the depressive symptoms are not severe enough to warrant a diagnosis of MDE. A careful history may elicit not only the precipitant of this disorder, but also earlier disappointments or losses in relationships that make the patient's current reaction more understandable, as the earlier disappointments sensitized the patient to further loss.

Antidepressant medication is rarely indicated for ADDM. What is indicated initially is an ongoing attempt on the part of the physician to support the patient through the crisis and to help him find a solution to his problem, or to support him and help him grieve his loss (Steinberg, 1989). If the patient's symptoms become unsupportable on an outpatient basis – if, for instance, he becomes suicidal, severely agitated, or more severely depressed – consultation with a psychiatrist and possibly admission to a psychiatric unit may be appropriate.

The diagnosis of PDD is appropriate when a patient experiences prolonged, if fluctuating, depressive mood for a period of at least two years with symptoms not severe enough to warrant a diagnosis of MDE. These patients are chronically miserable; often a personality disorder can be concurrently be diagnosed. In fact, it is often apparent that these patients' characteristic maladaptive patterns of interpersonal behavior contribute to their misery. The same criteria for psychiatric consultation and psychiatric admission apply here as in patients with ADDM, *as does the very low likelihood of their being admitted to hospital, even when it is indicated. Patients with PDD form a middle group between MDE and ADDM. Some may benefit from antidepressant medication, but most or all of them will require some form of psychotherapy.*

The same supportive approach should be followed with patients with PDD as has been referred to above (Steinberg, 1989), although these patients differ: instead of having one identifiable precipitant, they will have experienced a multitude of difficulties in their relationships and functioning over a period of years. In patients with PDD who have few realistic opportunities for change in their life, especially if their depressive symptoms approach the severity required for a diagnosis of MDE, an antidepressant may be considered in addition to a supportive psychotherapeutic approach. (Of course, patients with MDE who are appropriately treated with antidepressants also deserve the same supportive psychotherapeutic approach.) *Psychoanalytic psychotherapy or psychoanalysis should be considered for all patients who suffer from PDD and MDE. The amenability of patients to these treatments is not specific to diagnosis. The first introductory chapter provides lists of prognostic criteria regarding suitability for these treatments. Many patients with ADDM also can benefit from at least a short period of psychoanalytic psychotherapy.*

"*DEPRESSIO SINE DEPRESSIONE*" (DEPRESSION WITHOUT DEPRESSION, OR MASKED DEPRESSION)

Sometimes a patient may not complain overtly of depressive mood or describe depressive symptoms. Nevertheless, the family physician may experience some concern regarding depression, for example, if the patient has physical complaints that do not appear to correspond to a recognizable medical illness. In some cultures, it is common for patients who eventually can be diagnosed as depressed to present with somatic symptoms. This has become an important consideration, given the extent of immigration to Western nations of people from other cultures. Alternatively, the physician might find herself feeling very sad when meeting a patient when she was not feeling sad before, and is aware of no particular reason why she should feel sad then. Feeling sad under these circumstances may be an indication that the patient is struggling with sadness that for some reason he cannot bear to experience, somehow locating his sadness in his physician. In my opinion, this usually happens when the depressive mood is quite severe, or the patient's capacity for tolerating depressive mood is very low. A rather dramatic example of why this might be so is a patient whose father committed suicide when he was depressed, so feeling depressed might be very threatening to the patient. Many patients have less catastrophic reasons for having difficulty tolerating painful feelings. The physician experiencing sadness with a patient without knowing why might gently inquire if he is feeling depressed. Alternatively, she might suggest that there is a feeling of sadness in the room, and ask the patient for his thoughts about this.

Cognitive Behavior Therapy (CBT)

CBT is a time-limited, structured, symptom-oriented manualized psychological treatment provided on an individual or group basis for many conditions, first used to treat depression. CBT confronts a patient's cognitive distortions and maladaptive behaviors, challenging negative thought patterns, and promoting the development of new information-processing skills and coping strategies for current problems. CBT is a directive treatment. Specific phases of the treatment are outlined; homework often is given. The goal of CBT is symptom reduction, improved coping skills, and healthier thinking and behavioral patterns. CBT can be useful with patients who are not interested in or capable of understanding the basis for their depression, but want tools to help them feel better. The unconscious significance of patients' thoughts, feelings, and impulses, and how they contribute to patients' problems, is not considered in CBT.

PSYCHOANALYTIC (PSYCHODYNAMIC) PSYCHOTHERAPY

Some patients with ADDM and most patients suffering from PDD will not respond to the family physician's supportive approach. Other such patients may improve symptomatically, but the physician or patient may become aware of maladaptive patterns of behavior or difficulties in relationships that do not change during the physician's supportive treatment. Consultation with a psychiatrist familiar with the indications for psychoanalytic psychotherapy and psychoanalysis is a considerable advantage in these cases. When a patient has refractory depressive symptoms, the consultant may suggest another psychological treatment to address these symptoms. As well, patients who have symptomatically improved with the supportive approach the family physician offers may benefit further by a better understanding of the motivations for their repetitive maladaptive behavior (in the case of patients suffering from PDD who also have significant personality disturbance or a personality disorder), or of their sensitivity to the precipitant that resulted in a depressive reaction (in the case of ADDM).

Of course, many patients suffering from MDE, in addition to being treated with antidepressant medication, can similarly benefit from psychoanalytic psychotherapy or psychoanalysis. Psychotherapeutic treatment can help such patients become more aware of their contribution to becoming depressed, including repetitive maladaptive behaviors, and learn some of the latter's antecedents in their earlier life. The most powerful mechanism for this kind of learning is in examining how these patterns of relationship are repeated in the relationship between analyst/psychotherapist and patient (the transference) as the experience is here and now, happening in the consulting room, where the individuals involved are able to talk about the experience.

Family physicians generally are not trained to perform psychoanalytic psychotherapy. Formal training in psychoanalysis or psychoanalytic psychotherapy is undertaken by a minority of mental health professionals. Unfortunately, one of the major determinants regarding whether a patient is referred for psychoanalytic psychotherapy or psychoanalysis is the referring source's familiarity with such treatments, and her having a basis for believing that these treatments are beneficial. This is problematic because very little is taught in medical school or in family medicine or other specialty residencies about these treatments. Unfortunately, residencies in psychiatry in present times offer limited theoretical teaching and practical training in these treatments, and it is a small minority of psychiatrists who undertake psychoanalytic training. Fortunately, with increasing awareness of the limitations of antidepressant medications and short-term, manualized symptom-focused psychotherapies, there is some increased awareness of the value of psychoanalytic psychotherapy and psychoanalysis.

Patients likely to benefit from a psychoanalytic psychotherapy and psychoanalysis should be identified both because other treatments may not be as beneficial, and because the personality changes resulting from these therapies can protect the patient from further depressive episodes. That is, psychoanalytic therapies are a form of secondary prevention. As mentioned above, the goal of psychoanalytic psychotherapy is not a *restituo ad integrum*, restoring the patient's original condition, but the setting in motion of a new process of thinking and feeling that is intended to be ongoing for the patient's entire life, which involves continuous growth beyond the patient's premorbid state. This is one of few situations in medicine where the patient may not only be relieved of his complaints, but is helped to develop a process of ongoing improvement beyond his premorbid state.

CONCLUSION: AVOIDING "MISDIAGNOSIS"

For terminological clarity, ideally the term "depression" should be reserved for patients with MDE. This usage is impractical because our colleagues, not to mention our patients, will continue to use "depression" to denote a symptom, a syndrome, a reaction to loss, or even a variation of normal mood. I suggest that family physicians should bear in mind the distinction between various types of "depression," and limit the prescription of antidepressants to that minority of their patients who are most likely to benefit from them. (The latter group are ones most closely approximating the DSM-5 description of MDE and some patients with PDD, as noted above.) Appropriate psychotherapy without antidepressants should be prescribed to patients in whom antidepressants are not indicated, although it may be tempting to prescribe antidepressants in the hope that it will help the patient. Many patients will share this hope, or even demand an antidepressant. *Of course, there may be a transient placebo effect when an antidepressant is prescribed to a patient for whom it is not indicated; I believe our patients deserve more than that.*

It may support the family physician in resisting a request for antidepressants that are not indicated to know that in my experience of doing psychiatric consultations in a general hospital intensive care unit, by far the greater number of antidepressant overdoses are taken by patients with rather severe personality disorders in whom antidepressants were at best questionably indicated. These patients usually appeared also to be suffering from ADDM, or from PDD. Such patients, who sometimes pressure their physician to prescribe medication, or for whom their physician hopes to find a quick remedy because of the discomfort or trouble this type of patient causes her, often show by their effect on the physician that they are unlikely to have a depressive condition amenable to antidepressant treatment. *That is, the physician's awareness of her feelings about the patient, the physician's countertransference, gives her a hint about the degree of disturbance of the patient's personality and of the patient's difficulty in interpersonal relationships.*

A patient with MDE having reduced energy and self-esteem is unlikely to pressure his physician to do anything. A physician is likely to feel compassion for such a patient. On the other hand, the discomfort that some patients with personality disorders can induce in us sometimes results in our prescribing a drug to relieve us of our discomfort with the patient, or to satisfy the patient's demands and get the patient off our back. It is nevertheless in the interest of such patients that we persevere in our attempts to help these patients find a constructive solution to their problems, protecting them from the danger of overdose, and reserving antidepressant medications for those patients more likely to benefit from them (Steinberg, 1983a, 1983b).

When patients who have suffered from MDE or PDD have experienced what benefit can be expected from antidepressants and their physician's support, they may remain significantly depressed. Then consideration should be given to their suitability to undertake psychoanalytic psychotherapy or psychoanalysis. This is also the case for patients with ADDM or who have a personality disorder with depression whose depressive symptoms and mood persist after receiving symptomatic psychological treatments, such as CBT. A patient's suitability for psychoanalytic psychotherapy or psychoanalysis is not based on diagnosis. A patient's openness to understanding his suffering in psychological terms is an important criterion. However, with advances in these types of therapy, even that is a capacity that often needs to be developed during therapy.

REFERENCES

American Psychiatric Association (2013). *Diagnostic and Statistical Manual of Mental Disorders*, 5th edition. Arlington, VA: American Psychiatric Association.

Lehmann H (1985). Affective disorders: Clinical features. In: Kaplan HI, Sadock BJ (eds.), *Comprehensive Textbook of Psychiatry*, 4th edition. Baltimore, MD: Williams and Wilkins.

Steinberg P (1983a). Psychiatry of family practice. I. The problem patient. *Canadian Family Physician* 29:1942–1947.

Steinberg P (1983b). Psychiatry of family practice. II. Interviewing the patient. *Canadian Family Physician* 29:1953–1957.

Steinberg P (1989). Two techniques of supportive psychotherapy. *Canadian Family Physician* 35:1139–1143.

Weissman MM, Boyd JH (1985). Affective disorders: Epidemiology. In: Kaplan HI, Sadock BJ (eds.), *Comprehensive Textbook of Psychiatry*, 4th edition. Baltimore, MD: Williams and Wilkins.

CHAPTER 4

"MY PATIENT IS PSYCHOTIC": DEALING WITH A PATIENT WITH A PARANOID DELUSION ABOUT HER DISEASE

This chapter describes the management, utilizing psychoanalytically informed psychiatric consultation, of a patient who has managed a chronic medical illness well, but becomes delusional at the prospect of surgery.

CASE HISTORY

Mrs. A was a 74-year-old married patient, new to Dr. Z. She had emigrated from Europe years ago and maintained the customs of the old country. One of her three children lived in the same city. Mrs. A had long-standing non-insulin-dependent diabetes mellitus well controlled by glyburide 5 mg t.i.d. and a diet that she executed well. Before seeing Dr. Z, she was treated with perphenazine, an antipsychotic medication, for unclear reasons.

Mrs. A had bilateral cataracts and macular and retinal problems. One of her children called Dr. Z from out of town, complaining that Mrs. A had trouble with her eyes and needed surgery. Mrs. A said her previous family physician wouldn't listen to her. Contact between Dr. Z and him did not elucidate Mrs. A's condition beyond that Mrs. A and her doctor had an "impossible personality clash." Mrs. A's family knew Dr. Z, and recommended him, assuring her that he would listen to her.

Mrs. A was completely logical when discussing her medical problems, except regarding her eyes. She was as unhappy with the ophthalmologists she had consulted as she was with her former family doctor. She required cataract removal followed by retinal surgery. She was very upset about requiring surgery, and did not believe that cataracts were the real problem. Mrs. A seemed obsessed with the idea that her visual difficulties were the result of an incorrect prescription for eyeglasses that "closed" her eyes. Dr. Z found it impossible to elicit a medical history from Mrs. A about her eyes; she focused incessantly on her belief that her eyeglasses had harmed her.

Mrs. A's ophthalmologist said that he would not proceed with the proposed lens implant until Mrs. A accepted the need to have it before the retinopathy was treated. Mrs. A said that she completely accepted the need for the lens implant, but believed that the real problem was the series of "incorrect" prescription eyeglasses that had altered her vision. In describing this, she made bizarre references to the muscles closing the eyes that did not correspond to accepted anatomical knowledge. Mrs. A had her own quite fixed ideas about how these muscles function. Apart from the strange ideas about her eyes, Mrs. A displayed no other disorder of form or content of thought, no hallucinations, and was not otherwise paranoid. She was almost obsessive about her diabetes, keeping diaries of her diet and learning dietary substitutions, resulting in good control of her diabetes.

Whenever consulting Dr. Z, Mrs. A steered the discussion back to the subject of her vision several times. It was clear that her cataracts had to be removed and lens implants fitted before doctors could visualize the retinae for laser treatment. Because of the retinopathy, lens implants by themselves would not improve Mrs. A's vision; adjunct laser treatment might. The ophthalmologist understandably was concerned that surgery might precipitate a psychotic reaction. He requested a management plan to deal with this possibility before performing surgery, and refused to proceed until Mrs. A consulted a psychiatrist. *This ophthalmologist in my opinion demonstrated considerable discernment in recognizing the need for psychiatric consultation.*

Mrs. A's children indicated she had been better since meeting Dr. Z, who she believed listened to her. Dr. Z, however, believed she invested him with "magical" qualities. He presented Mrs. A's history to the psychiatric consultant during one of the regularly held seminars between the consultant and family physicians and residents.

COLLABORATIVE MANAGEMENT APPROACH

What is the family physician's role in managing a patient such as Mrs. A? He must understand both ophthalmological and psychiatric diagnoses. A good psychiatric formulation of the problem gives important clues for diagnosis, prognosis, and management.

The psychiatric consultant thought Mrs. A's standing prescription for antipsychotic medication suggested a history of psychotic symptoms or a vulnerability to psychosis. He agreed that Mrs. A was at risk of postoperative psychosis due to her distress about the prospect of surgery and her unrealistic beliefs about her cataracts. Contributing factors include Mrs. A's belief of her eyeglasses having damaged her, her unsatisfactory relationship with previous physicians, and sensory deprivation if both eyes were to be operated on simultaneously. Mrs. A's preoccupation with the damage from eyeglasses seemed to be a circumscribed delusion. Any previous history of psychiatric symptoms and treatment would be useful in assessing how likely a florid postoperative psychotic state would be.

The psychiatric consultant thought Mrs. A's meticulous approach to managing her diabetes and the resultant good control suggested that she was comfortable and effective in situations where she felt "in control." Given the paranoid nature of her delusion about her eyeglasses, it was understandable that she felt threatened by the prospect of surgery in which she would have no control at all, especially surgery performed by a member of the specialty she believed had damaged her eyes. The ophthalmologist's apprehension that she would be dissatisfied and inclined to blame him, whatever the results of the surgery, appeared well founded. The psychiatrist suggested helping Mrs. A somehow to feel in control of her ophthalmologic treatment, rather than experiencing herself as the passive victim of surgery, which would likely increase her paranoid symptoms. He suggested that Dr. Z describe to Mrs. A in considerable detail exactly what would happen in the hospital, repeating himself as necessary, to ensure that Mrs. A felt well informed about all aspects of her treatment. In effect, Dr. Z would reinforce reality for Mrs. A. Dr. Z would function as an emotional support, a positive attachment, and an auxiliary ego. The latter involves enhancing Mrs. A's perception of reality, playing down her paranoia by focusing attention away from it and on to more realistic concerns, such as the real hospital environment Mrs. A would find herself in. The psychiatrist thought it was important for Mrs. A to experience herself as an active part of the treatment team. He asked Dr. Z to discuss with Mrs. A's family her special needs for emotional support and for reinforcing the realistic aspect of her hospital stay. Dr. Z was to encourage their sensitivity to Mrs. A's fears. The psychiatrist also met with Mrs. A's nursing team to inform them of her sensitivities and advise them on the best psychological approach to nursing care of her, along the collaborative lines suggested to the surgeon and Dr. Z.

DIAGNOSIS AND MANAGEMENT

The provisional diagnosis was delusional disorder. There was no evidence of an organic mental disorder. The psychiatrist suggested a prophylactic increase in Mrs. A's antipsychotic medication; it might be necessary to discontinue it preoperatively if its anticholinergic effects interfered with surgery. Unilateral cataract removal was suggested to obviate the stress of temporary blindness, especially dangerous for this paranoid patient, whom it would threaten more than the average patient (Weisman & Hackett, 1958). Cataract surgery was arranged with Mrs. A's agreement. A week before the operation, she canceled it. Neither she nor her family approached Dr. Z during the ensuing seven weeks. Mrs. A then agreed to the cataract surgery without explaining her changing her mind. She underwent the surgery, did well, and stayed in hospital overnight because of concern about her diabetes. She was supported by her family and Dr. Z. She demonstrated no psychiatric symptoms after the operation. *In retrospect, it would have been instructive and likely helpful to medical management if the reason for Mrs. A's decision to proceed with surgery was ascertained. Perhaps it was just that in canceling the surgery and then deciding to proceed, Mrs. A experienced personal agency about the decision, which made the surgery feel less threatening. Merely having her explain her reason to her physician may have left her feeling better understood and respected.*

DISCUSSION

Steinberg (1988) describes adverse psychological reactions to surgery, including preoperative psychotic symptoms (see Chapter 10). It is generally thought to be unproductive to argue with an individual about a delusion. Delusions are fixed and serve important psychological functions, for example, the projection of hostility that isn't consciously acceptable to the patient. *(Projection involves the experiencing in someone else's mental contents, such as a thought, feeling, fantasy, or impulse, that the individual finds unbearable to recognize in himself. So, for example, an envious person, rather than experience his own envy, may feel that someone envies him, and may accuse them of this.)* Rather than arguing with a patient about a delusion regarding illness, a physician can disagree respectfully with the patient, indicate what his understanding is about the reality of the patient's condition, and describe his recommendations for treatment and the basis for these recommendations, and add that the patient (presuming he is competent) has the right to refuse a proposed treatment.

Patients who are suspicious or frankly paranoid are very frightened, however frightening they at times may appear to their caregivers. *In fact, sometimes the best clue about how a patient is feeling is how he makes his physician feel. If you feel threatened, perhaps your patient is feeling threatened too. Your feeling threatened, for example, may represent your patient's unconscious communication to you about how he is feeling. Much more is communicated between people, including physicians and their patients, than can be represented in words. Other means of communication include tone of voice; physical mannerisms, such as hand movements; eye movements; and the presence of physiological accompaniments of emotions, such as sweating, facial flushing, pallor, or tremor, to mention but a few.* With patients who are suspicious or paranoid but not frankly delusional, it is essential to describe in meticulous detail the expected benefits and potential risks of treatment, the possible and likely adverse effects of not having the treatment, and the specific techniques of the proposed procedure. It is equally important to describe the milieu in which the procedure will occur, for example, day surgery or an inpatient surgical unit, to minimize the unexpected and reduce the patient's feeling helpless and out of control. *With this you are attempting to mitigate the characteristic fear and sense of helplessness that these patients feel.* This is in the context of an important relationship, the physician–patient relationship. Of course, as suggested above, when people on the treatment team are apprised of the patient's special psychological needs and how to approach them, chances of a positive outcome are improved. Several weeks may elapse before the patient feels comfortable enough to agree to surgery.

A meticulous explanation of what will happen to the patient after surgery is as necessary as it is before surgery. The patient's family should be involved in preoperative discussions and should be present immediately before and after surgery. Medical and nursing personnel, no matter how friendly and supportive, are no replacement for individuals to whom the patient has long been attached, especially if the patient is paranoid. Of course, if there appears to be active distrust or hostility between the patient and family members, judgment would have to be exercised regarding the degree of the family's involvement. Emphasizing the importance of the family's support does not diminish the importance of the patient's ongoing relationship with the family physician. Patients will benefit from knowing that their primary physician is involved at all stages of treatment.

It is always gratifying and often useful to understand, with some confidence, the meaning of a patient's symptom. This is possible only when sufficient information is available, which was not the case with Mrs. A. Nevertheless it is tempting to formulate hypotheses about what Mrs. A.'s visual impairment meant to her, to the extent that she accused doctors of causing it through prescription of eyeglasses. An individual with paranoid tendencies is vigilant in order to forestall expected attacks. Weakened vision interferes with one's vigilance. Mrs. A might have thought that in being prescribed eyeglasses, she had been weakened and made more vulnerable. She may have thought that it was a sign of weakness and vulnerability to require help, including medical treatment. This is consistent with her very successful management of her diabetes, over which she may have felt she had complete control. Mrs. A's belief that she did not need cataract surgery, and that the real problem was improper eyeglasses, raises the question of whether Mrs. A was competent to agree to surgery. In practice, this was a moot point because part of the psychological approach to treating her was to discuss repeatedly the benefits and risks of having and not having the treatment. This is how to test a patient whose competence is being questioned (Ben-Aron & Hoffman, 1990). It would be inviting a postoperative, if not a preoperative, psychosis, potentially with violent or self-destructive behavior, to declare this patient incompetent and attempt to treat her surgically over her objections, even with the agreement of her next of kin. The ophthalmological benefits of treatment would be outweighed by the negative psychological consequences, including a loss of trust in the physician–patient relationship.

Mrs. A appears to have dealt with the pain of the loss of her vision by finding an enemy in the environment. She thus appears to have been unable to cope with the sadness inherent in grieving such a loss. One could surmise that her difficulty in containing painful feelings like grief and sadness was based on her never having experienced an early relationship in which she was able to learn how to bear such feelings by having them borne for her by a parent who could allow him- or herself to feel Mrs. A's feelings as a child, bear the feelings without fleeing from them, and convey in a manner tolerable to the young Mrs. A the experience of these feelings so Mrs. A could develop a similar capacity to bear such feelings. This is how the minds of infants and children grow, by having an adult caregiver, traditionally a mother at first, able to experience what the child feels, and articulate it back to the child. Rather than feeling grief and sadness, Mrs. A experienced suspicion and fear. She was in more of a paranoid than a depressive stance. Unfortunately, her suspicions and fears made it more difficult for her to experience her medical caregivers as acting in her interest, and, ironically, interfered with her accepting treatment that could reverse the cause of some of her grief.

The understanding of how children's minds grow described above reinforces my opinion that there being a full-time parent in the home during a child's earliest years is preferable to the child being sent when very young to an institution such as a daycare facility. This is a politically sensitive comment to make because, especially given current economic conditions, and, sometimes the material expectations of families in the West, it is accepted that both parents work, with children cared for during the day outside the home until they can attend school. This may be practically necessary, but is not necessarily best for the development of the child's mind. A potentially healthier alternative would be for a family friend or relative well known to the child, such as a grandmother, to take care of the child. This is rarely practicable, given the high mobility of families and the need of even grandmothers to work.

PSYCHIATRIC LIAISON WITH FAMILY MEDICINE

At some university teaching family medical centers, psychiatric consultation to family physicians in a liaison model is provided (Steinberg, 1987). Consulting psychiatrists do not necessarily interview patients themselves, but have cases presented by family physicians and residents, sometimes with videotaped patient interviews. A discussion regarding diagnosis and management follows. We believe this is an effective teaching device and a cost-effective way of providing psychiatric consultation for some patients, especially when referral to a psychiatrist may entail an undesirably lengthy wait. The effectiveness of this model is based partly on the ongoing working relationships that develop between the family physicians and consultants involved. This "liaison" model of psychiatric consultation to family medicine facilities is recognized. Oken (1983) contrasted psychiatrists' consultation and liaison roles using Hackett's (1978) simile about a fire-fighting rescue squad: a consultation service puts out the blaze and returns home, whereas a liaison service also sets up fire prevention programs and spots potential areas of conflagration. Oken suggests that the liaison psychiatrist should be concerned with the operation of psychological and social factors in every illness, because understanding any illness requires a synthesis of biological, psychological, and social factors.

The liaison psychiatrist's continuing presence and free access to all patients in the medical setting enable her to identify the operation of psychosocial issues even among patients in whom these are not apparent or have no seeming consequence for the current episode of illness, or who are not immediately troublesome. The consultant psychiatrist, in contrast, is called in to deal with overt, aberrant behavior and to identify and treat psychiatric disorders. Williams and Clare (1981) reject the "replacement model" of consultation (in which psychiatrists replace general practitioners as doctors of first contact for patients with psychiatric disorders) as uneconomical and impractical. They also reject a second model, increased referral (in which general practitioners refer more patients to psychiatrists while still retaining the primary care role) because of the consequent undervaluing of the general practitioner. They describe the liaison and attachment model as being the preferable form of contact between general practitioner and psychiatrist, claiming that it should improve continuity of care, promote awareness of the problems facing each discipline, and widen the skills of each professional group. They describe three forms of liaison: a psychiatrist consulting in an outpatient clinic on general practice premises; a consultation service in which a psychiatrist is present only in an advisory capacity; and an educational situation in which a psychiatrist visits a general practice regularly to take part in lectures or seminars. *This could be incorporated into contemporary shared care models that do not always offer all three forms of liaison.* Tyrer et al. (1990) suggest that the main elements of these three forms can be combined in a comprehensive model in which collaboration between primary care and psychiatric teams is the important element. The original liaison model is based on collaboration between generalists and specialists (Brooke, 1967; Gibson et al., 1966; Lyons, 1969). Tyrer's data demonstrate the relationship between the introduction of general practice psychiatry and a reduction in the use of inpatient psychiatric services, and suggest that, as primary care liaison becomes established, this relationship becomes even more marked. They conclude that liaison with general practitioners mobilizes the considerable resources of primary care to focus more on treating the mentally ill, with a resulting decrease in the need for hospital treatment.

In the family medical center in which I served as consultant, I was well known and involved in several ways. In addition to meeting the family medicine staff in teaching seminars 20 half-days yearly for 12 years, I performed psychiatric consultations for the family physicians in my hospital office, sometimes accompanied by the referring family medicine resident. I collaborated in writing peer review publications with family medicine consultants, and formally supervised residents in psychotherapeutic assessment techniques and ongoing psychotherapy. In my role as coordinator of the liaison psychiatric service for the tertiary care teaching hospital to which the family medical center was attached, I collaborated with family medicine staff in the assessment and treatment of hospitalized patients on medical, surgical, and obstetrical units for whom a psychiatric consultation was requested.

I believe that the combination of consulting, teaching, and clinical experiences in which I was associated with the family physicians and their residents enhanced the influence I had on the provision of family medical care. Of course, the influence went both ways: the educational experience between consulting psychiatrist and family physician is mutual. A psychiatrist offering liaison to a family medicine unit has many learning opportunities not available to psychiatrists who limit their work to hospital units or outpatient offices. Consultation/liaison psychiatrists must respond to the practical and often urgent needs of family physicians, in contrast to the less pressured (in some ways) work of outpatient psychotherapy or the more controlled environment of an inpatient psychiatric unit. They learn about family medicine, and are challenged to apply psychiatric and psychoanalytic knowledge to that setting, which can be relatively unfamiliar territory, unless they previously practiced as family physicians. Psychiatrists also must respond to the challenge of becoming part of a team whose training and orientation are different than theirs. These aspects of psychiatric liaison to family medicine offer opportunities for psychiatrists to enrich their work and their learning about themselves, about what they and psychiatry can offer (see Chapter 6), and about what their and its limitations are. Lastly, liaison work not only provides better patient care but also gratifying and mutually supportive professional relationships to those involved.

DEALING WITH SUSPICIOUS PATIENTS

Historical antecedents of a suspicious, fearful, or paranoid attitude in patients include:

1. When a child realistically has much to fear and be suspicious about, for example, a violent father, even if beatings are infrequent. It is especially difficult for a child when he doesn't know why he is being beaten. Unpredictability adds to the fear and need for vigilance.
2. When the child's temperament makes him vulnerable (a higher than average sensitivity), favoring his interpreting experience as traumatic that other children may not experience as such.
3. If parents are excessively suspicious and fearful, the child may identify with this attitude. This occurs most poignantly when a child's parents are suspicious of him.

Of course, combinations of the above factors may occur. Fear, suspiciousness, and vigilance cover a wide range of clinical presentations from mild personality traits manifested only under stress; through a more consistently paranoid attitude to the world, which represents paranoid personality traits, or, if it significantly interferes with an individual's reality testing, functioning and/or relationships, a paranoid personality disorder; to the acute or chronic paranoid symptoms of delusional disorder, or paranoid schizophrenia, often with threatening hallucinations.

A comment about defenses in people with paranoid characteristics: psychological mechanisms of defense are unconscious attempts to reduce anxiety and other painful feelings. To the extent that an individual is paranoid, he is frightened and feels helpless. He often reacts with anger and hatred. All these feelings are painful to experience in oneself. Projection is a frequent defense among paranoid individuals. The paranoid individual projects his hatred on to others, seeing them as hating him, which only increases his fear, sense of helplessness, and hatred, in a vicious cycle. The suspiciousness that characterizes paranoid individuals isolates them, reducing the likelihood that they can reassure themselves about their fears and suspicions with a realistic appraisal of their environment. In order to maintain some experience of the environment as positive, paranoid people sometimes split their perception of individuals in their environment, idealizing some and devaluing others. This represents a projection of a split in their unconscious internal images of others, and probably of their unconscious images of themselves, into good and bad parts. Unfortunately, this unrealistic evaluation of others interferes with the individual's capacity for judging people, so the paranoid individual, either in being suspicious of everyone, or in arbitrarily being suspicious of some and not others, renders himself less capable of identifying who he realistically needs to be cautious of, rendering him vulnerable to people who don't have his best interests at heart, another vicious cycle. To say that being afraid can be very frightening seems circular. One way of defending against an awareness of one's fear is to displace the fear from someone whom it might be appropriate to fear to someone whom one does not need to fear. Again, this renders the individual using this unconscious mechanism more vulnerable than he otherwise would be.

REFERENCES

Ben-Aron MH, Hoffman BE (1990). Assessments of competence to consent to medical treatment: A balance between law and medicine. *Medicine and the Law* 9(5):1122–1130.

Brooke A (1967). An experiment in GP/psychiatrist cooperation. *Journal of the Royal College of General Practice* 13:127–131.

Gibson R, Forbes JM, Stoddart IW, Cooke JJ, Jenkins W, McKeith SA (1966). Psychiatric care in general practice: An experiment in collaboration. *British Medical Journal* 1:1287–1289.

Hackett TP (1978). Beginnings, liaison psychiatry in a general hospital. In: Hackett TP, Cassem NH (eds.), *Massachusetts General Hospital Handbook of General Hospital Psychiatry.* St. Louis, MO: Mosby, 1–14.

Lyons HA (1969). Joint psychiatric consultation. *Journal of the Royal College of General Practice* 18:125–127.

Oken D (1983). Liaison psychiatry (liaison medicine). *Advances in Psychosomatic Medicine* 1(1):23–51.

Steinberg P (1987). Broader indications for psychiatric consultation. *Canadian Family Physician* 33:437–440.

Steinberg PI (1988). Psychiatric complications of surgery in the male. *Canadian Journal of Psychiatry* 33(1):28–33.

Tyrer P, Ferguson B, Wadsworth J (1990). Liaison psychiatry in general practice: The comprehensive collaborative model. *Acta Psychiatrica Scandinavica* 81(4):359–363.

Weisman AD, Hackett TP (1958). Psychosis after eye surgery: Establishment of specific doctor/ patient relationship in prevention and treatment of "black patch delirium." *New England Journal of Medicine* 258:1284–1289.

Williams P, Clare A (1981). Changing patterns of psychiatric care. *British Medical Journal* 282:375.

CHAPTER 5

HOLDING PATIENTS WITH MEDICATION: USING NEUROLEPTICS AS AN ADJUNCT TO PSYCHOTHERAPY IN PATIENTS WITH SEVERE PERSONALITY DISORDERS

Although Freud did not believe that patients with psychotic conditions could be treated with psychoanalysis, in the decades following his death, analysts in the United Kingdom and the United States undertook this very demanding work (Bion, 1967; Rosenfeld, 1965; Searles, 1965; Segal, 1957; Sullivan, 1962). This involved, among other things, dealing with very disturbing countertransference experiences. That is, it was impossible for analysts to treat these severely ill patients, who themselves experienced very intense painful and frightening feelings and disturbances in their thought processes, without experiencing these feelings and disturbances of thinking themselves. Issues that become evident in treating patients with psychotic disturbances include the deficient development of the capacity to symbolize, a part of the psychotic patient's mind attacking his capacity to think, the need for interpretation of pathological use of defenses, such as projective identification and splitting, and the patient's effort to drive the analyst crazy. These psychotic patients undertaking psychoanalysis in the mid twentieth century were treated without benefit of antipsychotic medication, which was being developed concurrently.

The finding that patients with psychotic disorders have a non-psychotic part of their personality led to the understanding that neurotic and apparently normal individuals (including physicians!) also have a psychotic side to their personality. From this one may conclude that individuals are found along a spectrum of mental health, between functioning at one extreme at a very psychotic level, and at the other extreme at a relatively healthy level. As well, people are not fixed at any given point of the spectrum, but fluctuate, depending in part on the extent to which they experience wholesome support from their environment, and the extent to which they are exposed to stresses, including traumatic experiences, loss, isolation, and unconscious intrapsychic conflict. The understanding that each individual has a psychotic and non-psychotic part to her personality makes so-called borderline conditions more understandable. Rather than having to divide individuals in a binary fashion regarding whether they are psychotic or not, we can understand that people can, on the basis of both constitutional factors and early traumatic experiences, have a greater or lesser propensity to psychotic functioning, which can be exacerbated by stress. This is not a difficult concept to accept. After all, it is clear that some prominent public figures are capable of denying reality. Even if these individuals are lying and really do understand reality, the lie involves a perversion of thinking (Chasseguet-Smirgel, 1985) that can be considered psychotic in nature.

Advances in psychoanalytic understanding of more severe pathologies, with corresponding changes in technique (Stone, 1954), have made it possible to treat patients with a much broader range of disturbances initially thought to be beyond the range of psychoanalytic treatment, including not only patients with psychotic symptoms, but also patients with borderline, narcissistic, schizoid, paranoid, and other personality disorders, psychosomatic disturbance (McDougall, 1989), paraphilias (sexual perversions) (Chasseguet-Smirgel, 1985), and patients with substance addictions and traumatized patients.

Given therapists adequately trained in treating patients with severe personality disturbance suffering from the above conditions, a significant percentage of these patients could be treated with psychoanalysis or psychoanalytic psychotherapy without adjunct treatment with neuroleptic medication. Obviously, not all patients with severe mental disturbance need, want, or can benefit from psychoanalysis. Family physicians, psychiatrists, and other physicians, as well as non-medical mental health professionals, offer supportive relationships and possibly some form of counseling to patients with disturbances of thinking to help them cope better.

It is important to distinguish between psychotherapies such as psychoanalysis and psychoanalytic psychotherapy, where significant growth in the patient's personality and improvement in her functioning in her relationship to the world is anticipated, from counseling, in which the patient is helped to continue with the same coping mechanisms, and is provided with encouragement, practical advice, and emotional support. I wish to emphasize a point. I am not suggesting that all severely disturbed individuals can be treated successfully with psychoanalysis or psychoanalytic psychotherapy. However, it is important that physicians know that effective evidence-based treatment that offers expectation of improvement in functioning is available to patients who otherwise might be treated with medications or forms of psychological support, of which the only benefit can be to reduce symptoms and at best restore the patient to her previous level of functioning.

Some patients who have personality disturbance suffer from disorders in the form or content of their thinking, in their regulation of affect, or in their capacity to contain their impulses. These disturbances can be significant enough to interfere with progress in various forms of psychotherapy. Clearly they also interfere with these patients' conduct of their lives, including their capacity for intimate relationships and productive work. My experience with patients in a psychiatric day treatment program (DTP) suggests that small doses of atypical neuroleptics can help to relieve the symptoms of these patients and allow them to benefit from psychodynamic group psychotherapy. Further research is needed to determine whether this benefit will obtain in other modalities of psychotherapy and in patients being provided emotional support by family practitioners. Research is also needed to determine to what degree improvement is due to medication and to psychotherapy, and whether at some point after completing psychotherapy, patients might stop taking neuroleptics without experiencing symptomatic relapse. It is important for clinical and medico-legal reasons to review the serious side effects of neuroleptic medications with patients and to monitor patients for side effects.

The patients in that DTP generally suffered from personality disorders of moderate to severe degree, usually severe enough to render them unable to function in competitive employment or to establish or maintain long-term relationships. Although most of them suffered from symptoms of a concomitant Axis I disorder, most frequently major depressive disorder, none were floridly psychotic. Nevertheless, many had significant disturbances of their thought processes. These included the maintaining of mutually contradictory beliefs or thoughts without awareness of the contradiction; beliefs that were obviously false but did not qualify to be called delusions; a tendency to dissociate or derail thinking when an emotionally intolerable thought was approaching consciousness; and abrupt changes of subject to avoid articulating an emotionally disturbing thought. Other disturbances in thinking included twisting the meaning of a word the therapist used to render meaningless what she was trying to express; hairsplitting about the meaning of a word until what was emotionally important about the discussion was lost; and responding in a tangential or irrelevant manner to the discussion. Lastly, these patients could have disturbances of their thought content, becoming paranoid or grandiose when under stress, including the stress of interpretations or confrontations in the group.

> *These patients' difficulty with affect regulation was manifest by volatility of affect, with patients rapidly becoming upset, enraged, despairing, or elated; affective numbness, with patients characteristically demonstrating and/or feeling little affect, or becoming affectively numb when an emotionally disturbing thought arose; or a characteristically superficial expression of affect that was unresponsive to current circumstances, for example, consistently appearing cheerful or calm. Difficulty containing impulses often was manifest by a tendency to action rather than reflection on how one felt and discussion of what was transpiring in one's inner experience. Some patients would abruptly leave a group that was upsetting them, quit DTP impulsively, not show up for groups, or become enraged in a group and express it in an intense manner. Sometimes patients acted in impulsive and destructive ways outside of DTP, leaving their partners, getting into physical fights, or relapsing into substance abuse. The motivation of these patients to explore their inner world generally was low when they were admitted to the program.* We found that progress in psychodynamic group psychotherapy is fostered in some of these patients with the use of low doses of atypical antipsychotics to improve thought processes, affect regulation, and impulse control (Steinberg et al., 2004).

DTP offers both unstructured psychotherapy groups and semi-structured groups in which an activity is used to introduce a theme about which the patients may do psychotherapeutic work. The theoretical emphasis of the program is psychoanalytic, with a strong emphasis on confrontation, limit setting, and interpretation.

Between one and four of about 35 DTP patients had a significant disturbance in the form or content of their thinking. Many more had disturbances in their affect regulation, and/or in their capacity to contain their impulses, rather than acting on them without reflecting on them. These disturbances interfered with the patients' progress in therapy, and were often difficult to categorize diagnostically (American Psychiatric Association, 2013). They did not represent a brief psychotic episode, although many of our patients received a diagnosis of borderline personality disorder. The disturbances of thinking did not appear to be transient reactions to stressful events, but rather represented the individual's characteristic mode of thinking, although the disturbance could become more pronounced when the individual was under stress, including the stress of attending DTP. This also was true of the patients' disturbances of affect regulation and impulse control. Frequently accompanying the disturbance in thinking was a disturbance in affect regulation; these individuals became intensely angry and even paranoid, or overcome by sadness, weeping uncontrollably. Their affective responses made it difficult for them to remain involved in the psychotherapeutic process. These patients did not experience other psychotic symptomatology, such as delusions, hallucinations, or Schneiderian criteria (Kaplan & Sadock, 1995) of schizophrenia. None of these patients ever had an acute psychotic episode or required hospitalization for acute psychiatric symptoms. While some of these patients' presentations suggested schizotypal personality disorder, they were not eccentric in other ways, did not usually demonstrate other schizotypal traits, and had not received such a diagnosis prior to attending DTP.

We found that low-dose neuroleptic treatment enabled these patients to benefit from involvement in psychodynamic group psychotherapy. Although no literature was found describing the use of neuroleptic medications as an adjunct to group psychotherapy, or to psychotherapy in general, there is such evidence for the treatment of psychotic patients. Frosch (1983) describes the nature of psychotic defenses, the state of the ego and its functions, and the ego's position vis-à-vis reality. He also describes approaches to the psychoanalytic treatment of psychosis. Beitman (1996) addresses the integration of pharmacotherapy and psychotherapy, examining studies involving psychotherapy during randomized controlled medication trials, considering psychotherapeutic aspects of pharmacotherapy, and addressing the meaning of medications during psychotherapy. Several authors have treated schizophrenic patients with psychotherapy and medication (Feinsilver & Yates, 1984; Rock, 1970).

CLINICAL EXAMPLES

Violet was a 31-year-old cleaner living in a common-law relationship. Although well educated and articulate, she went off on tangents, leaving behind the subject being discussed. Sometimes she made inappropriate, bizarre comments unrelated to the topic being discussed. She evinced no insight into the effect on others of this. For example, when angry, she told other group members, "I feel like killing you all," in a neutral tone of voice. She mentioned feeling like mutilating people in public places, and showed no awareness of how this admission might affect other group members. When she said something untoward, it appeared to be unconsciously provocative.

Violet was treated with olanzapine 5 mg qhs. This produced a considerable improvement in the organization of her thinking. Her tangential associations almost disappeared, and she only infrequently made comments that seemed unrelated to the subject at hand. She stopped making bizarre and upsetting comments. Violet was able to do psychotherapeutic work on her tendency to be provocative and on what motivated it, which she had appeared unable to do before taking the olanzapine.

Adam, a married 33-year-old middle manager in a large corporation, is an especially articulate and intelligent individual, diagnosed with narcissistic personality disorder. Although there was no indication of a diagnosis of bipolar disorder, his manner of presenting himself was unmistakably grandiose. He found it difficult to tolerate confrontations in groups, which frequently resulted in his becoming angry and paranoid, expressing unrealistic suspicions regarding the motivations and behavior of many people, including other group members. Sometimes he became angry enough to stomp out of the room in the middle of a group. He would return the next day calmed down, but unwilling to discuss what had resulted in his leaving. Adam was treated with risperidone 1 mg qhs. This was followed by a complete cessation of his paranoid reactions, with more ability to contain himself when angry and discuss what made him angry.

Hazel, a 47-year-old married librarian, displayed a variety of disruptive behaviors and intensely expressed emotions in the group. In the assessment interview she began pulling her shirt off, exposing her chest, and became intensely angry at the therapist's instructing her to "keep her shirt on." *(It only occurred to me on reading the nth draft of this chapter that that phrase could help in understanding the motivation for Hazel's behavior!)* When sad, Hazel would weep uncontrollably in the group, disrupting her own and the group's work. Sometimes her anger had a paranoid flavor; it was difficult or impossible to reason with her. Hazel's thinking also became quite tangential when she was discussing anxiety-provoking material. Sometimes she appeared to have difficulty distinguishing fantasy from reality. She presented material in a disorganized manner. Hazel was treated with quetiapine 25 mg qhs. This was followed by a rapid modulation of her affects, to the extent that she was no longer overwhelmed by either sadness or anger. Her work in groups no longer was interrupted by uncontrollable affects. Her thinking became more organized, and her speech completely coherent and goal-directed. Paranoid ideation was no longer evident. Hazel completed DTP having made excellent use of the groups, and continued on quetiapine upon discharge. We were not aware of any of these patients suffering from side effects from their small doses of atypical neuroleptics.

DISCUSSION

Attempts to use psychodynamic psychotherapy and psychoanalysis to treat severely disturbed individuals, including individuals with psychotic illness, are well documented (Arieti, 1955; Frosch, 1983; Marder, 2007; Searles, 1986; see also Chapter 4). These treatments make considerable demands on the patient to integrate a combination of secondary process and creative primary process thinking, which is challenging work for anyone (Dorpat & Miller, 1992). It is particularly difficult for these patients, with their limited capacity to recognize reality, to maintain an integrated sense of their identity and to contain their uncomfortable affects and impulses. A significant number of DTP patients appeared so stressed by the psychodynamic approach, or to suffer from symptoms so severe, that their ability to benefit from group therapy was compromised. A small dose of neuroleptic medication enabled them to function better in psychotherapy and to derive more benefit from it.

These patients appear to have a borderline or psychotic personality organization (Kernberg, 1984; McWilliams, 1994). They were given a variety of diagnoses, none of which adequately described my patients' conditions. They could be overwhelmed by intense affect such as rage, sadness, or guilt, which paralyzed them in psychotherapeutic work. They could have a disorder of their thought processes, resulting in their engaging in tangential thinking, or experiencing transient or persistent disturbances of thought content, such as paranoid tendencies that made them litigious when threatened, or having a tendency to speak and behave impulsively or destructively to ward off painful affect. Small doses of atypical neuroleptics, such as 1.25–5 mg olanzapine, 6.25–25 mg quetiapine, or 1–2 mg risperidone, effected a significant change in these patients' mental status, and appeared to enable them to persist in constructive psychotherapeutic work that they couldn't accomplish without medication. These patients did not exhibit florid psychotic symptoms and did not need, and often did not tolerate, higher doses of neuroleptics. Often these disturbances were not identified in our 1½-hour intake session. The tendency to thought disorder usually showed up in Rorschach testing if it was undertaken while patients were in DTP.

RESEARCH POSSIBILITIES

The observations represented by the case data discussed here have implications for psychotherapeutic treatment of patients with severe personality disturbance in all forms of psychotherapy and also, I believe, for patients displaying these symptoms who are not receiving psychotherapeutic treatment. A small dose of neuroleptic medication may enable patients with the difficulties described to engage more productively in any modality of psychotherapy based on any theoretical approach, including a system-based family therapy, a cognitive behavioral individual or group therapy, or a psychoanalytic individual therapy. The ability of these patients to be actively involved in psychotherapeutic treatment in general is improved with the prescription of low-dose neuroleptic medication. The functioning of these patients outside DTP appears to have improved by administration of small doses of neuroleptic medication, unrelated to the therapeutic benefits of psychotherapy.

Our experience raises a question regarding to what extent psychotherapy helped these patients, and to what extent the patients' improvements were attributable to neuroleptics. Future research regarding this might compare the results of psychotherapy alone with the results of neuroleptic medication alone, and the results of combined treatment. Clinical experience suggests that combined treatment is most beneficial. It seems very unlikely that treatment with the neuroleptic medication alone would be as effective as treatment with combined treatment in this population. Some disturbances of thinking, affect regulation, and impulse behavior might improve with medications alone. However, the interpersonal learning and the improvement in and development of the capacity for abstract thinking that can take place in DTP would not occur, and the patients' improvement would be symptomatic only. There is no reason to believe that this improvement would be maintained if the neuroleptic medication were withdrawn. While it is possible that the environment might positively reinforce the more constructive behavior demonstrated while patients are taking neuroleptics, it appears more likely that this would be the case were the patient also to attend DTP. Ideally, patients who benefited from psychotherapy would build on their experience in DTP and continue to learn in interpersonal situations with or without ongoing psychotherapy. Eventually the neuroleptic medication might be withdrawn without a relapse of the symptoms prompting its prescription.

In the clinical situations described here, patients generally were not followed after discharge. They were referred back to the referral source, usually a family physician, psychiatrist, or mental health professional. If the patient of a family physician required continuing treatment by a mental health professional, an appropriate referral was recommended to the former. If a patient required ongoing psychiatric consultation, that was recommended. Research following patients after discharge from a DTP is valuable in determining progress in these different circumstances (Piper et al., 1996).

REFERENCES

American Psychiatric Association (2013). *Diagnostic and Statistical Manual of Mental Disorders*, 5th edition. Washington, DC: American Psychiatric Association,

Arieti S (1955). *Interpretation of Schizophrenia*. New York: Basic Books.

Beitman BD (1996). Integrating pharmacotherapy and psychotherapy: An emerging field of study. *Acta Psychiatrica Belgica* 96:201–217.

Bion WR (1967). *Second Thoughts*. London: Karnac.

Chasseguet-Smirgel J (1985). *Creativity and Perversion*. London: Free Association Books.

Dorpat T, Miller M (1992). *Clinical Interaction and the Analysis of Meaning*. Hillsdale, NJ: Analytic Press.

Feinsilver DB, Yates BT (1984). Combined use of psychotherapy and drugs in chronic treatment-resistant schizophrenic patients. A retrospective study. *Journal of Nervous and Mental Disease* 172:133–139.

Frosch J (1983). *The Psychotic Process*. New York: International Universities Press.

Kaplan H, Sadock B (eds.) (1995). *Comprehensive Textbook of Psychiatry*, 6th edition. Baltimore, MD: Williams and Wilkins, 170, 2003–2011.

Kernberg OF (1984). *Severe Personality Disorders*. New Haven, CT: Yale University Press.

Marder SR (2007). Integrating pharmacological and psychosocial treatments for schizophrenia. *Acta Psychiatrica Scandinavica* (Suppl) 102:87–90.

McDougall J (1989). *Theatres of the Body: A Psychoanalytic Approach to Psychosomatic Illness.* New York: Norton.

McWilliams N (1994). *Psychoanalytic Diagnosis.* New York: Guilford Press.

Piper WE, Rosie JS, Joyce AS, Azim HA (1996). *Time-Limited Day Treatment for Personality Disorders: Integration of Research and Practice in a Group Program.* Washington, DC: American Psychological Association.

Rock NL (1970). Long-term psychotherapy utilizing trifluoperazine in a psychotic preschool child: A case study. *Journal of Nervous System Disease* 31:546–549.

Rosenfeld HA (1965). *Psychotic States.* London: Hogarth Press.

Searles HF (1965). *Collected Papers on Schizophrenia and Related Subjects.* London: Hogarth Press.

Searles HF (1986). *My Work with Borderline Patients.* Northvale, NJ: Jason Aronson.

Segal H (1957). Notes on symbol formation. *International Journal of Psycho-Analysis* 38:391–397.

Steinberg PI, Rosie JS, Joyce AS, O'Kelly JG, Piper WE, Lyon D, Bahrey F, Duggal S (2004). The psychodynamic psychiatry service of the University of Alberta Hospital: A thirty year history. *International Journal of Group Psychotherapy* 64:521–538.

Stone L (1954). The widening scope of indications for psychoanalysis. *Journal of the American Psychoanalytic Association* 2:567–594.

Sullivan HS (1962). *Schizophrenia as a Human Process.* New York: Norton.

CHAPTER 6

WHAT PSYCHOANALYSIS AND PSYCHIATRY OFFER TO MEDICINE

I have not needed to add much to this chapter because the original paper largely discussed what psychoanalytically informed psychiatry offers that is useful to family physicians and specialists. This is especially the case regarding understanding a patient's unconscious motivation that contributes to an adverse reaction to illness or its management, understanding a patient's unconscious psychological contribution to the illness itself, and understanding difficulties in physician–patient relationships and the relationships amongst hospital staff or between staff and patients. Other areas in which psychoanalytic thought has an important contribution include the psychiatric assessment of outpatients, and the provision of personal psychotherapy and psychoanalysis to physicians who require these treatments.

WHAT PSYCHOANALYSTS AND PSYCHOANALYTICALLY INFORMED PSYCHIATRISTS OFFER TO PSYCHIATRIC AND MEDICAL MANAGEMENT

Communication and understanding between psychoanalysts and physicians often are less than optimal. Many physicians, including psychiatrists, have a limited understanding of what psychoanalytically informed psychiatrists do, and what psychoanalysis and psychoanalytic psychotherapy can offer their patients, or which of their patients are likely to benefit from these treatments. Physicians sometimes expect too much from psychoanalytically informed psychiatrists, or too little. The latter have the potential to offer physicians assistance in many facets of medical care. They can provide a psychoanalytic understanding of unconscious factors influencing not only the patient's behavior, but also the behavior of the medical and allied staff. The latter may be important when a patient is considered difficult to manage. The difficulty may include stirring up dissension among the medical and non-medical staff on an inpatient unit, which, if not addressed, can perpetuate the difficulties they are having with the patient, resulting in disharmony among the staff that can become very destructive. This is covered in detail in Chapters 15 and 16.

Psychoanalytic understanding of psychiatric inpatients is useful in providing a formulation, that is, an understanding of how the patient got to be who and how she is at the moment of clinical presentation, regarding both symptoms and personality, taking into account biological, psychological, and social factors. This is necessary for developing a rational management plan. Psychoanalytically informed psychiatrists can provide a similar psychodynamic understanding in outpatient assessment and follow-up of patients with psychiatric disorders, which is similarly essential in formulation and management planning. They also can offer help in handling difficulties in doctor–patient relationships based on their understanding of the patient's unconscious motivations and on the physician–patient relationship dynamics, taking into account considerations of transference and countertransference.

Piper et al. (1996) note that collective disturbances in psychiatric partial hospitalization day programs occur when there is covert conflict among staff members, which is difficult to resolve when there are no institutionalized meetings allowing all staff members to discuss conflicts openly. This applies not only in day programs, but also in partial hospitalization evening programs and outpatient clinics. O'Kelly and Azim (1993) argue that the designated leader of the milieu is in the best position to lead the staff relations group of an intensive milieu therapy program, and should model openness without burdening staff members with inappropriate self-disclosure, allowing and encouraging direct expression of anger towards the leader by the staff members, and facilitating the support of confrontation by staff members of each other. "The extent to which staff members' conflicts are dealt with in the staff member–staff member relations group determines the staff members' empathic availability to the patient group. Such empathy works against the vicious circle of escalating projective identifications between staff members and patients, which fuels the collective disturbances" (Piper et al., 1996: 23) within the intensive program. This applies to other treatment milieus such as inpatient psychiatry units, or, for that matter, any hospital inpatient unit.

Psychoanalytically informed psychiatrists also can provide assistance in the management of medical and surgical patients with adverse psychological reactions to illness and management, and in patients in whom psychological factors are influencing the course of illness. Understanding the unconscious basis for a patient's untoward reactions to illness and management can be a first step in helping physicians to overcome what otherwise might become an impasse in the management of these patients. The understanding psychoanalytically informed psychiatrists can bring to bear on the workings of the patient's unconscious mind and how the patient's unarticulated unbearable emotions or unthinkable thoughts may be expressed in somatic complaints or even in precipitation or exacerbation of diagnosable medical disease can provide an understanding of psychological factors in some patients' illness, to the extent that the illness has a psychological contribution. Often these patients are identified as having "psychosomatic" disturbance, but with a limited understanding of the psychological basis for this disturbance. Here a psychoanalytically informed psychiatrist has a unique contribution. Of course, I am not suggesting that all patients considered to have a significant psychological contribution to their illness should have a psychoanalytic treatment, although there is a substantial literature demonstrating how psychoanalysis or psychotherapy can benefit many such patients (Taylor, 1987). However, the opinion of a psychoanalytically informed psychiatrist regarding a patient's unconscious unmet needs, unarticulated emotions, and/or unconscious conflicts may help a physician to treat such a patient. (This is elaborated on in Chapters 7, 10, and 14.)

A service psychoanalysts can offer to psychiatrists and other physicians who undertake psychotherapy with their patients is ongoing psychotherapy supervision. This can be helpful to physicians even when the psychotherapy they are offering is not psychoanalytic in nature, as exploring what is transpiring between physician and patient that may be outside of the physician's awareness can be useful in any type of psychotherapy. This suggestion is not made from a position of superiority, but on the basis that two heads are better than one, and awareness that, in the stressful situation that psychotherapy often entails (to both therapist and patient), an outside observer may be able to see things that the therapist, at least at that time, cannot. Also, it is often very useful for a physician-therapist to explore the feelings she is experiencing with her patient with an experienced third party. Most psychoanalysts routinely obtain consultations or ongoing supervision with respected colleagues when this is needed. Part of the attraction of a psychoanalytic or psychotherapeutic career is the opportunity to continue growing professionally, as well as personally, throughout one's working life. That comes at the price of recognizing that sometimes one cannot do one's best work without the help of a colleague. Finally, psychoanalysts are available to provide psychoanalysis and psychoanalytic psychotherapy to physicians when the latter need it. The considerable stresses involved in medical practice are well recognized, as is the significant psychiatric morbidity among physicians, including depression, substance abuse, and very high suicide rates.

In medical settings, it is useful when the attending psychiatrist has some psychoanalytically informed training to apply in her daily work to enhance the provision of care. Psychiatrists have this training to a more or less limited extent. *Unfortunately, the current trend is to reduce the minimum required training in this area.* Optimally, a psychoanalytically informed psychiatrist can be utilized by physicians to enhance the care of their patients. This rarely is done, due to a lack of financial resources, lack of awareness of what psychoanalysts have to offer, and, sometimes, a prejudice that some physicians, including psychiatrists, have against psychoanalysis. Psychoanalysts must bear some responsibility for any prejudice against them as a group. However, this prejudice also may be on the basis of ignorance, or of physicians' feeling threatened by the subject matter of psychoanalysis, which involves the exploration of painful and frightening thoughts, feelings, and impulses that are uncomfortable to consider, especially if it strikes too close to home, bringing one uncomfortably close to conscious awareness of aspects of one's own personality, which is threatening.

Another basis of prejudice is contemporary society's preference for treatments that ostensibly offer quick, effortless, inexpensive, and complete relief from emotional pain. No reasonable clinician believes that such treatments exist. Psychoanalysis clearly is not quick or effortless, and is costly in terms of both the time and financial resources required to undertake it and regarding the emotional work it demands not only of the therapist, but also of the patient. Rather than offering complete relief from pain, it offers an opportunity to find more constructive ways of coping and living with pain, which is inevitable in life, and offers the opportunity for emotional growth that cannot be done on one's own, that ultimately can lead to adaptations involving less pain. Unfortunately, psychoanalytic (or psychodynamic) psychotherapy is often tarred with the same brush as psychoanalysis by people prejudiced against the latter. Psychodynamic psychotherapy generally is not quick (although there are some time-limited and short term therapies), but it is less expensive regarding what it demands of time and money, and in some jurisdictions is funded, sometimes partly, by the state.

DIFFICULTIES IN PSYCHIATRY

One might call psychiatry the Cinderella of medicine. Scientific developments in psychiatry occurred later than in other specialties. The ambivalence of other physicians towards psychiatry and its practitioners, which starts in medical school or earlier, is based on several factors. These include the competition between psychosocial and biological approaches, and among psychological schools, to explain psychiatric symptoms, a competition that often generates more heat than light. The subject of psychiatry can also be threatening, especially since unmet emotional needs, unconscious conflict, and disturbed interpersonal relationships are not limited to our patients (Freud, 1961: 22). A related factor is the ridicule to which psychiatric patients are sometimes exposed by society, and even, at times, by the medical profession. Another factor is that the benefits of psychiatric treatment are not always self-evident. The results of psychological treatments, especially the more complex ones, can be difficult to evaluate scientifically, which may cast doubt on their efficacy. The difficulties in establishing criteria for good or improved mental health make it difficult to assess the degree to which psychiatric services are being used effectively (Levitan, 1983: 26). *Questions posed regarding the validity of some research on the efficacy of psychoactive medications have not raised the esteem of psychiatry as a discipline in the eyes of the profession or the public. However, these questions are not limited to psychiatry, and apply to medicine in general.*

Finally, psychotherapeutic treatments involve the physician's personality to a much greater extent than biological treatments, although no reasonable clinician disputes the effect that the doctor–patient relationship in general can have on the course of illness. One cannot imagine anyone writing an article on what surgery offers to medicine, as it is obvious. This does not seem to be so with psychiatry. Physicians at times seem to expect little from psychiatry. .Many patients who could benefit from psychiatric consultation, for example, patients with postoperative delirium, are not identified or referred (Fisher & Gilchrist, 1993). In other situations, physicians seem to expect too much from psychiatric consultants and are inevitably disappointed.

Psychiatrists should be explicit about what psychiatric consultation and treatment offer in each setting where psychiatrists may be clinically involved. For example, the goals of a psychiatric hospitalization, or of psychotherapy, whether cognitive behavioral or psychoanalytic, should be explicit. Psychiatry as a discipline has fostered unrealistic expectations at times, for example, in the heyday of psychoanalysis, the 1950s, when more was claimed for this approach than could be fulfilled (Taylor, 1987: 38). Thus, medical practitioners have tended to perceive psychiatry from a split viewpoint, either idealizing or devaluing it (Grotstein, 1985: 9–12). Both these perceptions are unrealistic, and detract from the position of psychiatry in medicine. I wish to present psychiatry from a more realistic vantage point, and describe the aims and limits of what psychiatry can offer medicine.

ASSESSMENT AND MANAGEMENT

The most obvious service that a psychiatrist can provide his medical colleagues is assessment and management of patients with major psychiatric conditions. This is often associated in physicians' minds with inpatient care of patients with major psychiatric conditions, such as psychotic and affective disorders. Both the patients' and the referring physicians' expectations of psychiatric hospitalization would be more realistic if the goals of the hospitalization were explicit; for example, ongoing assessment of suicide risk, relief of psychotic symptoms, or providing support for patients with overwhelming symptoms such as depression or obsessions. *Unfortunately, as noted elsewhere in this book, patients suffering from the last two symptoms no longer routinely are offered psychiatric admission.* The shrinking of healthcare resources has been accompanied by a reduced availability of inpatient beds, making it necessary both to define for the patient the goals of admission, and to limit the indications for admission to cases in which it is absolutely required. It has been increasingly important for psychiatrists to communicate to referring physicians about which patients should be admitted, and what is expected during admission. It is equally important for referring physicians to discuss their expectations with the consulting psychiatrist. All this is especially important, given the need to admit not just patients with major psychiatric conditions with severe symptoms, but also those with personality disorders who are experiencing suicidal impulses and who cannot expect during their admission to undergo dramatic changes in their adaptive patterns. *Psychodynamic formulation, which is essential in psychiatric management planning, is based on psychoanalytic theories of development and personality. (See Chapter 14.)*

A second accepted function of the psychiatric consultant involves ongoing outpatient follow-up of individuals with psychiatric conditions. This may be similar to a medical model, especially in patients suffering from conditions such as schizophrenia, in which the mainstay of treatment is biological. *Of course, many patients with chronic major psychiatric conditions are now followed up in freestanding mental health clinics, and have a mental health case worker as their primary contact, with possible access to other professionals such as psychiatrists, social workers, psychologists, and nurses, when indicated.* At the other end of the spectrum are psychotherapeutic treatments. Some, such as cognitive behavior therapy and dialectical behavior therapy, are more structured and symptom-oriented, and resemble the medical model. Others, such as psychoanalysis and psychoanalytic psychotherapy, are less structured and seem unrelated to the medical model. These therapies should not be seen to be in competition, but to be complementary. Just as the most effective rheumatologist has many antiarthritic agents at his disposal, so the effective psychiatrist is prepared to tailor her management plan to each patient.

An unfortunate basis for some of the loss of credibility in psychiatry is the competition between approaches or even within different schools in each approach. It is important for the referring physician to know that the consulting psychiatrist recommends treatment on the basis of the patient's needs, as opposed to the psychiatrist's theoretical orientation. Implied in this is that psychiatrists often do not perform every treatment they prescribe. Nevertheless, a psychiatrist, having a medical background, specialist training in psychiatry, and adequate knowledge of psychological treatments, generally should be the most suitable mental health professional to suggest what is the best treatment for a patient, who may then be referred, for example, to a psychologist or social worker for the treatment to be applied. *I am afraid that the decreased availability of state-paid psychotherapists, especially psychoanalytic psychotherapists, and an increasing prejudice in psychiatry against psychoanalysis and psychodynamic treatments, at times may render this claim more idealistic than when it originally was written. In Canada, at least, the national licensing body for psychiatrists recently has reduced by 75% the previous minimum required training period for long-term individual psychodynamic psychotherapy. This has an impact not only on the number of psychiatrists who can provide psychoanalytic psychotherapy, but also on the familiarity psychiatrists have with this treatment, to know when it is indicated.* Physicians referring patients for psychotherapy must be aware of the realistic limits of even successful psychotherapy. At termination of psychoanalytic psychotherapy, patients may function better at work, in relationships, and in their ability to enjoy recreational pursuits. They may feel better. They may deal with their problems more constructively; this is different from not having problems. None of this implies that they will be new people. The patient who has undergone successful psychotherapy will be the same person, with a better awareness of her problems, and more constructive ways to cope with them, which should allow her to lead a more satisfying life. In addition, the patient who has had a good outcome in psychoanalysis has internalized the analytic process and can use it for the rest of her life in thinking about herself and her difficulties. This also is the case in successful psychoanalytic psychotherapies.

Physicians should be aware of the difficulties some patients have in accepting psychotherapeutic referral. One guide the physician may have in trying to understand this would be to consider her own reaction to the prospect of being referred for psychoanalysis or psychoanalytic psychotherapy. It is also helpful for the referring physician to be aware that, during the psychotherapy, the patient's negative transference (his negative feelings about his analyst/therapist) may manifest themselves in complaints to the referring physician about the latter. Although some of the complaints may be justified, it is in the patient's interest for the referring physician not to interfere with the treatment, but rather advise the patient to discuss his dis-satisfaction with the therapist. Transference aspects of the patient's dissatisfaction can then be explored, with resultant psychotherapeutic benefit. That is, to the extent that the patient is experiencing towards his therapist conflicts, impulses, and feelings that are primarily related to other important people in his life, this can be explored and interpreted in a way that is helpful to the patient in his relationships with others, including his family doctor. To the extent that the patient's concerns have a realistic basis, obviously this needs to be resolved with the ther-apist, and the meaning of the patient's concerns explored as well. Occasionally, the patient's complaints may require a discussion between referring physician and therapist to clarify the problem.

Family physicians more often require emergency psychiatric consultations than specialists. The indications for an emergency psychiatric consultation are limited, and include patients who are thought to be at risk for suicidal behavior, patients with psychiatric conditions who are thought to be at risk of harming someone else, and patients with newly diagnosed psychotic conditions. Another indication for emergency assessment involves patients with a psychiatric disturbance that renders them unable to care for themselves, to the extent that their health is potentially compromised, for example, a depressed or anorexic patient who is starving. An emergency consultation may be warranted because of the severity of the patient's symptoms, for example, a patient with severe panic disorder of acute onset.

Physicians should understand that what is accomplished in an emergency psychiatric con-sultation is limited, A decision must usually be made about whether the patient requires admis-sion, and whether to admit him involuntarily. Appropriate specific treatment will be provided for the presenting symptoms. The main management resource may be the temporary provi-sion of an environment where the patient is safe from self-destructive impulses; for example, a patient with a personality disorder experiencing suicidal ideation after the disruption of an important relationship. *(Such patients rarely are admitted now unless they are felt to be acutely suicidal.)* One cannot expect that ongoing problems in relationships or maladaptive patterns of behavior can be resolved in an emergency consultation or during admission to a psychiatric unit. Such problems may be identified, and sometimes a start may be made in therapy, but ongoing out-patient psychotherapy is the definitive treatment for these patients.

CONSULTATION FOR HOSPITALIZED PATIENTS

The psychiatric consultant is potentially an important resource to the attending physician caring for medical, surgical, obstetrical, and pediatric patients in hospital. Unfortunately, many patients who could benefit from psychiatric consultation are never seen by a psychiatrist during their hospital stay (Steinberg, 1987). Psychiatrists are often consulted when a patient already diagnosed with a psychiatric disorder such as schizophrenia is admitted to a medical or surgical unit This can occur without a specific indication for a psychiatric consultation, if medical, sur-gical, or nursing personnel are uncomfortable with psychiatric patients. This type of request parallels the lack of comfort psychiatric personnel feel when treating patients admitted to a psy-chiatric unit who also have medical and surgical conditions, resulting in a request for medical or surgical consultation, the need of which may be questioned by the consultant. These situations illustrate the need to improve communications between hospital psychiatrists and their medical and surgical colleagues.

There are other types of clinical situations where the attending physician will find a psychiatric consultation useful, even if the patient has no psychiatric condition. Patients may have an adverse psychological reaction to their illness or to treatment (Rodin, 1983; Steinberg, 1988). An example would be an adolescent diabetic struggling to become more independent of his parents, whose rebellion takes the form of a refusal to comply with diet and insulin management. Another group includes patients in whom psychological factors are felt to be influencing the course of illness either directly (Reiser & Bakst, 1975: 623), or through the patient's reaction, for example, with poor compliance with management recommendations. A third group involves difficult diagnostic situations where distinguishing whether a patient has a medical condition, a psychiatric condition, both, or a psychiatric condition complicating a pre-existing medical condition, is the challenge (Steinberg, 1994; Steinberg & Mackenzie, 1989). Examples include a patient presenting with somatic complaints who may have a somatic symptom (somatization) disorder or illness anxiety (hypochondriacal) disorder; a patient suffering from psychiatric symptoms who has intracranial disease without somatic symptoms; an individual with a history of depressive illness suffering from both hypothyroidism and depression; and a patient with a documented seizure disorder who is having pseudo-seizures. These situations are often challenging both to diagnose accurately and to manage effectively. Having a psychiatric consultant as part of the medical team can enhance management in these cases and is most effective in a hospital setting if one psychiatric consultant or a small group of consultants is interested in doing this type of work and identified as such to their medical-surgical colleagues. Examples of these situations are described in the consultation/liaison section of this book (Part II).

Areas in which psychiatric consultation is seen as especially important include neurology, where distinguishing between neurological and psychiatric problems can be a challenge; nephrology, in dealing with both psychological reactions to dialysis and psychiatric complications of impaired renal function; transplantation units, which may involve psychiatric input about patient selection, and psychological preparation for and management of adverse psychological reactions to transplants; endocrinology, in which diagnostic problems often present themselves; gastroenterology and dermatology, where there often is a psychological contribution to the patient's medical condition; and internal medicine, when there is a diagnostic problem in which psychiatric problems must be excluded, or to handle an adverse psychological reaction to illness or management.

OUTPATIENT MANAGEMENT CONSULTATION

Given the limited psychiatric resources available to many smaller communities, another useful role the psychiatric consultant can play involves one-time assessment of patients for an opinion about management, with referral back to the primary physician who will carry out the treatment. This is easiest with individuals who are likely to respond to medication and a supportive relationship with the referring physician (Steinberg, 1989). It is most helpful to the referring physician if the consultant specifies what issues he thinks may be important for patient and physician to discuss, and to what extent they should be discussed; for example, whether it would be helpful or potentially dangerous for the physician to offer an interpretation of the patient's unconscious motivation for a behavior. It can be especially helpful to delineate what types of difficulties the physician is likely to encounter in his relationship with the patient, and to outline an approach (Truant & Lohrenz, 1993a, 1993b).

Some patients present special challenges to physicians by virtue of the difficulties they create in all their relationships. Physicians of these patients often find that they are not exceptions, and are made uncomfortable by the intense if unaccountable reactions these patients have, which include both idealization and devaluation (Kernberg, 1984: 267). Consultation with a psychoanalytically informed psychiatrist can help the physician both identify such patients and find solutions to the dilemmas these patients pose. Family physicians often have to handle such individuals, as many specialists either never have enough contact with these patients to become so involved with them, or complete their consultation and refer them with celerity back to the family physician.

Another step in this direction is the provision of ongoing psychotherapy supervision to the attending physician. This is generally done by psychoanalytically informed psychiatrists, and undertaken by physicians with a special interest in this approach who believe that their patient population warrants such an investment. This form of continuing medical education can be rewarding to the physicians involved. Physicians justifiably feel more confident performing psychotherapy when they receive training that provides them with a rational theoretical approach, similar to feeling more comfortable performing surgical procedures for which they have been adequately trained. The relationship with the supervisor and what she relates of her own experience in psychotherapy can be supportive and instructive (Ekstein & Wallerstein, 1980). Psychotherapy supervision may be performed either individually, or in a group, with the supervisor meeting with several psychotherapists, one of whom presents a case for discussion (Balint, 1957; Steinberg & Shaw, 1989). A specific form of supervision by psychoanalysts for family physicians, Balint groups, is discussed in Chapter 2.

TREATMENT FOR PHYSICIANS

A final service that psychiatry may offer to medicine is more personal. The stresses of a medical career are well known, as are the high rates of suicide, divorce, and substance abuse among medical practitioners (Strain & Grossman, 1975: 31). To what extent these statistics can be attributed to the stresses of a medical career, and to what extent individuals predisposed to these unhappy solutions choose to become physicians, are important questions. It is safe to accept that the motivation to become a physician is usually complex. Psychoanalysis has shown how much of the motivation for important choices in life, including choice of life partner and choice of profession, is unconscious. These notions are not always palatable, but there is convincing evidence for them (Sussman, 1995). It is in the interest of both physicians and their patients that physicians who are under stress that they are unable to cope with, physicians who are suffering from anxiety, depression, or other psychiatric symptoms, and physicians who are troubled by their interpersonal relationships, know that psychiatric, psychoanalytic, and psychotherapeutic treatment is available. A trusted psychiatric colleague may provide psychotherapeutic consultation or refer the physician to another psychiatrist or psychotherapist. When the physician and psychiatrist or therapist are acquainted, this makes psychotherapeutic collaboration difficult or impossible. It is far preferable to be treated in psychotherapy or psychoanalysis by someone with whom you never previously have had a relationship. Some physicians may find consulting a psychiatrist, psychotherapist, or psychoanalyst to be either uncomfortable or even humiliating. These feelings themselves should become a focus for useful psychotherapeutic exploration. This discomfort seems infinitely preferable to the maladaptive types of destructive solutions mentioned, or to another destructive solution, sexual involvement with a patient (Steinberg, 1993).

CONCLUSIONS

I have tried to outline ways in which psychiatrists and psychoanalysts can help their medical colleagues. The nature of emotional problems, the inevitability of frustrations in important relationships, and the tendency of our patients to perceive us *in loco parentis* (and our tendencies to act thus) make it inescapable that at least some of these patients will have unrealistic expectations of their physicians. Perhaps most patients will have unrealistic expectations of us at some time. For physicians to have rational expectations of their psychiatric colleagues is an important factor contributing to effective consultee–consultant collaboration. The burden for this mutual understanding lies at least as much on psychiatric consultants as on referring physicians. Improved communication should lead to better care for our patients, more satisfying and less stressful clinical work, and more enjoyable professional relationships (Steinberg, 1983a, 1983b).

REFERENCES

Balint M (1957). *The Doctor, his Patient and the Illness*. London: Pitman Medical.

Ekstein R, Wallerstein RS (1980). *The Teaching and Learning of Psychotherapy*. New York: International University Press.

Fisher BW, Gilchrist DM (1993). Postoperative delirium in the elderly. *Annals of the Royal College of Physicians and Surgeons of Canada* 26(6):358–362.

Freud S (1961). Introductory lectures to psychoanalysis. 1: Introduction. In: Strachey J (ed.), *Standard Edition of the Complete Psychological Works of Sigmund Freud*, Vol. XV. London: Hogarth Press.

Grotstein JS (1985). *Splitting and Projective Identification*. New York: Jason Aronson.

Kernberg O (1984). *Severe Personality Disorders*. New Haven, CT: Yale University.

Levitan SJ (1983). Evaluation of consultation-liaison psychiatry: Better health at lower cost? In: Frankel SB (ed.), *Consultation-Liaison Psychiatry: Current Trends and Perspectives*. New York: Grune and Stratton.

O'Kelly JG, Azim HFA (1993). Staff–staff relations group. *International Journal of Group Psychotherapy* 43:469–483.

Piper WE, Rosie JS, Joyce AS, Azim HFA (1996). *Time-Limited Day Treatment for Personality Disorders: Integration of Research and Practice in a Group Program*. Washington, DC: American Psychological Association.

Reiser W, Bakst H (1975). Psychophysiological and psychodynamic problems of the patient with structural heart disease. In: Arieti S (ed.), *American Handbook of Psychiatry*, Vol. IV. New York: Basic Books.

Rodin GM (1983). Psychosocial aspects of diabetes mellitus. *Canadian Journal of Psychiatry* 28:219–223.

Steinberg P (1983a). The psychiatry of family practice: Personality disorders, Part I: The problem patient. *Canadian Journal of Psychiatry* 29:1942–1947.

Steinberg P (1983b). The psychiatry of family practice: Personality disorders, Part II: Interviewing the patient. *Canadian Journal of Psychiatry* 29:1953–1957.

Steinberg P (1987). Broader indications for psychiatric consultation. *Canadian Family Physician* 33:437–440.

Steinberg P (1988). Psychiatric complications of surgery in the male. *Canadian Journal of Psychiatry* 33:28–33.

Steinberg PI (1989). Two techniques of supportive psychotherapy. *Canadian Family Physician* 35: 1139–1143.

Steinberg PI (1993). Sexual abuse of adult female patients by male physicians. *Annals of the Royal College of Physicians and Surgeons of Canada* 26(4):2114.

Steinberg PI (1994). A case of paranoid disorder associated with hyperthyroidism. *Canadian Journal of Psychiatry* 39(3):153–156.

Steinberg P, Mackenzie RM (1989). A patient with insulinoma presenting for psychiatric assessment. *Canadian Journal of Psychiatry* 40:58–59.

Steinberg P, Shaw BR (1989). An evaluation of Balint training for psychiatric nurses. *Journal of the Balint Society* 17:28–32.

Strain JJ, Grossman S (eds.) (1975). *Psychological Care of the Medically Ill.* New York: Appleton-Century-Crofts.

Sussman MB (ed.) (1995). *A Perilous Calling: The Hazards of Psychotherapy Practice.* Hoboken, NJ: Wiley.

Taylor GJ (1987). *Psychosomatic Medicine and Contemporary Psychoanalysis*, Madison, WI: International Universities Press.

Truant GS, Lohrenz JG (1993a). Basic principles of psychotherapy. I: Introduction, basic goals, and the therapist's relationship. *American Journal Psychotherapy* 47(1):8–18.

Truant GS, Lohrenz JG (1993b). Basic principles of psychotherapy. II: The patient model, interventions and counter transference. *American Journal Psychotherapy* 47(I):19–32.

PART II

LEARNING FROM
CONSULTATION/LIAISON PSYCHIATRY

How much of what patients present to physicians represents emotional distress that patients are unable to formulate and articulate verbally, which often is expressed in somatic complaints or concerns about illness, when there is no evidence of disease, or in complaints far exceeding what one would expect, given objective evidence of disease? This is in addition to the overt unhappiness of which many patients explicitly complain. These patients often are investigated, with no medical diagnosis ever identified. How many medical treatments, prescriptions for medication, and investigative procedures and surgical operations are of questionable necessity, based on the patient's pressure on doctors to do something to relieve his disease, accompanied by the risk of potentially serious side effects and complications? How many antidepressants (hopefully mainly in the past, benzodiazepines) and narcotic analgesics are prescribed without adequate indications? The above management measures may permit the physician to feel she is doing something for the patient, and the patient to feel he is being treated for a treatable condition, with limited benefit to the patient beyond the time-limited placebo effect, but with potentially serious side effects and complications.

High substance abuse rates and high suicide rates among physicians, especially psychiatrists and ophthalmologists, are likely partly attributable to the stresses involved in the great responsibilities associated with being a physician in clinical practice. Another factor likely involves the question of who chooses to become a caregiver (Sussman, 1992). Application of psychoanalytic principles to medical care can reduce the stress of medical work by providing an understanding of patients and some practical approaches to the difficulties physicians face in their relationships with and management of their patients.

I hope non-medical health professionals also will find this section useful as regards considering the possibility that some of their patients' symptoms represent medical disease rather than psychological disturbance. We learn from our clinical practice; it can help keep us humble, and open to the possibility of error. Once I assessed a patient whose care was transferred to another psychiatrist. Back then, when I made such comparisons, I considered myself more competent than he. Nevertheless, it was he who identified the patient's porphyria, leading to appropriate medical treatment for a patient whom I accepted as having a psychiatric condition. In fairness, I interviewed the patient once briefly after an emergency admission, knowing that his care would be transferred. Nevertheless, the diagnosis slipped through my fingers, and fortunately was made by my colleague.

Looking back at a career of several decades, I have regrets about patients whom I haven't been able to help more, including the awareness that if I were treating them now, I believe I would do a better job than I was able to do then. Hirsch's (2008) *Coasting in the Countertransference* is relevant. This regret is balanced by my surprise when hearing from patients after many years about how they have done much better than I would have expected, and seemed to have benefited more from our work than I had thought. This is partly understandable in that, to the extent that psychoanalysis and psychoanalytic psychotherapy are successful, patients continue to grow following termination of treatment as they continue to utilize the thinking processes and access to their emotions they developed in treatment. This generally does not apply in other psychological treatments.

One of the challenges of starting a psychiatric consultation/liaison service is convincing hospital physicians that a psychiatric consultation has something to offer in the care of their inpatients. This process took years, especially with the psychoanalytically informed approach I took, which was hard for most of the referees to understand, and didn't always seem practical to them. Eventually I could identify a handful of internists who understood and respected my contribution to the care of their patients.. I found my understanding of psychoanalytic principles to be invaluable in my consultation/liaison work.

Now I regret not following up some of the patients I assessed in the consultation/liaison service. I could not have followed up more than a minority of them because of the volume of patients I assessed, and only some of them would have been appropriate for treatment with psychoanalytic psychotherapy, to which my outpatient practice was restricted. I realize now that one reason, apart from logistics, that I did not follow them up was my lack of confidence in dealing with these people, with their sometimes very significant psychological disturbance, often manifest in somatic symptoms. There was a realistic aspect to my lack of confidence, but I might have earned some sense of confidence in myself by working with these people, getting some supervision when I needed it, and gradually learning, with these patients, how to work with them in psychotherapy.

I wish to make explicit the distinction between a strictly consultation approach to psychiatric consultation to "non-psychiatric" inpatients, informed by psychoanalytic thought, and a consultation approach in which liaison between the psychiatrist and consultant is included. In the strict consultation approach, the consultee asks the consultant psychiatrist to assess one of her patients. The psychiatrist meets with the patient and provides the consultee with a written opinion about the psychiatric status of the patient. This might not only offer a diagnosis and management plan, but also address the possibility of the patient's having an adverse reaction to his illness or its management, or the possibility that psychological factors are affecting the patient's illness or its management, dealt with in Chapter 8. On the other hand, in a consultation approach that includes liaison, the consulting psychiatrist in effect becomes part of the medical or surgical team treating the inpatients. In addition to assessing individual patients, the consultant meets with the team on a regular basis to discuss concerns the team has regarding their patients. Questions may arise regarding whether the patient's hospital stay is complicated by the patient having a psychiatric disturbance, diagnostic difficulties when it is unclear if the patient's reason for admission represents a medical problem or a psychosomatic disturbance, in addition to concerns about whether psychological factors are contributing to the patient's illness or are complicating its management.

DESCRIPTION OF CHAPTERS

Chapter 7 describes patients suffering from "psychosomatic" disturbances, distinguishing somatization from conversion, and the origins of these conditions in early developmental difficulties.

In Chapter 8, I describe a liaison approach to psychiatric consultation, which increases the patient population who can benefit from psychiatric assessment during hospitalization for medical or surgical conditions or childbirth. This also broadens the scope of the psychiatric investigation of the individual patient. The meaning of the patient's illness to her, and her present methods of adapting to her illness, are important considerations. Unconscious concerns that interfere with the patient's compliance with medical management can be clarified, resulting in expediting management. Psychiatric consultation also is useful in preventing untoward psychological reactions to illness, if this is anticipated. This type of preventive consultation, often possible because of the physician's awareness of the psychological vulnerability of some of her patients, can result in reduced medical and psychiatric morbidity.

Chapter 9 deals with organizing one's thinking in diagnostically differentiating patients according to their symptoms. Some patients present with intuitive presentations, that is, with physical symptoms representing a medical condition, or psychological symptoms representing a psychiatric disturbance. Some patients' presentations are counterintuitive, such as a patient with a psychiatric disturbance presenting with physical symptoms, or a patient with a medical condition presenting with psychological symptoms. One also needs to consider the interaction between psychological factors and medical conditions and conditions presenting with disturbing or destructive behavior rather than symptoms.

In Chapter 10, four male patients with severe personality disturbance are described in whom surgery on their genital or perineal areas was followed or preceded by increased psychiatric symptomatology. What renders these men susceptible to psychiatric complications to surgery is explored. In the case where adequate historical detail was available, a psychodynamic formulation is undertaken, including the unconscious meaning of surgery to the patient. The propensity of these individuals to alternate between idealizing and devaluing their physicians is described. Suggestions on identifying and managing such patients are offered.

Readers might be surprised that a book about psychoanalysis in medicine would include chapters describing patients presenting with psychiatric symptoms who eventually are diagnosed with medical illness. However, a psychiatrist who also is a psychoanalyst must function as both in medical settings; sometimes psychoanalytic understanding can be used to clarify the existence of a yet-undiagnosed medical problem. If I could have read the following chapters, perhaps I would have avoided the mistake of assuming that my psychotherapy patient's intense bouts of panic were based on his psychological difficulties, and might have suggested earlier that he consult his family doctor, expediting his diagnosis of hyperthyroidism.

In Chapter 11, a patient with an undiagnosed insulinoma referred for psychiatric assessment illustrates the need for a high index of suspicion of organic mental disorder even in patients who have undergone extensive medical investigation. The diagnostic difficulties illustrate the need for persistence and cooperation between family physician and specialists in such cases.

In Chapter 12 a patient who presented with paranoid symptoms eventually was diagnosed with Graves' disease. This patient suffered concurrently from a delusional disorder and hyperthyroidism in a clear state of consciousness. This case underscores the need to maintain a high index of suspicion of possible medical conditions in patients identified as "psychiatric," especially in the presence of unexplained symptoms, and when there is a difficulty in communicating with the patient, for example, because of language differences. The importance of carrying out a careful physical examination on admission to a psychiatric unit is emphasized. Another indication for further medical investigation in a patient with psychiatric symptoms is the absence of a psychological explanation for a worsening of the psychiatric symptoms. A psychoanalytic approach to exploring possible psychological explanations is very useful in such cases. Additional thoughts are offered regarding the likelihood that trauma played a significant role in the genesis of the patient's psychiatric symptoms, which was not recognized at the time. I also describe psychoanalytic approaches to patients with psychotic symptoms.

Chapter 13 describes a woman referred for psychiatric consultation for "catatonia" who eventually was found to have an adrenal tumor. A high index of suspicion of organic mental disorder is necessary in medically ill patients, even when there is symptomatic evidence of psychiatric disturbance accompanied by many psychosocial stressors. A history of psychological stresses, no matter how severe and multiple, does not warrant concluding that symptoms that might represent either psychiatric disturbance or a medical disease are psychogenic and represent a psychiatric disorder; adequate medical investigation to rule out medical disease must be undertaken.

SOME ANECDOTES FROM MY EXPERIENCE IN CONSULTATION-LIAISON PSYCHIATRY

One of the attractions of consultation-liaison psychiatry is the wide variety of patients you encounter. With the exception of the psychoanalytic psychotherapy patient described below in The Skin and the Soul, I made no interpretations to the patients described below, as they had not undertaken to engage in psychotherapy with me. Nevertheless, my psychoanalytic understanding of their unconscious motivations helped inform my treatment of them.

Psychosis and Surgery

When I was an intern, I admitted a young man with acute schizophrenia to the psychiatric unit. He was floridly psychotic, with hallucinations and delusions. When he returned from a weekend pass. I discovered he had eaten a six-quart basket of cherries, including the pits. Shortly thereafter I diagnosed my first case of appendicitis. He was operated on and promptly transferred back to the psychiatric unit. What struck me was that my patient's psychotic symptoms were completely relieved for three days after the onset of appendicitis. This phenomenon is well documented but seems less well understood (Smadja, 2011). I don't know if confrontation with the reality of an acute abdomen and potential death is enough to temporarily relieve people of their psychotic symptoms. I have read that when there is a fire in a psychiatric ward, patients suffering from catatonic stupor, who are completely aware of their environment, do not respond with alarm and rush out of the ward, but have to be carried out. It was heartbreaking to see my appendicitis patient gradually relapse into his chronic schizophrenic state. There are limits to what we as physicians can do.

The Skin and the Soul[1]

The following vignette from a psychotherapy hour illustrates the adage "The skin is the mirror of the soul." The patient's dermatological symptoms may have disappeared on the basis of psychological changes she experienced. This session also shows that the effect on the therapist of

---

1   This excerpt is reprinted with permission; it originally appeared in the *Canadian Journal of Psychoanalysis* 2018; 26(2):150–172 (Steinberg, 2018).

psychotherapeutic work can be seen in his dreams. One theme of the therapy is a struggle for this young woman to assume personal agency over her life and experience herself as a separate independent individual.

Barbara dreamed, *I was staring in my reflection in a mirror. I saw that my blemishes were not so bad. I could live with them, and could do something about them if I wanted. Fred* [her boyfriend] *and his parents appeared. They did not seem in motion, like a snapshot.* This part of the dream was drab, dull, and gray. Barbara felt separate from her family and Fred, didn't have to deal with their issues, and felt optimistic and confident. The therapist suggested she seemed to accept herself in the dream. She compared a man she had met with Fred; she didn't feel anything special with either of them. Barbara used to feel she needed some kind of support from a man to feel good about herself. Now she didn't need that, so she wouldn't just accept a man who didn't feel right. She thought of a line in a song, "You can be happy." She described positive feelings bubbling up inside.

The mirror in Barbara's dream might refer to her feeling that therapy had helped her see she had some blemishes, but they were not so bad and could be worked on. In this session, the therapist noticed that Barbara's face was blemish-free. She had always had some minor blemishes until then. He did not know when this change had occurred. Could there have been a causal connection between her complexion improving and her accepting her internal "blemishes"? Or could his not noticing when the blemishes had disappeared represent some change in his attitude towards Barbara?

Then the therapist dreamed, *I was asked to see Barbara in consultation at the hospital. I neglected to ask about vegetative signs of depression.* A month after the therapist's dream, Barbara indicated she was very angry with herself, having exposed herself to the possibility of becoming pregnant having unprotected intercourse with her boyfriend one month previously. She felt ashamed, and agreed that she had been quieter in the previous month because she was afraid of the therapist's judgment. Therefore Barbara didn't talk about her concern about the risk of pregnancy until then. She mentioned, "To err is human," but didn't know the ending, "To forgive is divine." She indicated that, at the beginning of therapy, she wouldn't have said anything about exposing herself to the risk of getting pregnant, not trusting the therapist. Since his countertransference dream occurred when Barbara was exposing herself to this risk, he may have unconsciously understood that she was not telling him something, or that he was not hearing the gaps in what she was telling him. It is not clear to what extent this involved an active if unconscious communication to the therapist from Barbara. Perhaps his dream was an anticipatory dream indicating his unconscious awareness that Barbara was withholding something from him, which she would eventually tell him.

A Psychotic Reaction to Illness

I assessed a terrified psychotic woman in "terminal" congestive heart failure. I thought she was delirious from poor perfusion of blood to her brain, and ordered haloperidol 0.25 mg o.d., gradually increasing to t.i.d., afraid that even this tiny dose might push her into the next world. Not only did her psychosis clear, but her heart rate decreased, because, I believe, she was no longer terrified once the symptoms of delirium had decreased. She recovered from heart failure and was discharged from hospital. I saw her being presented in medical rounds nine months later. I observed no indication of psychosis. I wondered whether the haloperidol, in indirectly reducing her heart rate, may have saved her life, and that part of what had made her congestive heart failure "terminal" was the terror she experienced in her delirium.

Annoying Patients with Irrelevant Questions

A young man whose chief activity was riding motorcycles had been in a serious accident and incurred chronic pain. Although it didn't seem likely to be germane, I asked him, as I ask all patients when performing a consultation, if he had suicidal thoughts. He angrily said that he planned to go up north with his girlfriend and "fuck myself to death." That was his response to a question he felt was not relevant to his difficulties.

History by Tattoos

Asked to perform a consultation in a medical unit on a young man, I found he hadn't been informed of my visit. This is not uncommon when performing psychiatric consultations in hospital; psychiatrists, patients with psychiatric symptoms, and psychiatry as an institution are not always well regarded by medical colleagues. The patient reacted poorly to meeting me, and refused to provide a history. My efforts to get him to cooperate were unavailing. In desperation I observed that he had many visible tattoos on his arms. This was before tattoos had become commonplace; back then it was unusual to have tattoos except sailors and jail inmates. *Faute de mieux*, I showed interest in the tattoos and asked him about them. He brightened up and, dropping his sullen demeanor, seemed delighted not just to describe what the tattoos depicted, but also to outline his life circumstances when he acquired each of them, and to partially undress and show me all ten of his tattoos.

Each tattoo depicted an interpersonal loss, or was symbolic of one. This man experienced very significant early losses in close relationships that made him vulnerable to what seemed to be unbearable emotional pain when experiencing losses in adult life. He appeared to have found having a tattoo to symbolize each loss to be the closest he could come to articulating and accommodating to the loss emotionally. These losses, many of them related to his father or men representing his father, from whom he wanted the love and guidance he never received from his father, prevented him from trusting me enough to provide me with a history. This youth appeared unable to think of or express his emotional distress in psychological terms. He chose action, getting tattoos, to express them in a concrete way using his body as a canvas. The tattoos were there, ready to be interpreted, like conversion symptoms. The use of action, rather than words, is reminiscent of an infant, who can only scream and flail when he is in distress, not yet having developed the capacity for language and thinking that would be necessary to communicate on a more sophisticated level. As my patient's earliest traumata occurred before this period, his symptom, tattoos, were expressed in a non-verbal way, action. This is the patient I most regret not writing an article about. I regret not having the foresight to have recorded details of the tattoos, the stories he told me about each tattoo, and the specific interpretations I had about them.

Denial in Action

I have already described the man with a serious myocardial infarction, who was having a manic reaction to this illness, performing jumping jacks and other high-exertion exercises in a denial of what had happened. This was another patient who was expressing by action what he could not express verbally, like the tattooed patient.

Obstetrical Action

I rarely assessed obstetrical inpatients, given their brief stays and the usually happy circumstances that brought them to hospital. However, I did see a few patients who had delivered their babies at home into the toilet. These were usually psychotic women who until then had denied that they were pregnant. Their attitude towards their babies (and I think, themselves) was graphically illustrated by the manner of delivery. These babies survived physically, although I think they probably had a difficult life ahead of them emotionally, given their mothers' apparent attitudes towards them. To put it crudely, these women may have experienced their children as shit, unwanted material to be evacuated and disposed of. Sadly, I believe their attitude towards themselves was similar. They were referred on discharge for psychiatric follow-up and home visits by a nurse, particularly with a view to monitor and help them with their care of their children.

Conversion, Hypochondriasis, and Somatization

Ms. Q, woman in her late 60s, was a caregiver to older women. Her last client was a woman with hemiplegia from a stroke. Ms. Q presented with similar symptoms, although neurological examination was not consistent with her symptoms, and was within normal limits.

Ms. Q was obliged to take care of her mother in a way that was not in a child's interest. Her mother expected to be taken care of, rather than taking care of her daughter. This was true both concretely, with mother expecting to be served tea in bed from when Ms. Q was 6 years old, and emotionally, with mother expecting Ms. Q to listen to her complaints and worries, without providing an ear for what Ms. Q herself might need to talk about. Ms. Q, as a child, needed to repress her resentment of her mother out of conscious awareness, to be able to take care of her and maintain the hope that her mother would eventually provide some care for her. It was clear to her that if she were openly angry with her mother, her mother would only react negatively.

Ms. Q's unconscious resentment about her mother persisted, and was never resolved. It remained outside of her conscious awareness. She never had a chance to discuss it with anyone, and to reflect on how this ongoing early experience with her mother affected her life. This seems to have influenced her choice of professions. She never received any type of professional training, but chose to continue taking care of "mothers," that is, older women, devoting herself entirely to this work, never marrying or pursuing other gratifying social experiences or recreational endeavors. Her last client appears to have resembled her mother more than she could bear, in terms of her experience of the client's excessive demands and unreasonable expectations. Ms. Q's way of coping with her resentment of this client, that was amplified by resentment about spending a lifetime taking care of women who represented her mother, was to identify with her client, unconsciously imitating her client's symptoms in an attempt to secure for herself the care that she had longed for since she was a child taking care of her mother.

The above is a psychoanalytically informed formulation of Ms. Q's difficulties. Ms. Q obviously was not a candidate for psychoanalysis. I did not make any of these interpretations to her. My recommendation was for her to be gently encouraged to increase her activity and be given gradually more strenuous rehabilitation exercises. This combined with daily visits from me while she was in hospital provided enough support to help her recover her functioning from what back then was described as a "hysterical paralysis," but now would be diagnosed as a conversion disorder. Without adequate treatment informed by psychoanalytic principles, this patient might have ended up chronically "paralyzed," requiring institutionalization and nursing care for the rest of her life.

These days, patients are more sophisticated than they were in Freud's time, and we see far fewer patients with conversion symptoms. When patients have conversion symptoms, they often represent a complication of a legitimate medical condition, for example, pseudo-seizures in an individual with a legitimate seizure disorder.

Patients suffering from somatization (somatic symptom disorder) have physical complaints without evidence of medical disease, or have physical complaints far in excess of what would be expected, given the medical disease they do suffer from. Patients with hypochondriasis (illness anxiety disorder) are preoccupied with imagined illness without objective evidence of disease. Individuals with these diagnoses are thought to be functioning at a more primitive emotional level than what is represented by a conversion disorder, in that they are unable to express their psychological distress in psychological terms, using language. Their psychological distress is transformed into either physical symptoms or preoccupation with disease. Hypochondriacal and somatization symptoms are thought to be associated with very early childhood emotional traumata occurring before the infant has developed language and a capacity for thinking, necessary to be able to experience distress in psychological terms. Rather than experiencing emotions, they experience "proto-emotions," suffering in which the somatic and the psychological are not yet differentiated. This helps make the physical preoccupation and complaints, respectively, of hypochondriacal patients and somatizing patients more understandable. Chapter 7 deals with this at more length.

A Psychosomatic Solution

Once, as a medical student, I was called in the middle of the night to catheterize a man in acute urinary retention. I did not relish going through that process, and asked the four nurses who were gathered around the man, who was expected to urinate in a basin in bed, to leave us. I helped him walk to the bathroom, turned on the bath, asked him to think about Niagara Falls, and left him to urinate standing up, which he eventually did. Of course, I did not cure him of his prostatism; the combination of leaving him alone, the running water, and the suggestion of the mighty flow of Niagara Falls relaxed him enough to allow him to urinate, obviating the need for what otherwise would have been a technical procedure that neither of us would have welcomed in the middle of the night. I offer this as a trivial example of how psychological factors can affect even the mechanical functioning of the body, like a urinary obstruction. This was a psychosomatic event.

REFERENCES

Hirsch I (2008). *Coasting in the Countertransference: Conflicts of Self-Interest between Analyst and Patient.* New York: Analytic Press.

Smadja C (2011). Psychoanalytic psychosomatics. *International Journal of Psychoanalysis* 92(1):221–230.

Steinberg PI (2018). Dreams as indicators of the psychoanalytic treatment process. *Canadian Journal of Psychoanalysis* 26(2): 150–172.

Sussman MB (1992). *A Curious Calling: Unconscious Motivation for Practicing Psychotherapy.* Northvale, NJ: Jason Aronson.

CHAPTER 7

PSYCHOANALYTIC APPROACHES TO PSYCHOSOMATIC MEDICINE

People calling someone a pain in the neck or the ass or describing feeling their heart is breaking or that they've been kicked in the gut are expressing emotions through reference to their bodies. People often experience negative feelings somatically when these feelings are hard for them to accept, for example, anger results in tension in the neck or jaw, resulting in a headache. The anger one can't accept consciously is experienced instead as muscle tension. An individual might have a conflict about anger, for example, if to him, anger and violence unconsciously are equivalent. This might occur in an individual whose father beat him every time the latter became angry at him. However, someone may be conflicted about being angry at a certain person, or under certain circumstances, for example, if he believed being angry wasn't compatible with loving his wife. Under both these circumstances, the affect of anger does not have an outlet in emotional experience. Various options are available to cope with this "homeless" affect. Some individuals attempt to relieve themselves of an unwanted feeling through addictive behaviors like substance use, or overeating; compulsive behaviors such as overworking, video-game playing, or shopping; promiscuous sexual behavior; or physical violence, such as physical abuse of partners or children, or of strangers, fighting in bars. The psychosomatic alternative to these behaviors, which are frequently destructive, as an outlet for "homeless" affect is that the affect is transduced into the body and experienced as a somatic experience, often pain. This chapter deals primarily with psychosomatic conditions in which what cannot be articulated in the mind becomes expressed in the body.

"PSYCHOSOMATIC" CONDITIONS AND CONVERSION

I believe it is relevant to outline a psychoanalytic approach to psychosomatic medicine because many physicians are not familiar with this. First, I will distinguish between conversion symptoms and somatization symptoms.

Fischbein (2017) describes somatization as a primitive defense potentially appearing in any clinical picture, as a state of tension is diverted into the body. Somatization constitutes the reappearance of a residue of an infantile experience predating the acquisition of the capacity for symbolization. "Symbolization" refers to the capacity, acquired in the first years of life, to articulate thoughts, feelings, impulses, and wishes in words. Prior to this, an infant is "preverbal," not yet capable of expressing these mental contents in words. Individuals who in their first years lack caregivers who adequately foster the development of this capacity are left with deficiencies in or an inability to symbolize. This renders them vulnerable to somatization, to their experiencing uncomfortable mental contents, including unconscious emotional conflicts, unbearably painful or unacceptable feelings, unthinkable thoughts, or unmet emotional needs, in their bodies, rather than experiencing them as conscious thoughts, feelings, and impulses. Somatization does not symbolically represent these mental contents, as do conversion symptoms; it only gives them expression.

Taylor (2010) emphasizes the role of trauma in deficiencies of development of symbolization, concluding that the capacity for symbolic functioning enables humans to cope with the physical and mental pains that everyone encounters throughout life. This capacity collapses when adults experience massive psychic trauma, or when children experience serious traumatic events with no parent able to contain the overwhelming feelings and render them bearable for the child. When one can't mentally represent the unbearable emotional states, they are dissociated, split off from conscious awareness, but may return as somatic illness. Psychoanalytic therapy of psychosomatically ill patients requires identification and experiencing of dissociated emotional states so that unsymbolized trauma, with the aid of the analyst's capacity to contain and symbolize, can be transformed into the patient's psychic structure. The traumatized individual, then, can experience and articulate the painful thoughts and feelings associated with the trauma, so they no longer are expressed through the body.

Patients who somatize are not able to convert sense impressions and proto-emotions, the infantile precursors of emotions, into thoughts associated with emotions. These sense impressions and proto-emotions are not differentiated from each other and build up, like toxic substances that have to be evacuated. One target of such an evacuation is the patient's body.

> If the mind proves unable to dispose of the accumulation of stimuli by transforming them into dreams, … thoughts … [or] hallucinations … this overabundance of stimuli will bombard the body … such … that one of its parts will go mad. The mad part of the body will then give rise to what we call "psychosomatic disorders."
>
> (Meltzer, 1982: 334)

The body is a vessel into which emotional pain that an individual can't experience and articulate in words is evacuated, because of a lack of the capacity to symbolize. The body adapts to this evacuation through the experience of somatic complaints, called somatization. This process involves emotional experience being split off from one's capacity to think, disavowed, and projected into the body. At times this process is not limited to the subjective experience of somatic symptoms (categorized in DSM-5 as somatic symptom disorder, illness anxiety disorder, or conversion disorder), but involves actual tissue changes, constituting a medical disease (categorized in DSM-5 as psychological factors affecting other medical conditions).

As opposed to somatization, conversion symptoms are physical symptoms that cannot be explained by the presence of medical illness, although they imitate it, such as subjective paralysis without objective signs of paralysis, and are found to symbolize an unconscious conflict or repressed affect. An unconscious conflict can result in a conversion symptom (Fischbein, 2017). A symptom takes on different symbolic meanings based on what it refers to. It summons up scenes from other times in the patient's life, and is connected with people significant to the patient. The function of the symptom is to maintain the unconscious conflict or repressed affect unconscious, while permitting it some expression. That a patient creates a conversion symptom implies some degree of capacity for thinking; the patient can unconsciously articulate the conflict verbally. Otherwise, he would not be able to represent it with a symptom symbolizing the conflict or unmet need. That is, the conflict or unmet need must be thought of before being repressed out of conscious awareness (unlike in somatization, described above).

For example, a patient once complained of pain in the shoulders. His physician could find no evidence of shoulder pathology. Detailed history revealed how much of a burden he felt had fallen on him from his family of origin. One could interpret his shoulder pain as symbolizing this burden. Psychoanalytic psychotherapy explored his conflict between "shouldering" the burden to relieve his family of their difficulties, and wishing to be relieved of having to devote his life to helping them. Treatment involved him experiencing intense emotions regarding his experience of his family as a burden, and increased understanding of how this had affected his life in the past and present. This was accompanied by gradual relief of his shoulder pain as he decided to limit the energy devoted to his family. Eventually this patient felt that the analyst and psychotherapy were burdensome to him (transference); this needed to be worked through as well. (See Chapter 9 for a patient with a similar complaint and psychodynamics.) Fischbein (2017) describes a patient with shoulder pain who felt everyone was offloading obligations on to her. She associated to caryatids, statues of women that hold up the façades of old buildings, saying that she had to "shoulder" the weight of her relatives' needs. To summarize, a conversion symptom expresses through the body the perception of a problem, the realization of its conflicting aspects, and the possibility of assigning meaning to them within the subject's life history. With somatization symptoms, the conflict or unmet need cannot be thought of, and therefore no meaning can be assigned to the symptoms. Somatization symptoms must be distinguished from psychosomatic symptoms, which involve organic pathology, while somatization symptoms do not. However, both groups of these conditions involve theoretically greater disturbance in the capacity to think and contain painful emotions, as opposed to conversion disorder.

PSYCHOSOMATIC CONDITIONS

I am indebted to McDougall (1989) for the following observations about psychosomatic patients. Everyone tends to somatize, to experience in the body what cannot be experienced in the mind, when internal or outer circumstances overwhelm our habitual ways of coping. Some adults can function psychologically like infants who cannot use words to think with, and respond to emotional pain only psychosomatically. Since infants have intense somatic experiences from the beginning of life, long before they have any clear representation of their body image, they experience their own and their mother's bodies as an indivisible unit. Some adults continue to unconsciously experience their body limits as ill-defined or unseparated from others, and never develop a sense of separateness from others, or a capacity to experience emotions as emotions. In these individuals, painful emotional experiences with significant others, or with anyone who reactivates a memory of early emotional trauma, may result in a psychosomatic reaction. Psychosomatic research emphasizes the psychosomatic patients' unavailability of conscious experience of their emotions, lack of imaginative capacity, and difficulty in verbal communication. McDougall observes, "*not all communications use language*. In attempting to attack any awareness of certain thoughts, fantasies, or conflictual situations apt to stir up strong feelings of either a painful or an overexciting nature, a patient may … produce a somatic 'explosion' [*sic*] instead of a thought, a fantasy or a dream" (1989: 11; italics in original) that an individual with more access to his inner life might experience.

Everyone uses action at times instead of reflection when their usual defenses against mental pain are overwhelmed. Instead of experiencing an uncomfortable feeling, as noted above, we might overeat, consume an excessive amount of alcohol, take a drug, be involved in a car accident, or fight with our spouse. These are examples of "expression in action," through which one *disperses* emotion rather than thinking about the precipitating event and the feelings connected to it. Such phenomena also include psychosomatic expressions, where the action takes place in the patient's body, for example, exacerbations of inflammatory bowel disease, asthma, ischemic heart disease, or peptic ulcer.

Conversion symptoms, in contrast, refer to dysfunction when a body part or sense organ assumes an unconscious symbolic meaning. There is no physiological damage; the affected organ displays a symptom without the signs expected to accompany such a symptom. On the other hand, symptoms such as reduced or absent sexual desire, constipation, indigestion, and insomnia, in the absence of identifiable organic illness, are not typical of conversion symptoms, such as paralysis or interference with vision or hearing. While the former symptoms result from unconscious anxieties about conflict, emotional attachments, and sexual desires, they also are frequently associated with aggressive and sadistic impulses. In all of these cases, the mind employs the body to communicate something, preventing forbidden impulses and wishes from being fulfilled or unbearable feelings from being experienced consciously.

With access to a patient's unconscious fantasies, one can distinguish between symptoms that refer to a neurotic condition, based on an unconscious conflict, for example, about aggression, such as a conversion disorder, and those associated with a more profound disturbance, related to deficits of mental development where the individual has not developed a capacity to contain thoughts or impulses that are experienced as too threatening, or painful emotions that are felt to be overwhelming. The latter situation makes one vulnerable to a psychosomatic reaction, bypassing the mind that is not capable of containing what feels unbearable.

McDougall employs the symptom of erectile dysfunction to distinguish between a conversion disorder representing an unconscious psychological *neurotic conflict*, and a psychosomatic symptom, representing a psychological disturbance based on a *deficit* in the provision of the infant's early needs, resulting in disturbance in the development of the capacity to articulate thoughts and feelings. As an example of a conflict, some men suffer from severe erectile dysfunction whenever they want to make love. For one patient, all women who interest him sexually unconsciously represent his mother, so any woman he is interested in becomes forbidden as an object of desire, and other men, as representatives of father, may be feared as potential castrators (punishers). This is a classical example of an oedipal conflict. In this situation, the man's impotence is a protective device; the patient "castrates" himself to protect himself from "father" castrating him for his sexual interest in "mother." In this way, the conversion symptom is a solution to the unconscious conflict. "Neurotic fears are typically aroused when the normal adult right to pleasure and sexual love relations or to narcissistic satisfaction in work and social relationships [are] unconsciously contested and therefore punishable" (McDougall, 1989: 17).

On the other hand, another man suffering from erectile dysfunction might discover that he fears he might lose a sense of his body limits while making love and disappear inside his partner, thereby becoming her, losing both his sexual identity and his identity as an individual. Such fantasies enter the more primitive territory of psychotic anxiety. Traces of these archaic fears are found in every individual's unconscious mind; they are the fears and wishes of babies. When these archaic fears, dating back to a preverbal time before they could be experienced and expressed in language, are re-experienced, as in this second example of erectile dysfunction, the outcome (the symptom) is considered a psychosomatic symptom rather than a conversion symptom, based on a deeper psychological disturbance.

In psychosomatic manifestations, the physical damage often is real. The meaning of the symptoms is of a pre-symbolic (unrepresented verbally) order that circumvents the use of words. The thought processes of the psychosomatic sufferer frequently appear to have drained language of its emotional significance. McDougall (1989) considers all cases of physical injury or ill health in which psychological factors play an important role as related to psychosomatic phenomena, including accident proneness; reduction of immune function when an individual is under stress, making one more vulnerable to infectious disease; addictions, a psychosomatic attempt to deal with conflicts and unmet psychological needs by temporarily blurring the awareness of their existence; and patients suffering from allergies, heart and respiratory illnesses, gynecological disturbance, and other maladies whose onset or reappearance is related to events of psychological importance to the patient. I would add that many dermatological and gastrointestinal symptoms often have a psychosomatic component. All patients somatize at one time or another, particularly when stressful events override their usual ways of dealing with mental pain and conflict. McDougall describes patients who react to almost every emotionally arousing situation, particularly those that mobilize anger or separation anxiety, by becoming ill. She found, in some of these patients, an unconscious need to preserve their illness, not only as a reassurance of their body limits, but also as proof of psychic survival.

"Operatory thinking" (Marty & de M'uzan, 1978) is thinking marked by a pragmatic and emotionless way of relating both to oneself and others. These patients describe themselves or others without any expression of feeling. They treat potentially traumatic events with unusual insensitivity, eliminating recognition of inevitably ensuing overwhelming emotions. This increases their psychosomatic vulnerability; what isn't experienced emotionally may be expressed somatically. The term "alexithymia" (Sifneos et al., 1977), literally "no words for feelings," refers to people without words to describe their emotional states. They are unaware of the latter or are incapable of distinguishing one emotion from another. They may not distinguish emotions from physical sensations such as hunger. For them, feelings are experienced as overwhelming, too exciting, or terrifying. They also have psychosomatic vulnerability, appearing to refuse knowledge of their psychological suffering, dispersing their experiences, which are unavailable for thought, and experienced somatically.

These reactions to psychological stress are defensive measures against inexpressible pain and fears of a psychotic nature, such as the danger of losing one's sense of identity, of becoming mentally fragmented, or going crazy. Such individuals may present with somatic symptoms while being unaware of psychological suffering. Frequently these patients have experienced an early psychic trauma (Taylor, 2010) that may lead to primitive forms of anxiety. McDougall (1989) notes that infants send signals to their mothers on an ongoing basis regarding their needs and dislikes. To the extent that a mother is free from distracting internal pressures (such as excessive anxiety or depression, or delusions or hallucinations), she will be in close communication with her infant, and in touch with his signals. If internal distress prevents her from "receiving" and understanding her baby's cries, smiles, and gestures correctly, the mother may do harm to the baby "transmitter" by superimposing her own needs and wishes on him, oblivious to his needs and wishes, creating ongoing rage and frustration in him. The baby may protect himself against overwhelming storms of affect by transducing the affect into his body.

Some patients employ a disguise of pseudo-normality not to think or feel too deeply about emotional pain and conflict that they might otherwise experience as unbearable and mentally disorganizing. They do not connect their physical symptoms with emotionally disturbing experiences. All physicians are familiar with patients who present with somatic complaints in the absence of diagnosable disease, who clearly are emotionally upset. These patients appear heedless of physical and psychological indications that something is amiss. Perception of these indications is not consciously registered and subsequently blocked from conscious awareness. (In repression, by comparison, the disturbing thought or feeling is experienced and then rendered unconscious.) In these patients, any memory of the disturbing experience is eliminated. Individuals who have developed a personality organization based on unconscious conflict between different structures in their mind create a protective structure in the form of a psychological (neurotic) symptom to deal with emotional pain or psychic conflict (that has been repressed), which protects them from the pain or conflict being manifest somatically. In psychosomatic afflictions, a regression to more primitive forms of relationship between body and mind occurs, related to the lack of differentiation between physical and emotional experience in infants. A similar process occurs in individuals using addictions as a way of dispelling mental suffering. In them, the normative development of differentiation between physical and emotional experience in infants never adequately occurred, resulting in a deficit related to the infant's emotional needs not sufficiently being met.

Some allergic, gastric, cardiac, and other reactions may be an expression of the individual's attempt to protect himself from early unmet longings for love or a lack of a sense of intactness that are felt to be life-threatening, similar to an infant's experiencing the threat of death. To achieve this purpose, when these patients feel threatened, similar to infants, a primitive message of warning to the body bypasses the use of language, preventing the individual from thinking about the danger. This may result in psychosomatic disturbance, for example, ulcerative colitis, asthma, eczema, or urticaria.

> Alternatively, the psychic message might result in increased gastric secretion, heightened blood pressure, or quickened pulse rate, or ... may give rise to disturbances of such normal bodily functions as eating, sleeping or eliminating ... In the somatic sphere a complex body–mind reaction also tends to be ... repeated ... when certain relationships with significant others are felt to be threatened.
>
> (McDougall, 1989: 28)

Emotional arousal is not recognized in a symbolic way, that is, through language, which would have allowed the emotion-laden representations to be named, thought about, and dealt with by the mind. Instead, it is automatically transmitted by the mind to the body in a primitive non-verbal way, such as flight-or-fight impulses, producing a psychosomatic symptom.

The symbolic nature of neurotic symptoms (related to unconscious mental conflict) that are created from repressed verbal thoughts does not have a counterpart in psychosomatic symptoms. With severely somatizing patients there is frequently a pseudo-normal communication with the rest of the world; words are divested of their emotional counterpart, at least in that sector of the personality that is constantly seeking to eliminate recognition of primitive anxieties. Although many psychosomatic symptoms may rapidly lead to death, in contrast to conversion symptoms, which are purely symbolic and rarely cause physiological damage, these psychosomatic symptoms also represent an attempt to survive unbearable psychological experience. Secondary damage is possible with conversion symptoms. (For example, the pseudo-hemiplegia of a hysterical paralysis may result in muscle wasting.) In psychosomatic patients who undertake psychoanalysis, the goal of the treatment is slowly to transform the mute and mysterious messages contained in psycho-somatic processes into verbal communications that can be reflected on.

To the infant, her mother and herself make up one whole person. So psychic life commences with the experience of merging, leading to the fantasy that there is only one body and one mind for two people. The mother is the total environment for the infant. Many suggest that deep in our unconscious there is a longing to return to this illusory fusion and become again part of the omnipotent mother universe of early infancy, where there is no frustration, responsibility, or desire. However, in such a universe, there is no individual identity, so the fulfillment of such a longing would mean the loss of personal identity, of psychic death, which is terrifying.

The fantasy of mother and child having one body originates in intrauterine life. The wish to regain this experience is central to the psychic life of the neonate. The baby's cries induce the mother to re-create the illusion of oneness, using the warmth, rhythm, and protective closeness of her body, as well as her voice. In maintaining this illusion, she enables the neonate to take in an internal image of the maternal environment, bringing comfort, and enabling him to fall asleep.

Equally important is the baby's need for separation. If a mother has her own difficulty with separation, she may have difficulty with her infant's need to relinquish her physical presence in order to sleep. This may precipitate a psychosomatic disturbance of infancy, the baby with insomnia who can only sleep in his mother's arms. When the mother–child relationship is good enough, the infant will progressively differentiate between her own body and her first representation of the world, mother's breast. Concurrently, the psychological gradually becomes differentiated in her mind from the somatic.

Graeme Taylor (1987) outlines a psychoanalytic understanding of connections between early unmet emotional needs leading to structural deficiencies in one's personality, unconscious conflict, and psychosomatic disturbance. Taylor provides a cogent history of developments in psychosomatic medicine and the empirical evidence demonstrating the effects of psychological disturbance on the body, including its predisposition to, precipitation, and perpetuation of medical illness.

> [P]eople with a high susceptibility for developing physical disease suffer from psychological *deficits* rather than (or in addition to) specific psychological conflicts … a different model of psychopathology is needed to understand the complexities of their psychic disturbance. While disease-prone individuals sometimes … resemble people with borderline or narcissistic personality organizations … the psychological disturbance is often localized and masked by areas of apparently intact functioning.
>
> (Taylor, 1987: 5)

Recent greater focus is on the importance of the early mother–infant relationship for the development of psychosomatic unity and a healthy personality. Psychobiological research and observational studies of infants confirm that deficiencies in the infant's earliest relationships result in developmental defects that reduce the individual's capacity to self-regulate essential psychobiological functions, predisposing the individual to bodily disease.

Episodes of illness occur in clusters when individuals are having major interpersonal difficulties or experiencing their life situations as threatening or unsatisfactory. Taylor notes an association between loss of important relationships and the onset or exacerbation of disease in individuals who couldn't cope psychologically with loss. Leukemia and lymphoma frequently develop when an individual is depressed and struggling to cope with the loss or separation of a key person. Similarly, some patients with ulcerative colitis who have an intense dependency on a mothering figure experience the onset or exacerbation of the colitis, accompanied by feelings of helplessness and depression, when this relationship is threatened or disrupted. Subsequent studies demonstrate that threatening losses and symbolic losses as well as actual losses can have a similar effect. Another study showed that, for 41 of 42 hospitalized medical patients, actual, threatened, or symbolic loss, as well as feelings of helplessness and hopelessness, preceded disease. Many of these patients had suffered similar losses of or separations from important figures of their early years, and were thought to demonstrate uncompleted mourning and lifelong feelings of unsupported dependency needs.

Taylor (1987) also describes the occurrence of sudden cardiac death in predisposed individuals who experienced disruption in an important interpersonal relationship, noting that loss in a relationship often contributed to the emotional disturbance during which an ischemic stroke occurred. Emotional upsets due to violent arguments, and threatened separation from family members, were found as significant in precipitating congestive heart failure. Loss of relationships commonly precedes onset or exacerbation of medical disease, including ulcerative colitis, diabetes mellitus, bronchial asthma, multiple sclerosis, and cancer. Recovery from disease often is associated with the restoration of a lost relationship or replacement with a substitute relationship. There exists considerable evidence that bereavement can lead to increased morbidity and mortality.

Taylor's observations as a consultation psychiatrist in a general hospital coincide with mine: "object loss [the object of one's love] frequently plays an important etiological role in the onset or exacerbation of disease" (1987: 46). He describes evidence for a direct brain–immune system pathway that can be influenced by emotional stress, and a change in endocrine and immune function with loss of important relationships. He also describes increased susceptibility to disease in infants who experience chronic maternal deprivation, consistent with Spitz's (1945) linking hospitalism with increased infant mortality. Spitz quotes from a Spanish bishop's 1760 diary "En la Casa de Niños Expósitos el niño se va poniendo triste y muchos de ellos mueren de tristeza." (In the orphanage, children become sad, and many of them die of sadness; my translation.) Taylor (1987) notes that in infants and children with deprivation dwarfism, which resembles idiopathic hypopituitarism, children with this failure-to-thrive syndrome:

> show abnormal growth hormone responses and typically come from chaotic home environments and impoverished parent–child relationships ... [G]rowth is resumed when these children are admitted to hospital and provided with a playful and attentive relationship with a nurse. The interactions within such a relationship presumably help regulate the production of growth hormone.
>
> (Taylor, 1987: 130)

Taylor describes the mothers of children who will have psychosomatic disturbance as adults being unable to respond empathically to their child, using their child to compensate for something missing in their own emotional development, for maintenance of their own psychic equilibrium. The theory that psychological predisposition to disease is due primarily to psychic defects, rather than unconscious conflicts, provides a better explanation for some people's greater vulnerability to separation and loss of important relationships. "People with a high susceptibility to disease are lacking certain self-regulating capacities ... [T]he loss of an external regulatory [relationship] ... evokes feelings of helplessness and hopelessness which may develop into a full-blown 'giving up/given up' complex" (Taylor, 1987: 254), similar to patients with substance abuse or bulimia who try to utilize an external agent, such as food, alcohol, or drugs, to substitute for the self-regulatory system that never was internalized from the parents.

Taylor notes, "psychopathology connected with both sexual perversion and physical disease may be split off and *encapsulated* in a psychotic (or primitive destructive) part of the personality which is not readily accessible to the psychoanalytic process" (1987: 269; italics in original). This part of the personality is characterized by confusion between self and other, thinking at a pre-symbolic level, and employment of primitive defense mechanisms such as splitting and projective identification, which are used to discharge unbearable tensions and fantasies into the analyst. "[D]ependent people have suffered deficiencies in their earliest object relationships;

their inner worlds lack adequate representation of a well-functioning [mother–child] unit that normally would substitute for the external mother [in her absence] and provide self-regulatory functions. To compensate for this, many of these people retain a symbiotic relationship with their mother or form a substitute symbiotic ... relationship with" an important figure in adult life. If this figure is unavailable, the regulation inherent in the relationship is removed, and the individual is "at greater risk for developing physical disease following separation and object loss" (Taylor, 1987: 285).

Psychoanalytic/psychotherapeutic treatment of these patients must take into account the deficits in their early relationships, which are reflected in their internal world, and in the quality of their current relationships, upon which they rely for psychobiological regulation. These patients are more vulnerable to psychological and physiological dysregulation when interpersonal relationships do not provide what these patients need psychologically. These individuals unconsciously choose life partners with whom they repeat their unsatisfactory early relationships with parents, creating a vicious cycle that perpetuates their disturbed internal and external regulating mechanisms. In the psychoanalytic treatment of these patients, the analyst assumes the role of a regulatory relationship. These patients often become dysregulated at times of separation from the analyst, such as vacations or even weekends. Some may develop physical illness at these times. (Balint (1957) opined that by far the most frequently used drug in general practice is the doctor himself.) The analyst's assuming the role of the regulatory relationship is necessary but not sufficient for the successful treatment of these patients. This likely is true, more or less, in all psychoanalytic/psychotherapeutic relationships, although in the latter this might not be recognized, unless the therapist has a psychoanalytic approach to understanding her relationship with her patient. Taylor has compiled compelling evidence demonstrating the connections between early unmet emotional needs that lead to personality disturbance, unconscious emotional conflict, and stress in adult life, and psychosomatic disturbance.

Maunder and Hunter (2008) suggest that adverse childhood experiences alter the relational world of children, inhibiting the development of secure attachment bonds. They survey evidence that attachment insecurity can impair physical health throughout the lifespan. They propose that insecurity in attachment contributes to risk of disease through several mechanisms, including:

(1) disturbances in arousal and recovery within physiological systems that respond to stress;
(2) physiological links between the mediators of social relationships, stress, and immunity;
(3) links between relationship style and various health behaviors; and
(4) disease risk factors that serve as external regulators of dysphoric affect, such as nicotine and alcohol.

(Maunder & Hunter, 2008: 11)

They conclude that the evidence that has accumulated to date suggests that early experience in relationships exerts effects on physical health throughout the lifespan.

Ferrari "takes the view that there is no such thing as the 'psychosomatic patient,' because he sees the question of the mind–body relationship and its dysharmonies as a general problem of the person's internal functioning" (quoted in Lombardi, 2016).

Space does not permit further descriptions of recent writing on psychosomatics and psychoanalysis. The following references are for those interested in further reading: Aisenstein (2008), Beutel et al. (2008), Blumenfeld (2006), Ginieri-Coccossis & Vaslamatzis (2008), Ikonen (2014), Katz (2010), Kohutis (2008), Kradin (2011), Kuriloff (2004), Lichtman (2010), Magnenat

(2016), Meares et al. (2008), Rodin & Zimmermann (2008), Roose (2014), Shapira-Berman (2018), Sklar (2008), Sloate (2008, 2010), Taylor (2008a, 2008b), and Yasky et al. (2013).

I was asked to see a hospitalized middle-aged man who would not cooperate in the management of his severe type 1 diabetes with medication, diet, and exercise, although he appeared reasonably intelligent. This resulted in repeated hospitalizations and dangerous hypoglycemic episodes. His endocrinologist referred him to me. For this patient, the endocrinologist represented a demanding and resentful father whom the patient was determined to resist and disobey, having felt under the thumb of his own father (by then long deceased), who was very controlling for many years. He seemed to need to oppose his father (whose latest incarnation, one of many, was his endocrinologist) in order to maintain a developing experience of separation from his father in becoming an individual with his own mind. Hence his lack of cooperation with the endocrinologist, who admittedly was quite particular about diabetic control, which exacerbated the patient's resistance. So this patient had a father transference to his endocrinologist that interfered with medical management. A couple of visits during which I interpreted to the patient his unconscious motivation for opposing his endocrinologist's suggestions resulted in the patient developing a more cooperative attitude regarding his treatment, which led to improved diabetic control without further psychiatric intervention. This is an example of a psychoanalytically informed psychiatric consultation, followed by a few short visits while the patient was in hospital, which positively influenced the patient's relationship with his attending physician and the medical outcome. It was the patient's insight into his reacting to his endocrinologist as if the latter were his controlling father, in the context of our brief relationship, during which the patient could feel understood and respected as an individual, that enabled him to cooperate better with his endocrinologist, and manage his diabetes better. Winnicott (1971), a pediatrician/psychoanalyst, described similar "therapeutic consultations" (of which he performed 10,000!).

This case illustrates the interaction of several potential factors contributing to improvement in this patient's medical and psychological status as a result of a psychoanalytic approach to understanding his psychosomatic status. The patient's better compliance with his diabetic regimen directly improved his serum glucose levels, reducing the risk of diabetic complications in the long term, in addition to obviating the day-to-day risks associated with hypo- and hyperglycemia. The resolution of his conscious conflict with his endocrinologist might be accompanied by reduced adrenal catecholamines and corticosteroids, which could have a directly beneficial effect on diabetic management. The resolution of conflict with his physician also could have a psychologically beneficial effect. Finally, to the extent that this patient's unconscious conflict with his father about authority was resolved (which very likely would require ongoing psychotherapeutic treatment for an optimum result), this would result, in addition to benefits in other areas of his life where interactions with authority have proven difficult for him, in more collaborative future interactions with medical caregivers. This is especially important in individuals with chronic medical conditions who have to work with physicians for their entire lives.

Today no reasonable person would suggest that psychological factors in themselves cause medical disease, or that these diseases can be cured by psychological treatments alone. A more balanced view would be that psychological factors in some cases may be involved in the predisposition, precipitation, and/or perpetuation of medical illness. A psychoanalytically informed psychiatric consultation may be helpful in managing these illnesses, and psychoanalysis or psychoanalytic psychotherapy may be helpful and sometimes necessary in the management of these patients.

REFERENCES

Aisenstein M (2008). Beyond the dualism of psyche and soma. *Journal of the American Academy of Psychoanalysis* 36(1):103–123.

Balint M (1957). *The Doctor, his Patient, and the Illness.* New York: International Universities Press.

Beutel M, Michal M, Subic-Wrana C (2008). Psychoanalytically-oriented inpatient psychotherapy of somatoform disorders. *Journal of the American Academy of Psychoanalysis* 36(1):125–142.

Blumenfeld M (2006). The place of psychodynamic psychiatry in consultation-liaison psychiatry with special emphasis on countertransference. *Journal of the American Academy of Psychoanalysis and Dynamic Psychiatry* 34(1):83–92.

Fischbein JE (2017). Configurations of time, the body, and verbal communication: Temporality in patients who express their suffering through the body. *International Journal of Psychoanalysis* 98:323–341.

Ginieri-Coccossis M, Vaslamatzis G (2008). *Journal of the American Academy of Psychoanalysis* 36(1):33–47.

Ikonen P (2014). On psychosomatic phenomena. *Scandinavian Psychoanalytic Review* 37(2):85–90.

Katz AW (2010). Healing the split between body and mind: Structural and developmental aspects of psychosomatic illness. *Psychoanalytic Inquiry* 30(5):430–444.

Kohutis EA (2008). Concreteness, dreams, and metaphor: Their import in a somatizing patient. *Journal of the American Academy of Psychoanalysis* 36(1):143–163.

Kradin RL (2011). Psychosomatic disorders: the canalization of mind into matter. *Journal of Analytic Psychology* 56(1):37–55.

Kuriloff E (2004). When words fail: Psychosomatic illness and the talking cure. *Psychoanalytic Quarterly* 73(4):1023–1040.

Lichtman C (2010). Psychosomatic medicine: A psychoanalyst's journey through a somatic world. *Psychoanalytic Inquiry* 30(5):380–389.

Lombardi R (2016). Primitive mental states and the body: A personal view of Armando B. Ferrari's concrete original object. In: Borgogno F, Lucchetti A, Coe LM (eds.), *Reading Italian Psychoanalysis*. London: Routledge.

Magnenat L (2016). Psychosomatic breast and alexithymic breast: A Bionian psychosomatic perspective. *International Journal of Psychoanalysis* 97(1):41–63.

Marty P, de M'uzan M (1978). Das operative Denken ("Pensée opératoire"). *Psyche –Zeitschrift für Psychoanalyse* 32(10):974–984.

Maunder RGJ, Hunter J (2008). Attachment relationships as determinants of physical health. *Journal of the American Academy of Psychoanalysis and Dynamic Psychiatry* 36(1):11–32.

McDougall J (1989). *Theatres of the Body: A Psychoanalytic Approach to Psychosomatic Illness.* New York: Norton.

Meares R, Gerull F, Korner A, Melkonian D, Stevenson J, Samir H (2008). Somatization and stimulus entrapment. *Journal of the American Academy of Psychoanalysis* 36(1):165–180.

Meltzer D (1982). Implicazioni psicosomatiche nel pensiero di Bion. [Psychosomatic implications of Bion's thought.] *Quademi di psicoterapia infantile* 7:199–222.

Rodin R, Zimmermann C (2008). Psychoanalytic reflections on mortality: A reconsideration. *Journal of the American Academy of Psychoanalysis* 36(1):181–196.

Roose SP (2014). Review of Huber D, Zimmerman J, Henrich G, & Klug G (2013). Comparison of cognitive-behavioural therapy with psychoanalytic and psychodynamic therapy for depressed patients: A three-year follow-up study. *Psychosomatic Medicine and Psychotherapy*, 58:299–316. *Journal of the American Psychoanalytic Association* 62(1):118–119.

Shapira-Berman O (2018). Psychosomatic symptoms as physical dreams: Emotional experiences given expression through the body. *Contemporary Psychoanalysis* 54(3):560–589.

Sifneos PE, Apfel-Savitz R, Frankel FH (1977). The phenomenon of "alexithymia": observations in neurotic and psychosomatic patients. *Psychotherapy and Psychosomatics* 28:47–57.

Sklar J (2008). Hysteria and mourning – a psychosomatic case. *Journal of the American Academy of Psychoanalysis* 36(1):89–102.

Sloate PL (2008). From fetish object to transitional object: The analysis of a chronically self-mutilating bulimic patient. *Journal of the American Academy of Psychoanalysis* 36(1):69–88.

Sloate PL (2010). Superego and sexuality: An analysis of a psychosomatic solution. *Psychoanalytic Inquiry* 30(5):457–473.

Spitz RA (1945). Hospitalism – an inquiry into the genesis of psychiatric conditions in early childhood. *Psychoanalytic Study of the Child* 1:53–74.

Taylor GJ (1987). *Psychosomatic Medicine and Contemporary Psychoanalysis*. Madison, CT: International Universities Press.

Taylor GJ (2008a). Frontline – Why publish a special issue on psychoanalysis and psychosomatics? *Journal of the American Academy of Psychoanalysis and Dynamic Psychiatry* 36:1–10.

Taylor GJ (2008b). The challenge of chronic pain: A psychoanalytic approach *Journal of the American Academy of Psychoanalysis and Dynamic Psychiatry* 36:49–68.

Taylor GJ (2010). Symbolism, symbolization and trauma in psychosomatic theory. In: Eisenstein M, Rappaport de Eisenberg E (eds.), *Psychosomatics Today: A Psychoanalytic Perspective*. London: Karnac.

Winnicott WD (1971). *Therapeutic Consultations in Child Psychiatry*. New York: Basic Books.

Yasky J, King R, O'Brien T (2013). Challenges in treating patients with psychosomatic disorders: Some patterns of resistance. *Psychoanalytic Psychotherapy* 27(2):124–139.

CHAPTER 8

PSYCHIATRY FOR THE MASSES: BROADER INDICATIONS FOR PSYCHIATRIC CONSULTATION

Before a psychiatric service with an organized liaison component is organized in a general hospital, psychiatric consultations usually are requested relating to a patient's psychiatric symptoms or diagnosed psychiatric condition. The request usually includes an explicit request for help in managing the patient's psychiatric symptoms. Often the consultee wishes transfer of the patient to the psychiatric unit. This type of referral represents a patient-oriented psychiatric assessment and management approach based on a medical model. It involves psychiatric assessment of the patient and management approaches directed solely at the patient.

A liaison model of psychiatric consultation has broader implications for both assessment and treatment. In this model the focus is expanded beyond the individual patient. Doctor–patient, nurse–patient, doctor–nurse, and patient–family relationships may be considered, as well as the ways in which the patient's social milieu (for example, her workplace) affects her medical recovery (Hackett & Weisman, 1960a, 1960b; Meyer & Mendelson, 1961; Miller, 1973a, 1973b; Ramsay, 1983). The effects on cerebral functions of intra- and extracranial organic pathology are other variables that may interact with psychosocial considerations. The liaison psychiatry model encompasses not only the treatment of overt psychiatric symptoms, but also the management of the patient's adverse psychological reactions to her illness and its treatment, and includes consideration of the physician's awareness of how the patient's important relationships, both present and past, including relations with caregivers, influence these reactions.

When a medical or surgical patient demonstrates florid psychiatric symptoms, it is routine to request a psychiatric consultation because of the severity of the patient's symptoms, or because of how much the symptoms interfere with the attending physician's attempts to treat the presenting illness. This chapter will provide some examples of patients' less easily recognized reactions to their illness that, if ignored, may interfere with treatment in hospital. These are cases in which a liaison psychiatry consultation might support (Steinberg, 1983a) the patient, expediting her medical progress, or even rendering continued medical treatment possible when the patient would otherwise refuse it. Adverse psychological reactions to illness or treatment sometimes can be predicted. It is in the patient's interest to have psychiatric involvement early, in order, when possible, to prevent severe reactions. In many settings, however, it is only when patients have had severe reactions that a psychiatrist is consulted. Employment of psychoanalytic principles enhances the psychiatric consultant's considerations of the patient's personality, the unconscious meaning of an illness or management plan to a patient, difficulties in staff–patient relations, the influence of the patient's family on the patient's illness and management, and other factors related to who the patient is as an individual.

Anxiety about illness may result in excessive activity (*sometimes representing a denial of illness, like the inpatient who was performing jumping jacks as a manic reaction to his severe myocardial infarction*), excessive invalidism, or failure to cooperate with medical treatment, all of which are maladaptive defenses against anxiety. Anxiety about illness may also result in changes in the patient's personality functioning, with resultant difficulties in personal relationships. Such emotional reactions to illness may adversely affect the course or management of the illness (Steinberg, 1983b). This is especially true if the patient's interpersonal difficulties relate to those in charge of his medical care. It may be difficult to identify patients who can benefit from psychiatric assessment if they do not display overt symptoms, but behavior suggestive of maladaptive defenses, changes in personality functioning, or difficulties in interpersonal relationships associated with medical illness will all alert the watchful physician (Reiser & Bakst, 1975). Patients may, for example, angrily threaten to discharge themselves against medical advice; refuse treatment without giving a rational reason; request inappropriate treatments or unnecessary extensions of hospitalization; exaggerate or minimize the expected effects of illness or their functioning; resort to doctor shopping; or attempt to persuade one member of the medical staff to reverse the management decision of another, without discussing the change with the other physician. All of these responses suggest that the patient's illness or the management situation is interacting with his personality such that his judgment is being unduly influenced by unconscious considerations. Such behavior usually reflects either established maladaptive personality patterns or changes in personality functioning as a reaction to the illness or its management.

A psychiatric consultation informed by psychoanalytic understanding of reactions to illness and treatment may clarify some of these unconscious factors. The patient can be encouraged to put into words the concerns being expressed by potentially self-damaging behavior. Verbal expression of these concerns may foster a patient's having a healthier approach to the illness and its management. In an adolescent diabetic whose illness is poorly controlled, emotional factors may directly affect blood glucose levels, interfering with the best possible diabetic control. In addition, unconscious factors may adversely influence the patient's self-administration of insulin. The inappropriate way in which the patient administers insulin to himself may be an expression of self-directed hostility displaced from an important, but frustrating, relationship. *That is, rather than experiencing and possibly expressing hostility to another person whom the patient finds frustrating, his hostility is unconsciously directed towards himself. This behavior (inappropriate self-administration of insulin) might also represent an age-appropriate striving for autonomy, however self-destructively expressed,* or a symbolic representation of the kind of care the patient feels that he has received from others important to him. It similarly could be a non-verbal attempt to procure more or better care from others, or to induce others to take responsibility for his care. The latter is more likely in a patient who is already experiencing difficulty in adjusting to the separation from parents that is expected to occur gradually during adolescence, and in whom issues of dependence/independence are conflictual (Rodin, 1983). In this situation, psychiatric consultation, with appropriate treatment recommendations aimed at short-term resolution of the patient's unconscious conflicts and difficulties with interpersonal relationships, may have an observable effect on the patient's medical progress.

As outlined in the introduction to this section, psychoanalytic understanding of the patients described below is applied in their psychiatric management. However, they are not treated with psychoanalysis or psychoanalytic psychotherapy, and interpretations of the unconscious source of their difficulties, with few exceptions, are not made to them.

DENIAL OF ILLNESS

Mr. A, a 62-year-old man with diabetes and peripheral vascular disease, was referred for assessment of his competence to consent to above-the-knee amputation of a gangrenous leg, having been admitted to hospital in a delirium secondary to sepsis and diabetic ketoacidosis. He previously underwent coronary artery bypass, aortofemoral bypass, and a partial foot amputation in the same leg. Mr. A appeared to employ denial in dealing with the implications of his illness and proposed surgery, saying that he couldn't predict what might happen if he refused the surgery, and describing the gangrene as "black skin."

Mr. A had apparently discontinued all medical care a year and a half prior to this presentation, disappointed with his physicians because his previous amputation did not "cure" his vascular disease. Moreover, he would not cooperate with the management of his diabetes, and neglected his personal hygiene at home. At the time of the partial foot amputation, he apparently had been advised to have an above-the-knee amputation, to which he refused to agree.

Mr. A appeared to be incompetent to agree to surgery, and seemed to be at high risk for a severe postoperative psychological reaction. He was treated with small doses of haloperidol for his agitation, and regular brief visits by the liaison psychiatry staff in an attempt to involve him in a relationship with a friendly, interested professional whom he might eventually begin to trust or at least talk to. His course appeared unaffected by this treatment, except that his agitation diminished. He died of sepsis in the hospital.

I believe it would have been worthwhile to investigate, with a psychiatric consultation during the earlier admission, Mr. A's resistance to the advice of his surgeon concerning the above-knee amputation. The compromise of effecting the partial foot amputation that Mr. A permitted did not deal with his apprehension about medical treatment, demonstrated by his eventual withdrawal from all medical care. Perhaps an attempt to understand Mr. A's reservations about the treatment he was receiving might have led to better compliance with his doctor's advice. This in turn might have decreased Mr. A's risk of morbidity (Steinberg, 1983b).

Although there was no overt evidence of paranoid symptoms, Mr. A appeared to lack trust in his physicians, both trust that they knew what was wrong with him, and trust that they would recommend what was best for him. *According to Erikson (1950), basic trust is the first "age of man," that is, the first emotional developmental challenge. Negotiating this stage satisfactorily is dependent in part on a good-enough fit between infant and early caregivers, and on the actual care the infant receives from them. If the fit and/or the care is unsatisfactory, adequate basic trust may not develop. This can affect the quality of an individual's relationships throughout his life. Situations in which an individual is dependent on another for care, of which the physician–patient relationship is a prime example, are especially sensitive ones for people in whom the development of basic trust has been limited. They need the physician's special attention regarding apprehension they may have about their illness and their need to rely on physicians to care for them. They may employ several unconscious mechanisms of defense to reduce feeling that they need their physician, such as denying the seriousness of their illness or their need for a specific treatment, especially an invasive one, such as surgery or an investigation that requires an intrusive procedure. Clearly, their need to defend against conscious awareness of their anxiety regarding the care they will receive from the physician can have a very high price, in that the physician's management of the patient may be compromised, leading to worsening of the illness, or even death. This often can be obviated when the physician is aware of the patient's sensitivities regarding dependence and trust, and comports herself in a manner reassuring to her patient. This usually cannot be accomplished through overt reassurance, but rather through more indirect means, described below. Robertson Davies (1958) provides an insightful description of this type of patient in his novel* A Mixture of Frailties.

One may have a high index of suspicion that one is dealing with such a patient when aware that the patient has suffered significant early trauma, especially in the form of traumatic separations, neglect, or overt abuse. For example, a patient may have lost a parent when he was a child, or have not been adequately cared for, been beaten as a child, or "just" been separated from his parents for a number of weeks in the early years of life. Sometimes one hears of infants being left to cry in their cribs for hours at a time, the family's and sometimes physician's philosophy being that the infant must "cry it out" or "should not be coddled." However, such relatively obvious elements of history often are unavailable, and the physician is left with the possibility of sensing, from his experience of and emotional reaction to his patient, that his patient may be having some difficulty putting herself under the doctor's care. (See Chapter 1.)

Such patients need their physicians to be more patient in explaining what is wrong with them and what treatment they need. They may require more information than the average patient, more reassurance about the outcome of treatment, and more repetitions of this than might be expected. Such reassurance should never go beyond what is realistic. It is more important to explore with these patients what their apprehensions are than to try to cover them up with blanket reassurances. (In psychotherapy and psychoanalysis, reassurance is rarely reassuring. What patients in psychotherapy find more reassuring is an exploration of what is bothering them in the context of the relationship with their therapist. However, it is legitimate for physicians to reassure their patients realistically about their illness, management plan, and prognosis, which they are qualified to do.)

Often a psychiatric consultation can clarify the unconscious basis for the patient's apprehensions, identifying the patient as someone who requires especially sensitive care to get the best medical outcome. It is usually not necessary, and often can be counterproductive, to interpret to the patient his difficulty with trust, or what the psychiatrist believes is the basis for it in the patient's early experience. Interpreting this unnecessarily may result in a paranoid reaction in the patient, who likely is unprepared for a confrontation about what he needed to render unconscious because it was intolerable for him to think about. Nevertheless, at times this is the only approach that can help the patient agree to appropriate treatment. The latter criterion must be given a high priority.

CULMINATION OF LOSSES AND ANTICIPATING THE NEED FOR REFERRAL

Mrs. B, an obese 54-year-old woman, was admitted to hospital with a rupture of an abdominal aortic aneurysm that had been resected. Femoropopliteal bypass grafting was performed the next day, but did not re-establish arterial flow to the left leg, which became gangrenous, requiring above-the-knee amputation a week later. Mrs. B's course in hospital was complicated by pressure ulcers and breakdown of her wound edges. Psychiatric consultation was requested after a brief psychotic episode two months postoperatively, shortly before a planned transfer to a rehabilitation hospital. Mrs. B's life was filled with losses that she described as "challenges" that she had had to meet, including the death of her mother when she was 20, at which time her father had required her support, but offered her little support in return; her daughter's death at the age of 14 months; the near-death by myocardial infarction of her 31-year-old son, and most recently, the prolonged separation from her husband during her current period of hospitalization. She indicated how very strongly this last separation affected her, particularly because of her earlier losses.

Mrs. B appeared very anxious about her transfer to the rehabilitation hospital, and about her belief that her physicians couldn't agree about the best treatment for her. She appeared to have fought off depressive feelings for most of her life by putting on a brave face that she could "take it," an assertion she often insisted on after her unexpected amputation.

The attending staff were prompt in requesting a psychiatric consultation after Mrs. B's brief psychotic episode. She was treated with small doses of haloperidol. The psychiatric consultant advised hospital staff to avoid any hint of indecision in her management planning, and instructed them to explain meticulously details of the management plan, and to support her in her lifelong defense of being "strong enough to take it." The psychiatric consultant reinforced this approach, admiring the patient for the strength that had brought her through so many difficulties.

In view of the many losses that Mrs. B had suffered, climaxed by the unanticipated loss of one of her legs, and of the anxiety that she expressed about her doctors' perceived disagreement and her planned transfer to a rehabilitation hospital, a request for a psychiatric consultation might have been considered on the basis of her anxiety, before she became psychotic. Her belief that her doctors disagreed about her treatment, perhaps based only on a clinical discussion held too close to the bedside, may have represented to her yet another loss: that of her physicians as people she could count on to do the best for her. *An earlier psychiatric referral might have helped to obviate the psychotic episode and expedite Mrs. B's accepting the need for transfer to the rehabilitation hospital.*

SPEEDY REFERRAL

Mrs. C was a 55-year-old, foreign-born widow hospitalized for treatment of Parkinson's disease. Despite several changes in medication, her many vague somatic complaints were not relieved. Her frustration and hostility prompted a psychiatric consultation.

Mrs. C appeared to the psychiatric consultant to be suffering from a prolonged grief reaction to the death of her husband four years prior to this presentation. She seemed to struggle between a stubborn need to remain independent, despite progressive debilitation with Parkinson's disease, and a widely unconscious wish for increased dependence on her daughters, despite a fear of burdening them. She also appeared unconsciously resentful of helping her daughters by babysitting. Her complicated grief appeared related to her feeling that her husband had forced her to immigrate and then abandoned her by dying. She blamed anything that went wrong on his insistence on immigrating. *This is an example of complicated grief related to ambivalence in the relationship with the deceased.*

Mrs. C was diagnosed as having a dependent personality, a dysthymic disorder, and an unresolved grief reaction. She was treated with doxepin 100 mg qhs, and with three visits of supportive psychotherapy in which she quickly sealed over (repressed out of conscious awareness) her ambivalent feelings about her husband. She said doxepin improved all her somatic symptoms, especially her headaches. The social work department was involved in assessing the family and in investigating whether improving communication between Mrs. C and her daughters might be helpful. Mrs. C refused further interviews during which problems with husband and daughters could have been explored.

Mrs. C's physician quickly concluded that her symptoms could not be explained by Parkinson's disease alone. In requesting a psychiatric assessment, she realized that her patient's difficulties with treatment that removed the majority of her complaints, without dealing with her conflict over her unmet dependency needs or the basis for her unresolved grief reaction, would not be adequate. Prompt psychiatric referral led to a psychoanalytically informed understanding of which of Mrs. C's complaints had a psychological contribution. With this understanding and appropriate medication, some of her symptoms were relieved, and unnecessary further medical investigation and treatment were avoided.

NON-SPECIFIC SIGNS

There are other non-specific signs suggestive of a patient having difficulty coping with illness or its management. One is the patient's asking the doctor repetitive questions about his illness that the doctor believes he already has answered. Here, the patient behaves as if he does not understand his doctor, despite apparent intellectual capability of doing so. Unconscious reasons can prevent a patient from understanding his physician's explanations about his illness. If this is investigated, clarification may provide psychological relief for the patient, reducing anxiety and improving the chances of compliance with management. An example is the pneumonia patient described in Chapter 1.

Another non-specific sign of a patient's failure to cope with illness is outright denial of the fact of illness. A patient may believe, for instance, that cancer is invariably fatal, and that a diagnosis of cancer guarantees a slow, inexorable, and painful death. If the patient's reaction is to deny that she has this illness, she may bring about just what she fears, by avoiding the treatment that offers a reasonable chance of preventing this outcome. Ascertaining the individual patient's beliefs about an illness may render a psychiatric consultation unnecessary, or make it clear that it is clearly indicated. This involves exploring with the patient the meaning to her of her illness.

The patient who jokes excessively with the medical and nursing staff, especially if the jokes refer to his illness, is probably experiencing a good deal of anxiety (Freud, 1905/1960). This anxiety may be with respect to the illness, the experience of being a hospitalized patient, needing to rely on the physician for care, or something completely unrelated to his illness, such as difficulties in his relationships at home or at work. It would be helpful for the physician to inquire into the basis for the patient's discomfort. This might result in the patient's relief in being able to tell someone what is bothering him. Then the physician can decide whether to manage the patient's anxiety himself or to request a psychiatric consultation. In patients with congestive heart failure, it is especially important to follow up any hints that the patient is unduly anxious, because anxiety can precipitate and exacerbate heart failure by several mechanisms (Reiser & Bakst, 1975). The introduction to this section describes such a patient.

Another situation that suggests that a patient has mixed feelings about his treatment arises when he in some way interferes with appointments for examinations, diagnostic tests, or specific treatment procedures. The patient may explain that he "forgot" the arrangement, giving no conscious indication of wishing to interfere with his management. This response is more striking when it happens in hospital, where the patient is at hand, but manages to be unavailable inexplicably when due to be taken to nuclear medicine, or to eat something "by mistake" on the day of planned surgery. These "mistakes" are evidence of a disturbance in the patient's thinking processes that may be specific to the current clinical situation, or may be characteristic of the way the patient responds to stress. The "mistake" is usually unconsciously mediated. The physician can use her own feelings of frustration, in the face of the patient's conscious good intentions, as a barometer to measure the likelihood that there may be more to the situation than meets the eye: the more frustrated she feels, the more important it is to follow up the feelings, asking the patient directly about his own feelings, and about what the patient anticipates the outcome of illness and suggested management to be (see Chapter 2). A psychiatric opinion may be indicated if the physician is not satisfied that she understands what is transpiring, or if she is sufficiently concerned about what she has found out to want advice about the patient's management. The doctor's feelings of frustration may also reflect difficulties in the relationships involving patient, nurse, and doctor. Psychiatric consultation may elucidate some of the patient's difficulties in these relationships and lead to management suggestions.

What something means to an individual is very personal and unique, and is based largely on that individual's unique experiences in life. The awareness that one's earliest years have the most impact on who one becomes did not originate with Freud. The Jesuits, centuries ago, concluded, "Give me the child for the first seven years and I will give you the man." The physician may not be able to elicit information about the patient's early relationship experiences, that could help him predict the patient's concerns about the care he offers. Without this information, the physician must find out what he can. Although the exploration of unconscious meaning has been developed by psychoanalysts, physicians still are able to attempt to explore the meaning to patients of their illness and proposed management, Simply asking a patient what his concerns are, and what he expects will become of him should he have the illness he is afraid of having or knows he has, can begin a fruitful discussion that may reassure the patient of support in the face of an illness, investigation, or treatment he fears. This is especially the case if he feels his doctor is able to understand how he feels, treats his feelings with respect, and is able to take them into consideration in treating him. The patient may find more reassurance in this kind of experience with his physician than any amount of more overtly offered reassurance, which often is given to ease the physician's, and not just the patient's, anxiety. Establishing a relationship characterized by an ongoing interest in what the patient's illness and management mean to him, and titrating explanations based on what the physician feels his patient can understand and bear to hear, can help enable the doctor–patient couple collaborate in a management plan, even when the medical prognosis is realistically unfavorable.

CONCLUSIONS

Anxiety and other adverse psychological reactions to illness and treatment can have both direct and indirect effects on medical morbidity and on the patient's ability to collaborate effectively with his physician in the treatment of his illness. Psychoanalytically informed psychiatric liaison can help to reduce medical morbidity and to enhance the treatment of medically ill patients. By anticipating problems before they arise, using their own knowledge of their patients, physicians may prevent some of this morbidity in their patients.

REFERENCES

Davies R (1958). *A Mixture of Frailties*. Toronto: MacMillan.
Erikson E (1950). *Childhood and Society*. New York: Norton.
Freud S (1905/1960). Jokes and their relation to the unconscious. In: Strachey J (ed.), *The Standard Edition of the Complete Psychological Works of Sigmund Freud*. London: Hogarth Press.
Hackett T, Weisman A (1960a). Psychiatric management of operative syndromes I: Therapeutic consultation and the effect of noninterpretive intervention. *Psychosomatic Medicine* 22(4):267–282.

Hackett T, Weisman A (1960b). Psychiatric management of operative syndromes II: Psychodynamic factors in formulation and management. *Psychosomatic Medicine* 22(5):356–372.

Meyer E, Mendelson M (1961). Psychiatric consultations with patients on medical and surgical wards: Patterns and processes. *Psychiatry* 24:197–220.

Miller WB (1973a). Psychiatric consultation I: A general systems approach. *The International Journal of Psychiatry in Medicine* 4(2):135–145.

Miller WB (1973b). Psychiatric consultation II: Conceptual and pragmatic issues of formulation. *The International Journal of Psychiatry in Medicine* 4(2):251–271.

Ramsay R (1983) Use and abuse of psychiatric consultation. *Medicine North America* 35:3328–3331.

Reiser M, Bakst H (1975). Psychophysiological and psychodynamic problems of the patient with structural heart disease. In: Arieti S (ed.), *American Handbook of Psychiatry*, 2nd edition, Vol. IV. New York: Basic Books, 618–624.

Rodin G (1983). Psychosocial aspects of diabetes mellitus. *Canadian Journal of Psychiatry* 28:219–223.

Steinberg P (1983a). The psychiatry of family practice: Personality disorders II: Interviewing the patient. *Canadian Family Physician* 29:1953–1957.

Steinberg P (1983b). The psychiatry of family practice: Personality disorders I: The problem patient. *Canadian Family Physician* 29:1942–1947.

CHAPTER 9

WHERE DOES MY PATIENT FIT IN?: ORGANIZING ONE'S DIAGNOSTIC THINKING IN DIFFERENTIATING PATIENTS ACCORDING TO THEIR SYMPTOMS

This is a method of organizing diagnostic thinking, based on patients' presenting symptoms. Patients may present with psychological symptoms and be diagnosed with a psychiatric disturbance. Similarly, patients may present with physical symptoms and be diagnosed with a medical condition. In these cases, diagnosis is straightforward. In less straightforward situations, patients may present with psychological symptoms, and have a medical condition accounting for these symptoms, resulting in a psychiatric diagnosis of organic mental disorder, in addition to the medical diagnosis. Patients also may present with physical symptoms for which there is a not medical diagnosis. In these situations, the patient may have a somatic symptom disorder (formerly called somatization disorder), illness anxiety disorder (formerly hypochondriasis), or conversion disorder (formerly hysteria), where the physical symptoms or preoccupations represent a psychological disturbance.

Sometimes a patient's medical condition may be affected by psychological disturbance, often related to personal loss, such as difficulties in a close relationship or at work, that adversely impact her psychological equilibrium. Precipitation, exacerbation, or perpetuation of the patient's medical condition may follow. Alternatively, a patient may have a negative psychological reaction to her illness or its management, resulting in psychiatric symptoms that further complicate the illness. Defining the patient's problems by considering the manner of symptom presentation is helpful in management planning.

Historically, physicians sometimes dismissed some patients as being crazy, neurotic, or attention seeking when they presented with physical symptoms for which there was no diagnosable medical condition. Sometimes they made denigrating descriptions of these patients, such as hypochondriacal or hysterical. Although publication of the *Diagnostic and Statistical Manual of Mental Disorders* (DSM-5) (American Psychiatric Association, 2013) is helpful in diagnosis and management planning, it relies on symptom clusters for diagnosis. This provides little understanding of patients beyond their symptoms. However, the *Psychodynamic Diagnostic Manual* (Lingiardi & McWilliams, 2017) takes a more comprehensive approach to diagnosis, informed by psychoanalytic concepts, one that invites physicians to understand their patients' cognitive, emotional, and behavioral characteristics. This includes patients' psychodynamics (consideration of unconscious motivations), psychic functioning, and quality of their relationships; their emotional tolerance, and expression and regulation of emotions; their capacity to observe themselves and others; unconscious mental mechanisms of defense; the ability to understand themselves and others; and their ability to cope. This takes account of the patient's personality, including personality disturbance and her unconscious experience of her disorder, including emotional and somatic states and patterns of thinking. Psychiatric diagnosis *per se* does not include the above considerations of personality, relationships, and patterns of thinking and emotional regulation, all of which lead to a more profound understanding of the patient's psychiatric disturbance.

ORGANIZING PSYCHOLOGICAL AND MEDICAL SYMPTOMS

When patients present with medical symptoms, this may, in a straightforward manner, be a manifestation of medical disease. For example, congestive heart failure may present with fatigue, pedal edema, orthopnea, and tachycardia, **1** in this chapter's Appendix. On the other hand, medical symptoms may be a manifestation of a psychiatric disturbance. In this case, a diagnosis of somatic symptom disorder, illness anxiety disorder, or conversion disorder may be appropriate. For example, somatic symptom disorder may present with multiple recurring physical complaints, associated with thoughts, feelings, and behavior about the somatic symptoms that are considered to be disproportionate or excessive. This would represent a counterintuitive presentation, **3** in the Appendix. Naturally, patients do not correspond exactly to our ways of organizing our thinking about them, and can present both with medical and psychological symptoms.

Psychiatric disorders may present in a straightforward manner with psychological symptoms, **2** in the Appendix. Medical conditions may also present in a counterintuitive fashion with psychological and cognitive symptoms that do not represent a psychiatric condition to account for the extent of the symptoms, but organic mental disorder, **4** in the Appendix.

Psychological disturbance can present with a psychiatric disorder (**2**) or by somatic symptoms in the absence of a medical condition that could account for the extent of the symptoms (**3**). A diagnosis of a somatic symptom disorder often would be appropriate in the latter situation. Naturally a patient may experience somatic symptoms that cannot be accounted for by the presence of a medical disease, and concurrently have a different medical condition unrelated to these symptoms. A patient with a somatic symptom disorder either does not have medical disease or has symptoms beyond those explained by the objective evidence of disease. A third possibility is that a patient has a diagnosable medical condition whose symptoms are in excess of what one would expect from the medical condition, and represents psychological disturbance exacerbating the physical symptoms of the medical condition. Conversion disorders often appear as a complication of a pre-existing medical condition. For example, pseudo-seizures are usually seen in patients with a seizure disorder. Here the seizure symptom is recruited, as it were, by psychological disturbance, to fulfill a psychological function, communicating the patient's unconscious psychological conflict or unmet psychological need. This conflict or unmet need results in limits in the patient's ability to deal with the current stressful situation (that precipitated the conversion symptom) more adaptively. Even if the seizure disorder is well controlled by medication, the patient may still exhibit symptoms of seizures, especially when confronted with situations that are reminiscent of the patient's conflict or unmet needs (**3**).

Psychiatric conditions, including psychotic disorders, mood disorders, anxiety disorders, and factitious disorders, sometimes present with some somatic symptoms. However, the chief complaints of these conditions usually are not somatic in nature.

Medical conditions can be precipitated, exacerbated, or perpetuated by emotional distress. For example, diabetic control can be compromised when an individual is very upset (Rodin, 1983). What causes the degree of upset is specific to the individual patient's personality. For example, an individual who has experienced significant traumatic separations in childhood likely is more vulnerable to becoming very distressed with a similar traumatic situation, such as a marital separation, in adult life. Identifying this patient's vulnerability can lead to a referral for psychoanalysis or psychoanalytic psychotherapy. To the extent that this treatment is successful, the patient becomes less vulnerable to significant upset when exposed to the subsequent separations and losses that are inherent in life, and consequently is less likely to experience compromised diabetic control when experiencing this type, or other types, of stress. Such patients also often have better diabetic control because, due to their psychoanalysis/psycho-therapy, they are better motivated to take care of themselves, and consequently manage their diabetes better. In addition, the reduced anxiety resulting from the psychoanalytic treatment directly improves their diabetic control, as, with less anxiety, there is less adrenal secretion of norepinephrine and corticosteroids.

The DSM-5 diagnosis corresponding to the situation where a medical condition is precipitated, exacerbated, or perpetuated by psychological factors is "psychological factors affecting other medical conditions," **5** in the Appendix. This diagnosis includes any medical condition in which emotional factors may play a contributing role, and is not limited to med-ical conditions that may have been identified as "psychosomatic" in the past (Alexander, 1987). However, the gastrointestinal tract and the skin are particularly vulnerable organs regarding their susceptibility to emotional factors impinging on their functioning, as is the vulnerability of individuals with asthma to having attacks precipitated by emotional disturbance.

Patients with a medical condition may experience psychological symptoms or exhibit unco-operative or self-destructive behaviors that suggest that these symptoms or behaviors represent an unconscious reaction to their illness or to their physician's management of it. This represents a psychiatric complication to medical illness, **6** in the Appendix. This may be diagnosed as an adjustment disorder, but patients have been observed to react to medical illness with a variety of psychiatric diagnoses, including psychotic disorders, obsessive-compulsive disorder, and con-version disorder. Of course, under stress, an individual's personality characteristics often can be exaggerated, so that an individual with, for example, obsessive-compulsive personality traits may appear more like an obsessive-compulsive personality disorder. In Chapter 10 I describe a man with a preoperative psychotic reaction to surgery. He interpreted his upcoming sur-gery as a deserved punishment. As suggested above, individuals have specific psychological vulnerabilities, based on their personal histories, which predispose them to react adversely to medical management, or even, in that case, to the prospect of surgery. In the Appendix, items **5** and **6** represent, respectively, the complication of medical conditions by psychological factors, resulting in additional or worsened physical symptoms, and patients reacting to medical conditions and their management with psychiatric symptoms.

The category in the Appendix called "conditions presenting with behavior rather than symptoms" includes two large diagnostic groups. I place addictions and "acting out" in the first group because they both involve behavior or physical actions as their overt symptomatic mani-festation. The behavior is motivated by psychological factors, such as intense longing, which in the case of addictive substances can include physical sensations, especially during withdrawal. McDougall (1986) notes that addiction refers to a state of enslavement,

> in many ways similar to the extremely dependent relationship of the nursling to its mother. For the enslaved addict, the addictive object – [be it] food, tobacco, alcohol, pharmaceutical products, or opiates – is … [initially] invested as "good" … its pursuit is experienced as vital to the subject's well-being … Yet once absorbed, the addictive substance is usually experienced as "bad."

> (McDougall, 1986: 66–67)

Some patients use action as a defense against unbearably painful feelings. These patients fre-quently have severe personality disorders or impulse control disorders. The behavior may con-sist of getting into a physical fight, impulsively buying very expensive items (such as a luxury car), overindulging in eating, alcohol, drugs, or promiscuous sexual behavior, or involvement in reckless or risky behaviors (such as dangerous sports activities or occupations). Excessive work either may represent a characteristic way of trying to avoid painful feelings, or may be episodic when one is under more stress. These all appear to involve an omnipotent defense against painful or frightening experiences, such as needing others, helplessness, being confronted with realistic limitations, sadness that one feels one cannot bear, the losses of aging, the loss or threat of loss of a relationship, illness, fear of death, or vocational frustrations. Omnipotence is an attempt to avoid the experience of vulnerability, and involves a denial or disavowal of some aspect of reality. This type of defense usually is destructive to the person employing it, and can seriously interfere with one's interpersonal relationships. Individuals who rely on this defense generally have never been adequately contained when they were infants. That is, their parents were not able to be in touch with their inner experience and help them bear their painful feelings, fostering psychological growth by identifying their feelings to them and providing a model of how to contain painful feelings in a constructive way. Frequently the individual ends up engaging in the same types of behavior that his parents modeled.

CONDITIONS PHYSICIANS FEEL MORE COMFORTABLE IN MANAGING

Medical education equips physicians to deal confidently with patients presenting in a straightforward manner, such as depicted in **1** and **2** in the Appendix, that is, patients presenting with physical symptoms representing medical disease, and patients presenting with psychiatric symptoms representing psychiatric disturbance. Organic mental disorder, represented in **4** in the Appendix, in which medical disease presents with psychological and cognitive symptoms, may be difficult to diagnose. However, once the diagnosis is made and the medical condition causing the symptoms has been identified, management is straightforward. In cases of psychological factors affecting other medical conditions, depicted in **5** in the Appendix, in which psychological factors influence the onset, worsening, continuation or (sometimes) improvement of medical conditions, the focus of most physicians is on the management of the medical condition. Physicians who take more interest in their patients as people are more likely to consider the contribution of psychological factors to the medical condition, which might result in them offering support, exploring with the patient the nature of the stresses he is under, and/or requesting a psychiatric consultation. The psychiatrist may explore in more detail what psychological factors are complicating the medical condition and provide appropriate psychiatric treatment, including psychoanalytically informed supportive psychotherapy, which is a supportive short-term therapy informed by psychoanalytic principles aimed at fostering the patient's recovery from the current illness by helping him deal with his feelings about whatever stress he is struggling with.

CONDITIONS PHYSICIANS FEEL LESS COMFORTABLE IN MANAGING

In my experience, physicians are less comfortable in dealing with conditions included in item **3**, such as somatic symptom disorder, illness anxiety disorder, and conversion disorder. These are conditions in which there is no definitive medical treatment. A psychoanalytically informed understanding of the patient may enhance management, and sometimes provide symptomatic relief, especially in cases of conversion disorder. Somatic symptom disorder and illness anxiety disorder frequently become chronic conditions that frustrate physicians looking for a definitive cure.

These "somatoform" patients frequently present difficulties to physicians in their management, which consumes much of their physician's time. Questionably necessary investigations, specialist consultations, and treatments may ensue. If the physician doesn't feel confident she has adequately investigated her patient, and cannot identify a medical condition to account for his symptoms, the investigation could continue indefinitely or periodically without benefit to the patient. On the contrary, such an investigation is likely only to convince a patient that he has a serious medical condition. Chapter 7 includes a psychoanalytic approach to understanding these patients' difficulties. Some may be treated by psychoanalysis or psychoanalytic psychotherapy. Here I emphasize the importance of the physician's needing to limit medical investigations and consultations with these patients once she is satisfied the patient is not suffering from an identifiable medical condition.

However, diagnosing somatic symptom disorder, illness anxiety disorder, or conversion disorder mustn't be done by exclusion. One must be able to identify clearly the psychological factors underlying the cluster of somatic symptoms, exaggerated preoccupation with illness, or loss of function usually imitating a neurological condition, for which no medical diagnosis is found, to explain the symptom or degree of severity of symptoms. For example, in one form of complicated grief, an individual reacts to the death of his spouse by experiencing symptoms of the deceased spouse's last illness. When investigation does not suggest that the surviving spouse has a medical condition, the alternative is that the patient is expressing his difficulty in grieving through the physical symptom, for example, chest and left-arm pain in an individual whose wife died of a heart attack. Given that complicated grief reactions usually occur in individuals whose relationship with the deceased was marked by considerable unresolved ambivalence, the physical symptom may also represent a self-punishment the survivor unconsciously metes out for his unfriendly feelings about the deceased. In this case, the complicated grief reaction takes the form of a conversion disorder. Once this diagnosis is made, the patient may be provided with an appropriate psychoanalytically informed psychotherapy to help him deal with his grief directly, rather than expressing it through somatic symptoms. Until this diagnosis is made, the alternative could be unnecessary medical investigations and ongoing suffering by the patient, whose real difficulty is never recognized.

Addictive behaviors, located in **7** in the Appendix, may be used by an individual in an attempt to escape from intense feelings that he experiences as unbearable. We all may eat, drink, or smoke more than usual when under stress. However, when individuals use action as their characteristic way of defending against emotional distress, they may remain unaware of this distress and the problems leading to it, and only are aware of the intense need for the substance or activity they use to disperse the distress, be it food, tobacco, alcohol, medication, opiates, or perverse or compulsive sexual behavior (McDougall, 1989).

Some individuals use other people as addictive "substances" to help tranquilize them or contain what otherwise feels unbearable. The addictive "partner" of such an individual is unaware of playing this role. Often it is people closest to the individual who are chosen for, and have chosen, this role. In this way, individuals who use people as addictive substances play out with their "partners" the roles of their inner world, which is composed of unconscious images of oneself and others. Addictive partners only transiently provide the comfort that the "addicted" individual demands. Ultimately what they offer isn't enough for the desperate, starving infant hidden within the "addicted" individual. The latter often makes the partner responsible for all of his pleasure as well as his pain, and may end up treating this partner as an object, like an addictive substance, as opposed to a separate individual with her own needs, wishes, aspirations, thoughts, and feelings. Of course, the person accepting the role of addictive partner also has unconscious motivations for doing so.

For example, a woman who was mistreated in childhood by her parents and consequently has an unconscious persecutory image of the other (a persecutory internal object) may, on an unconscious basis, choose a boyfriend whose personality corresponds to this internal object, and who treats her in a similarly abusive way. This parenthetically introduces the psychoanalytic idea that many of our important choices in adult life, including the choice of life partners and vocation, are largely determined unconsciously. This patient's clinging to her boyfriend in spite of repeated or ongoing abuse may frustrate the physician who is trying to help her escape from this destructive situation.

I also place patients with paraphilias (sexual perversions) in **7** in the Appendix. Although they certainly involve sexual *behaviors*, the primary symptoms involve the preoccupation with and intense longing for a very specific form of sexual activity, whether with another individual, an animal or inanimate object, or oneself, usually in a destructive way. The term "perversion" has been rejected because of its pejorative connotations. It derives etymologically from the Latin *perversio*, meaning "a turning about." I think one might accept the term "perversion" if it can be used not judgmentally, but rather as an indication of a "turning about" of the individual's thought processes. For example, Ogden (1996) suggests that an individual may employ a sexual perversion as a way of protecting himself against the terrifying experience of psychological deadness. "Compulsive erotization is understood as representing a method of creating an illusory sense of vitality." The individual defends against recognizing the experience of psychological deadness through "compulsively enlisting others in the enactment of exciting, erotized, and often dangerous substitutes for the experience of being alive" (Ogden, 1996: 1121).

Patients having paraphilias/perversions and addictive behaviors also comprise groups that physicians feel less comfortable in managing, largely because they are frustrated when treating these individuals. The current epidemic of opiate addiction has resulted in the establishment of organized addiction treatment facilities and recognized treatment regimens in many jurisdictions. Nevertheless, relapses are frequent, as are deaths by overdose, and many clinicians feel helpless (when not judgmental) in trying to manage these patients. Similarly, most physicians, in my experience, are uncomfortable treating patients with paraphilias/perversions. Many have difficulty not being judgmental about these patients. Most physicians, including psychiatrists, do not treat patients with paraphilias for their paraphilias, in any case. The majority of treatment conducted for paraphilias is behavioral in nature, performed usually by psychologists who specialize in treating these conditions. Psychoanalysis offers an approach that aims at understanding the unconscious motivations for paraphilias/perversions and addictive behaviors, and provides clinicians with an approach to dealing with their feelings about such patients, that is, their countertransference. Paraphilias/perversions generally are felt to be quite challenging to treat successfully. It is important to distinguish between an individual engaging in compulsive sexual practices with a regular partner and with whom he is in a relationship, or an individual engaging in compulsive sexual practices with a series of sexual partners, on the one hand, from an individual with a sexual perversion, which may also have a compulsive component to it. I will describe a psychoanalytic understanding of the origins of paraphilias/perversions and addictions in a forthcoming publication.

Another group physicians are less comfortable in managing, represented in **6** of the Appendix, are patients who react to their illness or to their physician's management of it with psychological distress or overt psychiatric disturbance. The latter situations are very important to identify. However, physicians generally are less well trained to diagnose and manage their patients' adverse psychological reactions to illness or its management than they are to diagnose and manage medical disease. When physicians do not identify these types of psychological reactions to illness and its management, these complications can interfere with optimum treatment of the patient. As well, a patient may suffer unnecessarily in a situation where some of his suffering could be relieved. In Chapter 1 I describe a patient with pneumonia who refused appropriate treatment, resulting in a worsening of the pneumonia and increasing anxiety on the part of the physician.

In addition to the need to identify psychological factors contributing to a patient's physical symptoms in the absence of a medical diagnosis, one is on safer ground in diagnosing a somatic symptom disorder, a conversion disorder, or an illness anxiety disorder when one can identify specific psychological factors that *predispose* the patient to reacting to the precipitating factor(s). In the case where the precipitating factor was a bereavement, one might expect this patient to have a previous history of loss of an important relationship in which the patient was also ambivalent. In other words, the diagnosis of conversion disorder is more convincing when the experience that triggered the onset of symptoms has a specific meaning for the patient based on previous experience. The symptoms of patients with somatic symptom disorder and illness anxiety disorder, however, do not symbolize the patient's unconscious conflicts or unmet psychological needs.

Mrs. Y was referred to me as she suffered from upper-back pain between her shoulders for which no medical explanation could be found. Her symptoms were temporally associated with her husband having taken on a much more demanding job, which resulted in his being absent from the home much of the time. Mrs. Y felt obliged to "shoulder the burden" and assume all the responsibilities of running the home and caring for their children, essentially without her husband's involvement. What meaning might the possible precipitant, her husband's being unavailable to help, have for Mrs. Y?

Mrs. Y was raised by parents who neglected her in many ways, essentially letting her raise herself. Although she was adequately provided for materially, she described her mother as preoccupied with cooking wholesome meals and keeping the house clean, and her father as preoccupied with his work. Neither parent showed interest in Mrs. Y as an individual, for example, by spending time with her in enjoyable pursuits, helping her develop her talents, exploring with her what she might be interested in both vocationally and recreationally, comforting her when she was in distress, and helping her with and teaching her how to resolve the concrete problems of everyday life. Mrs. Y's mother was so preoccupied with housekeeping that she offered little not only to Mrs. Y, but to her three younger brothers as well. Mrs. Y as a child was intelligent and capable enough (one could say precociously capable, based on having to fend for herself) to be able to "shoulder" some of her parents' parental responsibilities. She tried to provide her younger brothers with some of the companionship and assistance they all were missing in their relationships with their parents. As well, Mrs. Y was sexually abused by a relative and not protected from this by her parents, although there were considerable indications of the abuse that they might have noticed.

I understand this patient's experience of neglect and abuse in childhood as predisposing factors to her reacting to her husband's unavailability, the precipitating factor. As a child Mrs. Y never felt she could turn to her parents when confronted with situations that caused her distress, such as sexual abuse by a relative. She also believed her parents were busy with their own work. She felt obliged to shoulder the burden of bringing up herself and her brothers. When Mrs. Y's husband's new work circumstances obliged her to shoulder the burden of childcare and housekeeping alone, a sensitive nerve was struck that precipitated her symptom. In this case, her shoulder pain does suggest that shouldering the burden symbolizes her conflict, having to provide resources beyond what is reasonable, with a background of unmet needs of her own. Mrs. Y's shoulder pain represented a conversion disorder. One could understand it as representing her life-long conflict and an indication to her physician about her current difficulties, that she was feeling burdened and unhelped by her husband (the precipitating factor), as she once was by her parents (the predisposing factor). A symptom can also represent a solution, however destructive, to the patient's conflict. In that shoulder pain rendered Mrs. Y unable to carry out some household and childcare tasks, this enlisted her husband's help. Consulting her family physician, and ultimately a psychiatrist, made available medical care and understanding that Mrs. Y appears never to have experienced in her relationship with her parents, and, more recently, her husband.

An important concrete outcome of establishing a diagnosis of a "somatoform" condition is that an otherwise almost unending series of medical investigations, and even treatments with limited indications, can be interrupted. Only at that point may a management plan that includes a psychoanalytic understanding of the unconscious basis for the patient's undiagnosed physical symptoms be undertaken. Until then, the physician is in danger of being overwhelmed by a *furor diagnosticus,* or a *furor therapeuticus.* A psychiatrist employing a psychoanalytically informed approach to the understanding of undiagnosed physical complaints can help the attending physician with diagnosis and a management plan.

Lastly, physicians often are uncomfortable in dealing with patients having "psychological factors affecting other medical conditions," in which psychological factors influence the onset, worsening, or chronicity of a medical condition. In particular, the focus on physiology and etiology of disease in the training of physicians does not prepare us to consider psychological factors in the predisposition, precipitation, perpetuation (or improvement) of medical disease. These are situations in which a psychoanalytically informed psychiatric consultant, who can offer an opinion regarding unconscious psychological contributions to the patient's illness, can enhance the management plan.

Psychoanalysis or psychoanalytic psychotherapy addressing the unconscious conflicts and unmet developmental needs of selected patients with "somatic symptom and related disorders" (formerly somatoform disorders) may be followed by reduced somatic complaints, hypochondriacal symptoms, or conversion symptoms. Similarly, these therapies addressing the unconscious conflicts and unmet developmental needs of selected patients with "psychological factors affecting other medical conditions" may be followed by reduced symptoms of their medical condition.

FINAL COMMENT

The Appendix that follows is not an attempt to oversimplify a sometimes complicated problem. It is intended to indicate the various possibilities in our current diagnostic system. Of course, a patient may present with a combination of somatic and psychological symptoms, a situation that challenges the physician to discover which category/categories best describe(s) that individual's condition.

APPENDIX

This is a summary of the categorization I have attempted in this chapter.

INTUITIVE PRESENTATIONS

1 Physical symptoms: straightforward medical condition presenting with physical symptoms

2 Psychological symptoms: straightforward psychiatric disturbance presenting with psychological symptoms

COUNTERINTUITIVE PRESENTATIONS

3 Physical symptoms (formerly somatoform disorders): somatic symptom disorder (formerly somatization disorder), illness anxiety disorder (formerly hypochondriacal disorder), and conversion disorder (formerly hysteria): psychiatric disturbance presenting with somatic symptoms

4 Psychological symptoms: organic mental disorder: medical disease presenting with psychological and/or cognitive symptoms

INTERACTIONS BETWEEN PSYCHOLOGICAL FACTORS AND MEDICAL CONDITIONS

5 Physical symptoms: psychological factors affecting other medical conditions (formerly "psychosomatic" disorders): psychological factors influencing the onset or worsening of medical conditions

6 Psychological symptoms: patients reacting to their illness or to their physician's management of it with psychological distress or overt psychiatric disturbance

CONDITIONS PRESENTING WITH BEHAVIOR RATHER THAN SYMPTOMS

7 Addictive behavior (e.g. substance abuse, or "addiction" to work, a relationship, sexuality, or a recreational activity); "acting out" (feelings being expressed in destructive action, e.g. physical violence and criminal behavior, often seen in individuals with some personality disorders and impulse control disorders); and paraphilias (sexual perversions)

REFERENCES

Alexander F (1987). *Psychosomatic Medicine: Its Principles and Applications*, 2nd. edition. New York: Norton.

American Psychiatric Association (2013). *Diagnostic and Statistical Manual of Mental Disorders*, 5th edition. Washington, DC: American Psychiatric Association.

Lingiardi V, McWilliams N (eds.) (2017). *Psychodynamic Diagnostic Manual*, 2nd edition. New York: Guilford Press.

McDougall J (1986). *Theatres of the Mind: Illusion and Truth on the Psychoanalytic Stage*. London: Free Association Books.

McDougall J (1989). *Theatres of the Body: A Psychoanalytic Approach to Psychosomatic Illness*. New York: WW Norton.

Ogden TH (1996). The perverse subject of analysis. *Journal of the American Psychoanalytic Association* 44:1121–1146.

Rodin GM (1983). Psychosocial aspects of diabetes mellitus. *Canadian Journal of Psychiatry* 28:219–223.

CHAPTER 10

"THE MOST UNKINDEST CUT OF ALL"[2]: PSYCHIATRIC COMPLICATIONS OF SURGERY IN MEN

This chapter's title is incomplete, as the psychological trauma of undergoing surgery is broader than the title suggests. This chapter's content also applies to women's reactions to surgery on their breasts and genitalia, especially as it pertains to women's perceptions of their femininity and their capacity to bear children, and, more or less, to everyone regarding injuries, surgery on other parts of the body, and illness that can affect their perception of themselves and their bodies. As well, the personality disturbances that influenced the psychological reactions to surgery in the men I describe also tend adversely to affect individuals' attitudes towards their physicians in many situations, often with untoward results.

The "most unkindest" surgical cut men experience is in undergoing operations on their genital organs, rectum, anus, or perineal region. The genital organs, their "crown jewels," are highly valued as they affirm men's masculine identity and provide sexual pleasure. Although surgeons cut intending to cure, some men experience the cuts a scalpel inflicts as an attack on their body. Castration anxiety can readily be activated. Some men experience a pseudo-homosexual anxiety related to passive submission if the anus is penetrated. I first elaborate on these anxieties and describe their relation to psychiatric complications of surgery, including those that may occur in men following any type of surgery, and comment on the potential for unresolved conflicts from childhood relationships to be projected on to patients' relationships with their surgeons.

Much is written on the psychological effects of surgery, particularly on the female reproductive organs. Despite general recognition of the psychological significance of the male genitals, especially considering the heavy emphasis that classical psychoanalytic writers place on castration anxiety, I found little in the literature describing adverse psychological reactions of male patients to surgery on the genitals, perineum, and rectum/anus, or predicting in whom these reactions are more likely to occur. It is accepted that surgery on these areas, with surgery on the head, especially the face (Kaplan et al., 1980: 1735), renders patients more susceptible to adverse psychological reactions than surgery elsewhere.

Taylor (2016) describes varieties of castration experience and their relevance to contemporary psychoanalysis and psychiatry, showing how this "concept has broadened and is currently used not only to signify fear of damage to or loss of the genital, but also metaphorically to indicate a threat to or loss of any valued human characteristic or function" (2016: 39). I suggest that castration anxiety can represent a primitive fear of destruction, death, or loss of bodily intactness, and therefore the loss of the integrity of a sense of self, including gender identity. Taylor distinguishes between castration anxiety, referring to fear of future injury, and castration depression, referring to a reaction to an already-experienced injury. He emphasizes early trauma in intensifying castration anxiety, concluding, "with many traumatized patients, castration conflicts are in the foreground ... the therapist needs to focus on the patient's proneness to humiliation, powerlessness, and shame" (2016: 39).

I describe four male surgical patients with severe personality disturbance, in whom surgery on their genital or perineal areas was associated with increased psychiatric symptomatology, requiring preoperative or postoperative psychiatric assessment and treatment. In one case, surgical treatment was abandoned because the psychological risks were thought to

---

2 With apologies to William Shakespeare (1599: III, ii: 183).

outweigh the indications for surgery. In a case where adequate historical detail was available, the psychodynamics of the case, including the unconscious meaning of surgery to the patient, are formulated. Suggestions are made on how to identify and manage high-risk patients.

Existing literature stresses the need for preoperative psychological assessment. Studies of postoperative sexual dysfunction are not cited, as I deal with more severe, global psychiatric reactions. Psychological effects of neonatal circumcision (Even-Tzur & Hadar, 2019) also are beyond this chapter's purview. My patients correspond with Taylor's description (2016) of patients with conflicts regarding castration more metaphorically.

LITERATURE REVIEW

Several authors emphasize the importance to postoperative prognosis of the meaning the patient gives to surgery. Schilder (1942) stresses the significance of the body image that may be threatened by surgery. Deutsch (1942) elaborates on fear of anesthesia and loss of consciousness, relating this to early separation experiences and unconscious fear of death. She suggests that preoperative anxiety about being cut is related to castration and punishment fears. Abram (1975) indicates that surgery involves an invasion of the patient's body space, and a disruption of the boundaries of the body ego, requiring a voluntary suspension of ego functions when submitting to anesthesia. Kolb (1952) believes persistent phantom pain after amputation is associated with disturbed coping with loss, regarding this as an expression of anxiety over loss, or a manifestation of depression, and emphasized the need to mourn for the lost body part. Postoperative reactions are less frequent when patients perceive surgery as offering a benefit, like symptom relief or a more desirable body image.

Tichener and Levine (1960) write about surgery activating conflicts of aggression and dependency in patients. Meyer (1967) elaborated on the strength of transference fear, love, and hate directed at the surgeon, referring to the patient's interpreting surgery as castration, homosexual surrender, or as transformation or rebirth, with subsequent disappointment. Physicians are experienced as powerful transference figures; the stress of illness and surgery favors re-experiencing of conflicts in early relationships, especially in the psychologically vulnerable patient. Abram and Gill (1961) find that high preoperative anxiety, denial, and unrealistic expectations of surgery are followed by higher incidence of significant postoperative reactions.

Many stresses associated with surgery generally (Tichener et al., 1957) include: threat of death or bodily injury; pain; metabolic abnormalities; separation from family; financial hardship; and the forced dependency of the surgical setting. Threats of bodily harm and of separation tend to revive childhood fears of parental punishment and abandonment (Baudrey & Wiener, 1975), requiring the patient to tolerate an ambivalent attitude towards the surgeon, *the capacity to see the surgeon as both potential benefactor and malefactor.* Kernberg (1984) and Masterson (1981) suggest patients with more severe personality disorders lack this, relying on the primitive defenses of splitting and projective identification. *Such patients tend toward either idealizing the surgeon as all-benevolent or fearing the surgeon as all-malevolent, possibly moving abruptly from former to latter when disappointed.* Excessive use of these defenses interferes both with relationships on the ward and with the external support that these patients need. Kernberg describes ego weakness in these patients, which favors more extreme transference distortion in the relationship with the surgeon, and a reduced capacity to test reality accurately.

> *Erikson (1950) describes how basic trust develops in an infant's first months of life, depending largely on adequate parental care, given the infant's individual sensitivities. When this development is impaired, an adult is less able to trust a caregiver such as a physician or surgeon. She may either defend against awareness of her lack of trust by idealizing the caregiver or unrealistically devaluing him. Of course, the propensity for unrealistic idealization or devaluation, and the potential for an abrupt switch from one to the other, not uncommon in these types of patients, isn't restricted to situations involving surgery, but is seen in every clinical situation. Men undergoing genital surgery, however, are especially vulnerable to these reactions if they have significant personality disturbance.*

Operations on genital organs are especially prone to adverse psychological reactions (Schilder, 1942). Groves and Muskin (2019) comment on stresses of illness and hospitalization; attachment styles, personality types, coping styles, and defense mechanisms; and emotional and behavioral responses to illness. These authors address the meaning of illness to patients, which varies depending on his personality style, and outline expected responses to illness of many personality types. They describe expected countertransference responses and management "tips," taking the patient's personality into account. They outline mature, neurotic, immature, and psychotic defenses. This chapter is based largely on psychoanalytic concepts that are so familiar that their origin is forgotten and not acknowledged.

Sockalingam and Hawa (2019) describe perioperative psychiatric issues, including patients' fears about surgery, anesthesia, needles, and machines. They approach assessment phenomenologically, and management biologically. Their approach to preoperative anxiety includes providing information to reduce anxiety. They describe postoperative acute and post-traumatic stress disorder.

Guthrie (2019) describes supportive and problem-solving approaches and relational therapies in consultation-liaison psychiatry, including interpersonal therapy and psychodynamic interpersonal therapy. This combines elements of psychodynamic and interpersonal therapies, emphasizing getting to *know* someone as opposed to *knowing about* them. They describe cognitive behavior therapy and mindfulness-based stress reduction interventions. I note that psychodynamic and interpersonal therapy are based on psychoanalytic principles.

The article on which this chapter is based contains a larger literature review on psychiatric complications of surgery (Steinberg, 1988). I found no reference to adverse psychiatric reactions to surgery in Blumenfield and Strain's (2006) encyclopedic reference text on psychosomatic medicine.

APPROACH TO THE CASES

Little is written on how personality pathology of surgical patients interacts with the possible meanings to patients of surgery, increasing the likelihood of psychiatric complications. The psychoanalytic literature abounds with references to castration anxiety (Freud, 1957) and the Oedipus complex. There could be no more fertile ground for speculation on these subjects than the area of surgical procedures on male genitalia, which in fantasy, and sometimes in fact, involve castration or excision of a portion of the genitals. I concentrate on considerations of the patients' interpersonal relationships and capacity to form attachments (Bowlby, 1969).

The reaction of a patient to surgery, which precedes the surgery itself, depends partly on his self- representation and internal objects, that is, his unconscious view of himself and of others. This depends largely on his experiences in relationships with important others, beginning with parenting figures. To the extent that someone views himself as helpless, vulnerable, or likely to be attacked, he will tend to anticipate and interpret surgery as an attack. The more he unconsciously harbors hatred, envy, and other painful feelings he cannot bear to be aware of in himself, the more likely he will interpret surgery as motivated by hate or envy in his doctors. These feelings are mitigated by supportive and understanding relationships in the patient's current life, for example, with a partner, child, parent, family physician, or psychotherapist. The bedside manner of the surgeon will help determine the extent to which the patient perceives the surgeon as benign, intending to help him, as opposed to projecting a malignant internal object on to the surgeon, misperceiving him as an attacker or punitive. An individual who hasn't developed a positive and stable view of his masculine identity is more likely to experience genital surgery as an attack on his manhood. Someone raised by parents he experienced as intrusive may interpret anal surgery as an injurious penetration or even rape. These reactions depend partly on the sensitivity of the individual patient; some are more resilient than others. Resilience may be based on a patient's history of positive, supportive relationships in the past, on currently enjoying similar positive, supportive relationships, on the development of a positive and stable view of himself, especially regarding his masculine identity, on having satisfying and meaningful work and recreational involvements, and on his temperament.

A CASE OF MULTIPLE SURGERY

Mr. A was a 37-year-old office worker admitted to a general hospital psychiatric unit on an emergency basis for depressive mood and suicidal ideation. He had undergone surgery for a rectal fistula two days prior to admission, and surgery on his knee six weeks previously. He claimed not to be depressed postoperatively until his first bowel movement, which he had anticipated as being extremely painful. Three years before admission, Mr. A. experienced an episode of agitation and very short temper, related to the pressures of being promoted to office manager. He ultimately gave up this position and returned to clerical work. Six months before admission, he noticed a "nervous" tremor, began arguing more with his wife, and found that his four children were getting on his nerves. His family physician treated him for "depression" with diazepam, followed by increased depressed mood. Mr. A also had a history of alcohol abuse.

Mr. A described his mother as frightening when she was angry. His father was alcoholic and epileptic, occasionally violent, and afraid of his own temper. Mr. A had to "respect" his parents, whether he thought they were right or wrong. They tolerated no expression of opinion different from their own, and demanded his immediate, complete compliance. When Mr. A first talked back to his father when 15 years old, his father physically attacked him. Mr. A's closest relationship during childhood was with a female cousin, with whom he had sexual intercourse from the ages of 12 to 14. He described this as his closest relationship in the family; however, she died of cancer when she was 20. When Mr. A was 16, he attempted suicide by stabbing himself with a knife when his parents unjustifiably blamed him for breaking a piece of machinery.

Although Mr. A rarely socialized outside the home with his wife, he resented her visits to neighbors, but he never told her this. She generally overrode his decisions. His difficulty in disciplining their eldest son, who was bigger than he, led to his wife's assuming this responsibility. Mr. A believed he had to control his anger completely, lest he be overwhelmed by it and attack someone, which he had done in the past. He related his anger to resentment and emotional distance he felt between himself and the rest of the family, and to envy of his wife, who he felt was closer to the children and could express her feelings. His difficulties functioning as office manager seemed to have two related aspects: an aversion to assertiveness and what he perceived was the cruelty inherent in being the boss, and an identification with the workers, whom he regarded as mistreated, like himself as a child. I believe becoming manager reactivated his repressed hostility to his frustrating parents, especially his violent father. His solution, to arrange for demotion, involved escaping from the anxiety-provoking situation, but doing so in a way that devalued him. I believe this was determined by his hostile internalized parental images. *I also see this representing an identification, in his attitude towards himself, with his parents, and an example of repetition compulsion.* Mr. A clearly had similar difficulties in asserting himself with his wife and eldest son.

With this history, one might expect Mr. A to experience a primitive and frightening transference towards his surgeon, and be likely to interpret surgical intervention as a punishment or attack. The history of stabbing himself in particular suggests a hostile attitude towards himself that Mr. A internalized from his parents, and a warning to his medical caregivers that surgery might be interpreted by Mr. A as being motivated by a similar hostile attitude. That is, Mr. A would expect his surgeon to be motivated by the same hostile attitude towards him that his parents demonstrated, which he also directed against himself with the suicide attempt.

During admission, the surgical team treated Mr. A for incipient anal stenosis by progressive rectal dilatation. He experienced this treatment, made necessary by the rectal fistula surgery, as another aggressive intrusion on his body, comparing dilators to "medieval instruments of torture." Mr. A also was treated for recurrent balanitis by a urologist who recommended circumcision. The psychiatrist advised that circumcision not be performed, in that there was considerable risk of serious psychiatric complications. Mr. A, who had years previously had an inguinal hernia repair, was to submit to surgical procedures on what were increasingly psychologically sensitive areas: from groin to rectum to penis. While in hospital Mr. A recalled a dream in which he attempted intercourse with his late cousin, only to discover that his penis was missing. This suggested that he viewed the proposed circumcision as castration, especially as he consciously felt guilty regarding his "incestuous relations" with her. This was even more intense as he attributed her death to their sexual relationship. The balanitis responded adequately to non-surgical treatment.

As circumcision was unnecessary, one wonders whether Mr. A may unconsciously have influenced his urologist's recommendation to operate: that is, to castrate or punish him, reminiscent of how his parents controlled him, especially when frustrated with him. This is consistent with the history that Mr. A had at least five elective operations (including total dental extraction), for which there were no clear indications. *The dental extraction might be interpreted as an attempt to have himself "defanged."* Perhaps he unconsciously participated in the recommendation for circumcision, inviting the surgeon to help him control his hostility by "attacking" him surgically. *To the extent that this may have happened, it could represent the mechanism of projective identification. By this I mean that Mr. A influenced the urologist, in a manner outside the conscious awareness of both of them, to "attack" him surgically as a method of externalizing his own destructive impulses towards himself into the surgeon. I relate this to the way his parents attacked him whenever he became angry, and to his stabbing himself when unjustly accused by his parents.* This hypothesis is plausible with respect to the index admission, as Mr. A recently had been experiencing increasing difficulty managing his frustration with his wife and children. Apart from the practical implications, possibly unnecessary surgery, the tragedy of this is that it involves a vicious cycle, increasing Mr. A's frustration with the urologist as he relives his difficulties with his parents with him. Of course, Mr. A likely would deal with this frustration in a characteristic self-destructive fashion. *Menninger (1934) has commented on unconscious motivations for polysurgery, including avoiding facing something that one fears more than surgery; longing for a strong father, sometimes involving a belief that acceptance of love from a father is conditional on experiencing pain; and the wish to be castrated or attacked.*

> *In retrospect, I suggest that Mr. A's feeling that he had to be the "big man" at work in the managerial position resulted in his developing expectations for himself that he felt he could not meet. Perhaps Mr. A was afraid that he would treat his subordinates as his parents, especially his father, had treated him. In object relations terms, Mr. A appeared afraid of projecting an abused child self-image onto his subordinates, while identifying with an abusive, angry internal object based on his experience of his parents. He also may have projected the abusive internal object onto his superiors, afraid that he would not meet their expectations, and became afraid of their punitive response, identifying with his abused child self-image. An alternative hypothesis is that Mr. A equated success with overcoming and killing his father, and feared retaliation by someone representing his father, such as a superior.*

A CASE OF PROSTATECTOMY

My data on Mr. B, a 56-year-old married man, are very limited. I present this case to give an example of a severe psychiatric disorder exacerbated by urological surgery, where awareness of a patient's psychiatric history suggests the need for preoperative psychiatric assessment, rendering possible preoperative psychiatric management, including psychological preparation for surgery. Mr. B was admitted to the psychiatric unit complaining of intense fear and anxiety, having been treated for six weeks for similar symptoms at another inpatient facility without improvement. These symptoms had worsened since a prostatectomy three months prior to admission. He suffered several "breakdowns" over five years characterized by anxiety and depression. Treatment had included electroconvulsive therapy (ECT). He had received a disability pension for his psychiatric condition. He intermittently was employed as a janitor, but his functioning gradually declined. He had erectile dysfunction since the prostatectomy. On admission he seemed weak and fragile, although apparently in good physical health. He had some suicidal ideation, thought others were trying to harm him, and appeared suspicious.

Mr. B's presenting symptoms became more severe after admission. He developed auditory hallucinations of threatening voices. He was treated with amitriptyline and haloperidol. Remission of the acute symptoms followed within a few days. He was discharged with diagnoses of psychotic major depression and inadequate personality.

> *This patient's history of chronic depression and anxiety with "breakdowns", severe enough to warrant a disability pension, following a gradual decline in occupational functioning, suggests that he had a somewhat vulnerable image of himself as a man. Considering that, his physician might enquire about Mr. B's feelings about himself and about the planned prostate surgery. Mr. B's history of erectile dysfunction likely affected his sense of potency as a man; this was not explored. Some education regarding what to expect postoperatively, as well as sensitive explanation of possible surgical complications, from common and self-limiting postoperative symptoms to more serious ones, such as erectile dysfunction, in the context of an ongoing supportive relationship, probably in the best circumstances a trusted family physician, likely would*

have given Mr. B the best chance of recovering from surgery without major psychiatric complications. Mr. B's increased depression and anxiety, paranoid ideation and suspiciousness, culminating in auditory hallucinations, suggest that he experienced the prostatectomy as an attack.

A CASE OF UNILATERAL ORCHIDECTOMY

Mr. C was a 43-year-old married man with five children who complained of anxiety for eight weeks following unilateral orchidectomy for testicular cysts. He was also preoccupied with somatic concerns, a feeling of pressure in his head, and a constant awareness of his heartbeat. His agitation rendered him unable to work. Mr. C's suspicion that postoperative analgesics had damaged his brain was the first indication he might have thought that his physician was harming him.

Mr. C was neglected by his mother, who left him alone from the age of three, "shopping" for most of every day. His father's attention involved forcing Mr. C to comply with his expectations, such as practicing the guitar and public performances, and doing household chores. Mr. C's wife "wore the pants in the family." She appeared very protective of Mr. C, who described their relationship as "one body, split apart." Mrs. C appeared to be in charge of her husband, not just during his illness. She rarely would cook his favorite dishes, and only according to her own inflexible schedule. Mr. C's eldest daughter worked at an identical job as her father in the same office. She took over from him the responsibility of disciplining the younger children.

Mr. C gave a history of severe hypochondriacal reactions to previous operations, including excision of a normal appendix followed by abdominal complaints for two years. Exploratory laparotomy, inguinal hernia repair, and cholecystectomy were all followed by somatic preoccupations lasting for years, including perianal burning and pruritus. Mr. C had no history of previous psychiatric treatment. For several years he masturbated while watching through binoculars a neighbor couple having sexual intercourse.

During admission, Mr. C's inability to be appropriately assertive became obvious, as did his inability to engage in any form of psychological treatment. He felt supported only by interest shown in his somatic complaints and the willingness of the psychiatrist to find the "right medicine" for him. Many neuroleptics and antidepressants were tried before a combination was found that relieved his agitation and preoccupations without causing intolerable side effects. Mr. C viewed himself as the passive recipient of treatment, unamenable even to learning muscle relaxation techniques. It was impossible to explore with Mr. C the meaning to him of surgical excision of his testicle. However, his comment that his wife wore the pants in the family, his avoidance of sexual intercourse with her, and his general passivity supported a casual comment that he made about not feeling like much of a man, especially since the orchidectomy. This feeling seems to have been expressed by his somatic complaints. Discharge diagnoses were hypochondriasis (illness anxiety disorder), generalized anxiety disorder, and dependent personality disorder.

Mr. C's presentation, consisting of somatic concerns and some hints of paranoid ideation regarding the results of treatment, leave the impression of someone who has difficulty articulating his inner experience or expressing his conscious feelings, which are expressed in somatic terms. This became evident in Mr. C's inability to explore the meaning to him of the excision of a testicle, his unwillingness to pursue any psychological treatment, and his insistence on a medical solution to his symptoms. His history of hypochondriacal reactions and somatic symptoms after previous operations was a warning sign to his surgeon that surgery should be undertaken only if absolutely necessary. Careful psychological preparation, including repeated and detailed explanations of investigations, hospital and surgical routine, and what can be expected postoperatively, would be necessary to have the best chance of minimizing the expectable hypochondriacal reaction to surgery. The fact that the surgery literally involved a partial castration in an individual whose identity as a man appeared very compromised makes this preparation even more vital.

In addition, Mr. C's description of himself and his wife as "one body, split apart" leaves the impression of an individual with poor awareness of boundaries between himself and his wife, as though he experienced himself as merged with her, and possibly not responsible for, or able to conceive of, functioning as an independent individual. This and the history of voyeurism suggest a quite severe personality disturbance, making Mr. C all the more vulnerable to serious psychiatric complications following surgery, especially involving the genitals. This is consistent with the limitations experienced in Mr. C's ability to cooperate as an active partner with hospital treatment.

I suspect the description of early neglect by his mother and of coercive behavior by his father, although consistent with the rest of the history, may not tell the whole story of untoward early influences on Mr. C. Individuals with similar histories often are found to have experienced severe early trauma that could not be processed and/or severe ongoing unmet emotional and attachment needs as children, resulting in insecure attachment. Sometimes collateral histories elicited from family members provide a view of a patient's early life that the patient is unable to give his physician. This information is helpful in making psychodynamic formulations, including an assessment of the likelihood of severe personality pathology, which can facilitate hospital management of such patients.

A CASE OF RECTAL CARCINOMA

Mr. D, a 55-year-old bachelor, was admitted to hospital with a provisional diagnosis of rectal carcinoma. Two days after diagnosis was confirmed, and prior to the planned surgical treatment, Mr. D expressed his beliefs that the medical staff intended to hurt him and that his illness was divine punishment for previous transgressions. He also experienced command hallucinations instructing him to kill himself. He alternated between denying the seriousness of his illness and feeling that he inevitably would die.

Mr. D had worked intermittently at various security guard jobs over the years, but was currently unemployed. He lived in a boarding house for many years, his main social contact being the landlord. The boarding house was about to be closed. Mr. D had no other close relationships. He had a homosexual orientation that he had never acted on, believing that such impulses were wrong.

Mr. D was the last of ten children. He described his father as busy and unavailable, whereas his mother was strict and punitive. He had not been in contact with any members of his family for many years. Our diagnosis was brief reactive psychosis. Mr. D was treated with haloperidol. We advised the surgical team to confront his belief that his illness was punishment, provide a medical explanation for it, and attempt realistically to discuss his prognosis.

Mr. D briefly was transferred to the psychiatric unit because of suicide risk. It appeared inadvisable to explore Mr. D's belief that the rectal carcinoma was God's punishment for his homosexual orientation, in particular, for fantasies of having anal intercourse with young men.

Mr. D made a quick symptomatic recovery, and after two days appeared competent to agree to surgery. Nevertheless, he remained quite anxious about his prognosis, which was thought a bad prognostic sign psychiatrically. The psychiatrist agreed, however, that surgery should proceed in any case, as it appeared unlikely that postponing it further would reduce Mr. D's anxiety. The day after surgery Mr. D relapsed into a psychotic state with depressive and paranoid features. Haloperidol was resumed. He gradually became asymptomatic over a week.

This case must be considered in the context of its times, the 1980s, when prejudices against individuals belonging to sexual minorities were more widespread and socially acceptable, and therefore more openly expressed than currently. One could interpret Mr. D's believing that his illness was divine punishment, and his having command hallucinations to kill himself, as manifestations of a harsh, primitive superego. (The superego is the repository of one's standards and values largely internalized from parents early in life.) With an object relations perspective, one could interpret Mr. D's belief that medical staff intended to hurt him, and that his illness was divine punishment for previous transgressions, as representing a persecutory internal object, derived largely from early relational experiences that he had experienced as persecutory, amplified by societal prejudices against gays. Mr. D's persecutory internal object appears to have been projected onto God and his physicians. I believe that in such cases this is based not only on the infant's and child's projection of hostile impulses on to the early caregivers, but to a significant extent on real untoward experiences with them. His command hallucinations to kill himself could be interpreted as emanating from a murderous internal object that likewise was related to early adverse experiences (Ferenczi, 1929). I consider it fruitless to speculate about to what extent actual experience versus temperamental sensitivity plays a role in the development of such symptoms. Mr. D's alternation between believing he inevitably would die and denying the seriousness of his illness seems to represent despair and a manic defense against despair.

Mr. D's transitory work history at security jobs, current unemployment, residence in a boarding house with his main social contact being his landlord, and lack of any other close relationships leave the impression of a socially isolated individual functioning marginally socially and regarding employment. This likely represents significant personality disturbance, and is consistent with Mr. D's having enjoyed limited positive early relational experiences and chances for favorable development. His never having acted on his gay orientation, believing such impulses are wrong, suggests a life of sexual frustration and intense guilt; this and the history of command hallucinations suggests his having a primitive persecutory "super-ego" (Britton, 2004). Mr. D's landlord's intention to close down the boarding house would result in the loss of this important attachment for him, and the disruption of his home.

Mr. D's being the last of ten children, with a father experienced as busy and unavailable, and a mother as strict and punitive, suggests that he received limited nurturing during childhood years. This deficiency, and the lack of contact with any members of his family for many years, is consistent with the above hypotheses regarding his persecutory internal world, with little in the way of internal mitigating factors. It suggests limited closeness developing between him and his many siblings during childhood, and consequently minimal or absent emotional support from his siblings in adult life. Mr. D's belief that his rectal carcinoma was God's punishment for his gay orientation, and his fantasies of having anal intercourse with young men, leaves the impression that he believed that internal psychic experiences such as wishes and desires were sinful and deserving of extremely severe punishment. This primitive mode of thinking makes no distinction between mental contents and behavior, between internal and external worlds, and represents not only a symptom of acute psychosis, but also a generally disordered way of thinking.

Our advice to the surgical team and our own approach to Mr. D was based onbelieving that the best tack psychologically, given that surgery was necessary, was to reinforce reality regarding Mr. D's illness and treatment, offering a different explanation for the cause of his illness besides divine punishment for fantasies of having sinned. I think "confront" could be misunderstood. I did not intend to mean that Mr. D should be confronted about his delusional ideation, but rather that an alternative, non-punitive, medical explanation should be offered in its place, and that this be done in the context of supportive relationships with both the surgical and psychiatric staff. It is accepted that it is fruitless to argue with patients about their delusions.

Mr. D's relapsing into a psychotic state postoperatively confirmed the preoperative negative psychiatric prognosis. He may have interpreted the surgery as God's punishment, performed by God's representative, Mr. D's surgeon. We advised the surgeon to devote extra care in describing the indications for surgery, the pre- and postsurgical routine, and the expected outcome of surgery to Mr. D, both in the hope of mitigating the projection of an internal persecutor on to the surgeon, and hoping that attempting to establish some form of relationship between surgeon and patient that reinforced realistic considerations, along with the support that the psychiatric service provided (to both patient and ward staff), might favor a more positive psychological reaction to surgery. The results were less than we had hoped for, but might have been worse if no attempt had been made to take Mr. D's psychological state into account. Our support of the ward staff involved helping them understand how threatened Mr. D was by his illness and the proposed surgery, and how much he needed emotional support and help in maintaining some relation to reality. I thought it would have been preferable for the psychiatric consultant to have followed Mr. D after he was discharged from hospital, but resources for this support were unavailable, and Mr. D's long-term outcome remained unknown.

DISCUSSION

These patients had severe personality disturbances, likely at the level of severe personality disorder, with serious difficulties both in their interpersonal relations and in their internal worlds. They respectively exhibited (in alphabetical order) borderline; inadequate; narcissistic and dependent; and schizoid traits respectively. There is an indication in Mr. C of weak ego boundaries and a fantasy of merging regarding his feeling that he and his wife were "one body, split apart." Non-specific evidence of ego weakness is apparent in these patients' histories, including low tolerance for anxiety, impulsive behavior, such as Mr. A's suicide attempt, and lack of sublimatory channels for aggression, *such as a satisfactory sexual relationship in the context of a warm long-term relationship, enjoyable sports activities, or an absorbing and meaningful hobby. (By "ego weakness" I mean relatively poor capacity of the executive functions of the mind in adapting to the demands of external reality. "Sublimation" refers to the diverting of sexual and aggressive energy into socially acceptable, constructive vocational or recreational activities, such as a gratifying intellectual, artistic or other cultural pursuit in the context of a warm long-term relationship, enjoyable sports activities, or an absorbing and meaningful hobby.)* Neither Mr. A nor Mr. C enjoyed hobbies or pleasurable recreational activities. Episodes of alcohol abuse, a paraphilia (sexual perversion), and an attempted suicide also suggest difficulties in the modulation of aggression and other affects. Mr. B and Mr. D appeared to have maintained marginal or declining levels of occupational functioning.

These patients' histories contain several factors associated with increased risk of postoperative psychiatric morbidity: previous postoperative adverse psychological reactions; several operations with unclear indications; previous or ongoing psychiatric symptoms; and lack of family support. There also is evidence in these patients of serious difficulties in close relationships and serious emotional neglect in childhood (where the history was available). Mr. A, Mr. C, and Mr. D, about whom more historical data were available, appeared to have serious conflicts over aggression. Mr. A was so threatened by his hostility that he appeared to suppress all assertive impulses. Mr. C seemed to express his frustrations regarding his relationships through somatic complaints. Mr. D was a caricature of meekness, to the extent that his behavior suggested a characterological defense against aggressiveness. *Individuals who are anxious about their own aggression have a tendency to project it, that is, to see it in others rather than in themselves. To the extent that they do this, they become frightened of those in whom they see their own aggression. In extreme cases, this can involve delusions of persecution and auditory hallucinations.* Common also to these three patients is a history of poor sexual adjustment, including incest, voyeurism, or ego-dystonic homosexuality, about which all three admitted intense guilt and anxiety. None of these patients had a marital history (or, in the case of Mr. D, a history of a sustained gay relationship) characterized by satisfactory sexual functioning within the context of a stable relationship. The two patients who had children were described as ineffectual fathers and husbands, who alternately were ruled or supported by their wives and children.

Surgery on the genitals was interpreted by these patients in a concrete way as a further attack on their manhood, or, in Mr. D's case, as punishment for his "sinful" experience of his manhood. Surgery thus exacerbated these men's deficient experience of themselves being intact, functioning men having personalities in which their aggressive and loving impulses were integrated in the context of satisfying relationships. These deficiencies predisposed them to this way of interpreting surgery.

These patients spent between one and eight weeks hospitalized with disabling psychiatric symptoms that were precipitated or exacerbated by elective surgery on their genitals, perineum, or rectum, without psychological preparation. Considering the difficulties regarding dependency, aggression, sexuality, and interpersonal relationships in these patients, it is not surprising that they experienced serious psychological reactions to surgery. Their conflicts regarding sexuality and difficulty in fulfilling the role (in their eyes) of man in the family predisposed them to psychiatric complications, particularly to these types of surgery.

Family physicians and surgeons cannot be expected routinely to take involved preoperative histories of their patients' emotional adjustment or relationships, nor to make formulations regarding their interpersonal and intrapsychic difficulties. However, the traditional medical/surgical history could be adapted, especially when surgery on psychologically sensitive organs, such as the male genitals, anus/rectum, or perineum is contemplated. Physicians taking such a history are better positioned to know when to consult a consultation-liaison psychiatrist.

An important consideration is the physician's interest in the patient's reaction to proposed surgery. The physician having a high index of suspicion regarding the likelihood of an adverse reaction, based on previous knowledge of the patient and observation of him during discussion of surgery, is better equipped to predict problems before they occur, and so more able to prevent them. The physician's factual explanation of what the patient can expect from the operation, the expected benefits, risks, and suffering, is part of this process. This can reduce the patient's fear of the unknown, optimize chances for him to express his anxiety, whether realistic or not, and strengthen the physician–patient relationship.

Specific areas about which the doctor could enquire include: psychological reactions to previous surgical and medical treatment, and to hospitalization; the patient's capacity to deal with stress generally; availability to the patient of emotional support from family and friends; previous history of psychiatric disturbance; present psychiatric symptomatology; evidence of unrealistic beliefs about illness or of unrealistic expectations of proposed treatment; the patient's level of functioning at work, in relationships, and in recreational activities; any history of sexual disturbance; and how the patient feels about the proposed surgery. Also relevant would be the patient's refusal to undergo indicated surgery; deteriorating relationships between staff and patient, *or among the medical, surgical, psychiatric, and nursing staff;* a serious diagnostic problem in the patient, where the need for an operation is uncertain; and patients who show excessive or too little anxiety postoperatively (Cassem & Hackett, 1971; Hackett & Weisman, 1960; Janis, 1958; Kilpatrick et al., 1975).

When the family physician or surgeon cannot assess and manage the psychological aspects of the problem, psychiatric consultation is indicated. The ideal arrangement is having a consultation/liaison psychiatrist as an integral member of the surgical team. The psychiatrist's role includes assessing the readiness of such patients for surgery, suggesting where the indications for surgery should be reconsidered, and direct involvement as part of the surgical team, such as assisting in psychologically preparing the patient for surgery, and in providing psychiatric treatment as indicated postoperatively.

The most likely benefit of psychiatric liaison is that the surgical team would gain an awareness of some patients' needs for a supportive therapeutic relationship. When provided as part of the preparation for surgery, such support often obviates the need for later transfer of the patients to a psychiatric unit. This kind of supportive relationship can be provided by any interested and sensitive health professional on the team, sometimes with the guidance of a consulting psychiatrist (Kennedy & Bakst, 1966; Kimball, 1969).

Bion's contribution to group theory and practice (1961) is a valuable guide to what may befall any type of group, such as a clinical team, any working group in any field, or, for example, all members of an inpatient unit, including patients, physicians, nurses, other health professionals on the unit, and administrative and support staff. Bion described three "basic assumption" groups, which he named fight–flight, pairing, and dependency, These basic assumption groups can supplant the functioning of a work group, such that the main function of the group becomes defensive, involving avoiding learning something, or not carrying out the work of the group. Bion's formulation of how groups sometimes malfunction helps elucidate problems in relationships in a surgical unit, or problems in the relationship between the psychiatric consultant and the surgical unit, for example, a paranoid reaction on the part of the staff towards the consultant (or vice versa).

SUMMARY

Surgical procedures are a significant source of stress. Surgery on the male reproductive organs and adjacent structures appeared to be particularly stressful. Men with severe personality pathology that makes them especially susceptible to adverse psychological reactions to this type of surgery may be identified. The individual patient's capacity to tolerate the stress of surgery should be evaluated in an ongoing manner by the healthcare team from when surgery is first contemplated. In patients who are judged to be at risk for psychiatric disturbance, psychiatric assessment and appropriate psychological preparation may reduce the incidence of such complications.

> *Of course, the approach taken here, of considering both the meaning to the patient of his medical condition and of the proposed surgical intervention, is applicable to all clinical situations. I am suggesting that, although in general, men are more sensitive psychologically to conditions involving their genital and adjacent areas, and to surgery on these areas, nevertheless any individual may, for his own reasons, based on his earlier experiences and fantasies, react with a similar sensitivity to virtually any medical condition or management.*

REFERENCES

Abram HS (1975). Psychiatry and surgery. In: Freedman A, Kaplan F, Sadock B (eds.), *Comprehensive Textbook of Psychiatry*, 2nd edition. Baltimore, MD: Williams and Wilkins.

Abram HS, Gill BF (1961). Predictions of postoperative psychiatric complications. *New England Journal of Medicine* 265:1123.

Baudrey F, Wiener A (1975). The surgical patient. In: Strain JJ, Grossman S (eds.), *Psychological Care of the Medically Ill*. New York: Appleton-Century-Crofts, 123.

Bion WR (1961). *Experiences in Groups and Other Papers*. London: Tavistock Publications.

Blumenfield M, Strain J (2006). *Psychosomatic Medicine*. Philadelphia, PA: Lippincott and Williams & Williams.

Bowlby J (1969). *Attachment*. London: Hogarth Press.

Britton R (2004). Narcissistic disorders in clinical practice. *Journal of Analytic Psychology* 49(4):477–490.

Cassem N, Hackett TP (1971). Psychiatric consultation in a coronary care unit. *Annals of Internal Medicine* 75:9–14.

Deutsch H (1942) Some psychoanalytic observations in surgery. *Psychosomatic Medicine* 4:105.

Erikson E (1950). *Childhood and Society*. New York: Norton.

Even-Tzur E, Hadar U (2019). Castration, circumcision, binding: Fathers and agents of socially accepted violence. *Psychoanalytic Quarterly* 88(2):349–376.

Ferenczi S (1929/1994). The unwanted child and his death instinct. In: *Final Contributions to the Problems and Methods of Psychoanalysis*. London: Karnac.

Freud S (1957). Inhibitions, symptoms and anxiety. In: Strachey J (ed.), *Standard Edition of the Complete Psychological Works of Sigmund Freud. Vol. XX*. London: Hogarth Press, 82.

Groves MS, Muskin PR (2019). Psychological responses to illness. In: Levenson JL (ed.), *Textbook of Psychosomatic Medicine and Consultation-Liaison Psychiatry*. Washington, DC: American Psychiatric Association Publishing.

Guthrie G (2019). Psychotherapy. In: Levenson JL (ed.), *Textbook of Psychosomatic Medicine and Consultation-Liaison Psychiatry*. Washington, DC: American Psychiatric Association Publishing.

Hackett TP, Weisman AD (1960). I. Psychiatric management of operative syndromes. *Journal of Psychosomatic Medicine* 12(4):267–282.

Janis IL (1958). *Psychological Stress: Psychoanalytic and Behavioral Studies of Surgical Patients*. New York: John Wiley.

Kaplan H, Freedman A, Sadock B (eds.) (1980). *Comprehensive Textbook of Psychiatry*, 3rd edition. Baltimore, MD: Williams and Wilkins.

Kennedy J, Bakst H (1966). The influence of emotions on the outcome of cardiac surgery: A predictive study. *Bulletin of the New York Academy of Medicine* 42:811.

Kernberg OF (1984). *Severe Personality Disorders, Psychotherapeutic Strategies*. New Haven, CT: Yale University Press.

Kilpatrick DG, Miller WC, Allain AN, Huggins MB, Lee WH, Jr (1975). The use of psychological test data to predict open heart surgery outcome: A prospective study. *Psychosomatic Medicine* 37(1):62–73.

Kimball CP (1969). Psychological response to the experience of open heart surgery, I. *American Journal of Psychiatry* 126:3.

Kolb L (1952). Psychology of the amputee: Phantom phenomena, body image and pain. *Collected Papers of the Mayo Clinic* 44:586.

Masterson JF (1981). *The Narcissistic and Borderline Disorders: An Integrated Developmental Approach*. New York: Brunner/ Mazel.

Menninger KA (1934). Polysurgery and polysurgical addiction. *Psychoanalytic Quarterly* 3:173.

Meyer BC (1967). Considerations of the doctor–patient relationship in the practice of surgery. *International Psychiatric Clinics* 4:17.

Schilder P (1942). *The Image and Appearance of the Human Body*. London: Kegan Paul.

Shakespeare W (1599). *Julius Caesar*. Mowat BA, Werstine P (eds.), Folger Shakespeare Library. New York: Washington Square Press.

Sockalingam S, Hawa R (2019). Surgery. In: Levenson JL (ed.), *Textbook of Psychosomatic Medicine and Consultation-Liaison Psychiatry*. Washington, DC: American Psychiatric Association Publishing.

Steinberg PI (1988). Psychiatric complications of surgery in the male. *Canadian Journal of Psychiatry* 33(1):28–33.

Taylor GI (2016). Varieties of castration experience: Relevance to contemporary psychoanalysis and psychodynamic psychotherapy. *Psychodynamic Psychiatry* 44(1):39–68.

Tichener JL, Levine M (1960). *Surgery as a Human Experience: The Psychodynamics of Surgical Practice*. New York: Oxford University Press.

Tichener JL, Zwerling I, Gottschalk LA, Levine M, Silver H, Cowett A, Cohen S, Culbertson W (1957). Consequences of surgical illness and treatment. *Archives of Neurology and Psychiatry* 77:623.

CHAPTER 11

PSYCHIATRIC DIAGNOSIS IS NOT A DIAGNOSIS OF EXCLUSION: A PATIENT WITH INSULINOMA PRESENTING FOR PSYCHIATRIC ASSESSMENT

Insulin-secreting tumors may, with their hypoglycemic effect, produce symptoms of central nervous system dysfunction, including dizziness, headache, blunted mental acuity, confusion, abnormal behavior, convulsions, and loss of consciousness, as well as clouding of vision (Clarke et al., 1972; Comi and Gorden, 1987; Foster et al., 1987; Scholz et al., 1960; Schein, 1973). The symptoms of insulinoma often lead to misdiagnosis of a neurologic or psychiatric disorder. Twelve of 60 patients were initially diagnosed to have a neurologic or psychiatric disorder (Service et al., 1976). Temporal lobe seizures were most commonly diagnosed. One patient was admitted to a psychiatric unit for "hysterical" behavior. Other misdiagnoses included cerebrovascular insufficiency, multiple sclerosis, narcolepsy, and hysteria. Service et al. (1976) note that hypoglycemic episodes can also mimic psychosis and brain tumor. A patient experiencing a number of psychiatric symptoms was referred to psychiatry by a neurologist for treatment of his "psychiatric" condition.

CASE REPORT

Mr. F, a 42-year-old married welder, was referred for psychiatric consultation by a neurologist who believed he required psychiatric treatment. Neurologic examination, including computed tomography (CT) and nuclear magnetic resonance (NMR) scan of the head and sphenoidal electroencephalogram (EEG), were unremarkable. Mr. F gave a history of several episodes of a variety of symptoms, over a period of one year, each episode lasting for a few minutes to half an hour, marked by sudden onset and gradual relief. The episodes involved irrational automatic behavior and increased motor activity, with amnesia for the episodes. They sometimes were accompanied by nausea, pallor, and a fluctuating level of consciousness, sometimes preceded by dizziness and diplopia. Mr. F occasionally experienced staggering gait and slurred speech. Other symptoms included giving inappropriate answers to questions, and behaving in an uncharacteristically angry, uncooperative, and even threatening fashion. He sometimes felt people were "doing things" to him. He recalled one instance of echolalia and derealization, and frequently had diarrhea and was incontinent of urine during the episodes. No psychological precipitants, such as interpersonal disappointments, losses, or injuries to self-esteem, could be elicited from Mr. F. He appeared embarrassed about how others would view his behavior, and worried about its consequences.

During the episodes, Mr. F felt as if he were dreaming. The episodes were associated with being fatigued or woken from sleep. Once he drove his car down the street, and became disoriented, not knowing where he lived. He expressed a concern about whether he was being poisoned by materials he was exposed to at work, although he couldn't elaborate on this.

Mr. F had no history of head trauma. Past medical history included hiatus hernia. He consulted a psychiatrist at the age of 22 for anxiety and was treated by some form of psychotherapy with no medications.

Mr. F complained that communication with his wife had always been difficult, resulting in them making decisions on their own, creating mutual dissatisfaction. Detailed enquiry elicited no history of disturbed early family relationships.

No abnormalities of affect, thought process or content, or sensorium were observed during psychiatric examination of Mr. F. The most appropriate diagnosis appeared to be a transient delirium of unknown etiology, with temporal lobe epilepsy being the psychiatrist's favored diagnosis. Not satisfied that his symptoms represented a psychiatric disturbance or an adequately diagnosed medical condition, the psychiatrist referred Mr. F to a general internist. The latter initially diagnosed temporal lobe epilepsy. Eventually, however, Mr. F's episodes were related to a fasting condition, and hyperinsulinemia with hypoglycemia was documented. His paranoid symptoms were replicated in hospital during fasting hypoglycemia. They were relieved by glucose ingestion, fulfilling Whipple's triadic criteria for insulinoma. No tumor was found by arteriography, ultrasound, or abdominal CT scan. The insulinoma was identified when Mr. F underwent specialized investigation in another country, by transhepatic portal venous sampling, which indicated, employing differential insulin gradients, an insulin-secreting tumor in the pancreas head. A benign islet cell was surgically removed.

Mr. F.'s recovery was unremarkable. He experienced no further episodes of the symptoms initially prompting psychiatric evaluation.

DISCUSSION

This patient was assumed to be psychiatrically ill on the basis that no medical diagnosis accounted for his symptoms; a psychiatric disturbance was assumed as a diagnosis of exclusion. *This is a dangerous basis on which to proceed.* Psychodynamic formulation, in which the patient's psychiatric symptoms can be accounted for by a psychological explanation, is essential when attempting to explain somatic symptoms on the basis of psychiatric disturbance. Even with a formulation, this does not establish that the psychological symptoms represent a psychiatric condition. (See Chapters 12 and 13.) Psychodynamic formulation also is an essential part of any psychiatric assessment.

Psychiatric examination of Mr. F revealed some data suggestive of psychological disturbance, including paranoid ideation, ongoing marital difficulties, and a history of previous psychiatric treatment. However, no psychiatric data convincingly explained the patient's dramatic symptoms, which, if not organic in origin, would likely suggest a diagnosis of a dissociative disorder such as depersonalization/derealization disorder, or a psychosis. Specifically, no temporally related psychological precipitant could be identified. Nor was there evidence of secondary gain for the patient's symptoms, with symptoms offering concrete advantages to the patient accrued in the environment, or of primary gain for his symptoms, with a reduction of anxiety about an unconscious conflict or unmet need.

The symptoms did appear consistent with a diagnosis of transient delirium. The bizarreness and circumscribed nature of the symptoms raised doubts about etiology. The initial neurologic investigation ruled out intracranial and structural pathology; the possibility of extracranial pathology, for example, metabolic in nature, could not be excluded without further investigation.

The transience of Mr. F's complaints without concomitant anxiety, the history suggesting vascular or muscle problems, the marked personality change, and the incontinence are atypical for psychiatric illness, unless a diagnosis of conversion disorder was considered. This diagnosis also should be made on the basis of positive evidence, and usually would not be made initially at Mr. F's age.

CONCLUSION

A high index of suspicion about the possibility of organic etiology is necessary in cases with ambiguous presentations, especially when no psychological evidence suggests a psychiatric diagnosis, even if the patient has already been examined by a specialist who hasn't diagnosed a medical condition. The consultant psychiatrist is obliged in such cases to maintain and utilize the medical knowledge that his colleagues in allied mental health disciplines lack. He simultaneously employs psychiatric knowledge his medical colleagues don't possess to positively make or exclude psychiatric diagnoses. Psychiatric consultants are uniquely qualified, bridging biological and psychosocial disciplines. They are helpful when diagnostic problems arise.

This case also illustrates the persistence and cooperation between psychiatric and medical colleagues necessary to arrive at a satisfactory diagnosis and management plan in patients with ambiguous symptoms and rare conditions. The involvement of a family physician, neurologist, psychiatrist, general internist, endocrinologist, and surgeon was required, as well as that of a specialized international team. *Psychiatric diagnoses are not diagnoses of exclusion. The absence of an understandable psychological basis for a patient's psychiatric symptoms in the form of a psychodynamic formulation should prompt the continuation of investigation for a medical etiology of such symptoms.*

REFERENCES

Clarke M, Crofford OB, Graves HA, Jr, Scott HW, Jr. (1972). Functioning beta cell tumors (insulinomas) of the pancreas. *Annals of Surgery* 175:956–970.

Comi R, Gorden P (1987). Approach to hypoglycemia in adults. *Comprehensive Therapy* 13(3):38–44.

Foster D et al. (1987). Hypoglycemia, insulinoma and other hormone-secreting tumors of the pancreas. In: Braunwald E, Isselbacher KJ, Petersdorp RG (eds.) *Harrison's Principles of Internal Medicine*, 11th edition. New York: McGraw-Hill.

Scholz DA, Remine WH, Priestley JT (1960). Hyperinsulinism: Review of 95 cases of functioning pancreatic islet cell tumors. *Mayo Clinic Proceedings* 35:545–554.

Schein PS (1973). Islet cell tumors: Current concepts and management. *Annals of Internal Medicine* 79:239–257.

Service FJ, Dale AJ, Elveback LR, Ballard DJ (1976). Insulinoma: Clinical and diagnostic features of 60 consecutive cases. *Mayo Clinic Proceedings* 51:417–429.

CHAPTER 12

DIFFERENTIATING PSYCHIATRIC AND MEDICAL CONDITIONS: A CASE OF HYPERTHYROIDISM PRESENTING AS DELUSIONAL DISORDER

Psychiatric conditions are closely associated with thyroid disturbance. Psychiatric symptoms accompanying hyperthyroidism include reduced concentration, sleep disturbance, ideas of reference, derealization, disturbances of thought process, phobias, manic behavior, anxiety, dysphoria, emotional lability, and cognitive impairment. Ten percent of these cases become psychotic, usually with paranoid symptoms associated with delirium (Whybrow et al., 1969). Acute agitation may accompany thyroid storm. Hyperthyroidism sometimes presents, especially in the elderly, with a contrary, "apathetic" picture characterized by apathy, lethargy, weight loss, depression, and pseudo-dementia. Although studies suggesting that some personality constellations and conflicts are specific to hyperthyroidism (Wallerstein et al., 1965) have been criticized (Hermann & Quarton, 1965; Paykel, 1966), the concept of precipitation and exacerbation of thyrotoxicosis by psychosocial precipitants has some support. There also is increased awareness of individual adaptational styles to the disease (Flagg et al., 1956).

Hyperthyroidism may first present with psychiatric symptoms (McGaffee et al., 1983). Initially the most frequently reported psychosis associated with hyperthyroidism was manic-depressive psychosis. Other psychiatric presentations include simple, catatonic, and paranoid schizophrenia, psychotic depression, "functional psychosis," psychoses of undetermined origin, and organic brain syndrome (Hall, 1983). Other authors describe associations between thyroid disorder and affective disorder (Bauer & Whybrow, 1986; Cowdry et al., 1983; Garrett, 1985; Giannandrea, 1987; Joffe et al., 1988; Loosen & Tipermas, 1983; Rodin & Voshart, 1986), anorexia nervosa (Rolla et al., 1986), organic mental disorder (Folks, 1984; Lassen & Ewald, 1985), and panic disorder (Katerndahl & Vande Creek, 1983; Yeragani et al., 1987). Major depressive disorder and generalized anxiety disorder were the most common psychiatric conditions found in untreated hyperthyroid patients in three studies (Kathol & Delahunt, 1986; Kathol et al., 1986; Trzepacz et al., 1988). The psychiatric symptoms of the majority of anxious and depressed hyperthyroid patients in one study (Kathol et al., 1986) were relieved without addition of psychoactive drugs to antithyroid therapy. I found no description of hyperthyroidism and delusional disorder coinciding as with the following patient, who presented with symptoms of delusional disorder. Graves' disease ultimately was diagnosed during psychiatric hospitalization.

CASE HISTORY

Mrs. Z, a 42-year-old separated unemployed woman, immigrated to Canada from a country whose history involved trauma, including the torture, murder, and disappearance of many citizens perceived to be unsupportive of the government. Seven months prior to presentation, Mrs. Z was admitted to a psychiatric unit, believing she was being followed and vulnerable to attack. These fears increased over three weeks prior to admission. Mrs. Z spoke little English; it was difficult to obtain details about her fears. She resisted attempts to involve an interpreter in hospital. Interviews were conducted in Spanish by her psychiatrist, whose knowledge of Spanish was limited. Mrs. Z did not allude to the trauma in her homeland.

Mrs. Z expected to be killed by the people she feared, but couldn't indicate why she feared this, whom she feared, or how she would be attacked. Her beliefs about being watched and threatened were fixed and caused her great anxiety. She was fearful on the psychiatric unit, but not angry at and did not feel threatened by staff or other patients. She developed friendly dependent relationships with several nurses, although she occasionally appeared frustrated by their inability to appreciate how threatened she felt from people outside the hospital.

Three years prior to admission, Mrs. Z was hospitalized for five weeks in her country of origin for a psychiatric condition. Her symptoms included persecutory fears. She was treated with "medication." When she was a teenager, her father had been admitted for several months to a psychiatric hospital for an unknown condition. Mrs. Z had no significant medical history, and no physical complaints on admission. She had no family in Canada, apart from a brother she was not close to, who could offer little information except that she was more suspicious than usual.

Little information was obtained about Mrs. Z's early relationships, described in vaguely positive terms. She was married at 27, had no children, and left her husband six years later. She worked sporadically at clerical jobs throughout her life but usually was fired or quit, apparently because of difficulty getting along with coworkers and employers, of whom she was suspicious. She seemed socially isolated and quite querulous in her work relationships. She described her relationship with her ex-husband in vague and neutral terms, not suggesting that she left him because she was suspicious of him.

Mrs. Z appeared fearful and agitated on admission. Her behavior and affect were appropriate, considering her fears. She appeared to have persecutory delusions without hallucinations or a disorder of thought process. Consciousness was full and cognitive functions appeared intact. Her judgment was unimpaired in areas unrelated to her persecutory ideas. She had little insight into the delusional nature of these fears, although occasionally she called them "crazy." No abnormalities were identified on physical examination; routine investigations were within normal limits.

Admission diagnosis was paranoid disorder (now called delusional disorder). There was some evidence for a paranoid personality disorder. Mrs. Z's previous admission seemed likely to be for paranoid disorder. She did not appear to have symptoms suggestive of schizophreniform disorder. Since her anxiety was associated exclusively with persecutory delusions, a diagnosis of anxiety disorder was not considered. A diagnosis of organic delusional disorder was not considered on admission. Mrs. Z felt supported by the ward milieu. She initially was treated with trifluoperazine up to 40 mg a day and benztropine 3 mg a day. She gradually became less fearful, but her persecutory ideas were unchanged.

In the second week in hospital, Mrs. Z experienced episodes of intense agitation of several minutes to an hour in duration. No psychological precipitant was discovered to account for them. They clearly were more severe than her baseline persecutory anxiety, which in itself was considerable. These episodes gradually became more severe and frequent, despite gradually increasing doses of trifluoperazine. They were accompanied by palpitations, hyperventilation, and dizziness. Mrs. Z denied feeling more afraid of being attacked during these episodes. They appeared to have a different quality than her presenting complaints, with more intense agitation, despite no increase in persecutory fears. Repeat physical examination revealed tachycardia of 120 beats/min, blood pressure of 150/195 mmHg, bilateral mild proptosis, and bilaterally moderately increased tendon reflexes. Thyroid function tests were consistent with a diagnosis of hyperthyroidism. Consultation with endocrinology confirmed the diagnosis of Graves' disease and ruled out pheochromocytoma.

Mrs. Z's treatment with radioactive iodine was followed by gradual disappearance of the episodes of agitation. Although her fear of being attacked diminished during her nine-week hospitalization, she was never completely free from persecutory ideation, despite trials of four neuroleptics of different classes at doses higher than those of the trifluoperazine. Six months after discharge, Mrs. Z's family physician reported that she appeared similar to her premorbid state, did not voice paranoid ideas to him, and remained isolated socially.

DISCUSSION

Although paranoid symptoms have been described with hyperthyroidism, I found no other description of paranoid disorder occurring with hyperthyroidism, nor of paranoid symptoms occurring in a clear state of consciousness in hyperthyroid patients. No psychological explanation was available to account for Mrs. Z's episodic symptoms. Her attachments with hospital staff, particularly with her psychiatrist, were positive, despite her paranoid symptoms. A search for a medical etiology was undertaken to explain the episodes, rather than assuming the episodes were psychogenic as the patient ostensibly had a major psychiatric condition. Given her paranoia, one would expect Mrs. Z consequently to fear attack from the staff and react accordingly; one would expect a very negative transference to staff, characterized by fear, hatred, and suspiciousness. These predictions failing to occur made it difficult to explain all her symptoms psychologically. Medical investigation was undertaken to try to explain them physiologically. When a patient's symptoms cannot be explained by a psychodynamic formulation, a different line of investigation is warranted. We don't know if Mrs. Z suffered from a delusional disorder concurrently with Graves' disease, or whether her paranoid symptoms could be attributed entirely to hyperthyroidism, where a diagnosis of organic delusional disorder would be sufficient. I favor the former explanation for these reasons: (1) evidence of a similar condition in the past without evidence of hyperthyroidism at that time; (2) premorbid paranoid traits; (3) history of her father's admission, presumably for a major psychiatric condition; and (4) her ability to distinguish clearly the episodes that resulted in a diagnosis of Graves' disease, that were relieved by appropriate medical treatment, from the symptoms for which she was admitted, which were not entirely relieved during the admission.

It is possible that Mrs. Z's thyroid condition may have precipitated or aggravated pre-existing psychopathology. Psychiatric patients have a high incidence of undiagnosed medical conditions. The unexplained episodes of agitation, different from her presenting symptoms, raised the question of another diagnosis, especially as they appeared despite neuroleptic treatment. It is possible that the communication limitations imposed by psychiatrist and patient not sharing a fluent common language delayed the diagnosis of hyperthyroidism. *These days, with thyroid function tests being routinely ordered for psychiatric patients, the diagnosis would have been unlikely to be delayed in any case.*

It is unlikely Mrs. Z would be hospitalized today. As the observations that led to a diagnosis of hyper-thyroidism were made in her second week in hospital, she might have been treated on an outpatient basis for delusional disorder; the hyperthyroidism might not have been identified for some time. She may not have been provided with the degree of care necessary to identify her hyperthyroidism; observations Mrs. Z's ward caregivers made of her likely facilitated the diagnosis of hyperthyroidism.

At the time this treatment occurred, trauma was not as well recognized by mental health professions, including psychoanalysis. Much progress has been made since then. The psychiatrist himself was not aware enough of the history of this woman's homeland to understand the likelihood that she experienced significant trauma before emigrating. This might include threats to her life or to the lives of those close to her, and torture or murder of those close to her. There was no physical evidence that Mrs. Z herself had been tortured. Her living in a country where this abuse was occurring regularly would be traumatic in itself, and likely made a significant contribution to her paranoid symptoms. Considering that Mrs. Z likely experienced some form of trauma, her fears and suspicions do not seem as paranoid now as when she was treated, many years ago.

CONCLUSIONS

Undiagnosed medical illness must be considered when unexplained symptoms appear or persist in patients being assessed for psychiatric disturbance, even when the unexplained symptom is "psychiatric." This is especially true if no psychological explanation for the symptoms is found. No disturbances in Mrs. Z's ongoing relationships (in this case, with hospital staff) were temporally linked with the onset of her episodes of agitation. An obvious predisposition to psychiatric disorder, whether by history of previous disorder, family history, or premorbid personality, does not preclude the concurrent existence of a medical condition, nor does a well-established psychiatric diagnosis. The incidence of thyroid disease is high, and the association of it with psychiatric symptoms is common enough (McGaffee et al., 1983) that a high index of suspicion of thyroid disease must be maintained when assessing psychiatric patients. From this case one might also conclude that unexplained episodes of agitation in "psychiatric" patients warrant an investigation to rule out endocrine disorders such as hyperthyroidism, as well as pheochromocytoma, a much rarer condition. The clinician needs to be especially vigilant if the quality of the history available is limited by the patient's symptoms (for example, psychosis or cognitive impairment) or by language differences. This case also exemplifies the importance of careful physical examination on admission to a psychiatric unit.

An Afterword Regarding Psychoanalytic Approaches to Trauma and Psychosis

It is not generally known in the medical community, including psychiatrists, that from the 1950s, psychoanalysts have treated some patients suffering from schizophrenia and other psychoses. This provided these severely disturbed patients with an opportunity for improvement of their condition. Undertaking this type of work also offered these analysts the opportunity to learn more about primitive aspects of the mind. They included Harold Searles (1965) in America, and Hanna Segal (1957), Wilfred Bion (1967), and Herbert Rosenfeld (1965) in London. This was part of a movement that expanded the indications for psychoanalytic treatment to include patients with other severe mental disturbances, such as what were called psychosomatic disorders and perversions, severe personality disorders, including borderline, schizoid, and narcissistic personalities, and patients who have been severely traumatized, all of whom previously had been considered to be untreatable by most psychoanalysts. Bion's work (1957) led to the concept of a psychotic aspect of everyone's personality.

Much important psychoanalytic and psychotherapeutic work can be done with the primitive part of individuals' minds. Many individuals are conventionally very high-functioning in their work, and do not manifest the symptoms and behavioral disturbances of individuals with the above diagnoses, but nevertheless have significant disturbance that usually is evident in their relationships. One significant outcome of this work is that psychoanalysts are trained to recognize manifestations of the primitive side of their patients' minds. This can be useful in the practice of medicine in formulating a management plan, and when indicated, providing treatment for a patient whose physical illness appears to have a significant psychological contribution. Examples include individuals who have adverse psychological reactions to illness or treatment, such as diabetic patients who don't cooperate with diabetic management, and individuals whose disease is exacerbated by difficulties in their relationships or by a disturbance in regulating emotion, such as inflammatory bowel disease. A contemporary example of a patient with schizophrenia being treated by psychoanalysis with significant benefit is provided by the patient, the distinguished jurist Elyn Saks (2014).

There has been considerable development of psychoanalytic understanding of trauma and treatments for traumatized individuals based on psychoanalysis since Mrs. Z was treated. That development and the broadened indications for psychoanalytic treatment, including the treatment of patients with psychotic symptoms, today would lead me to explore the possibility of a psychoanalytic psychotherapy with Mrs. Z after her discharge from hospital. Mrs. Z's country of origin had experienced a national trauma when an elected government was overthrown and a military dictatorship established. This was followed by persecution of individuals considered to be enemies of the new government, including individuals identified as being left-wing in their political orientation, intellectuals, authors, scientists, and anyone else who, by their existence, threatened the government. Many individuals were known to have been murdered by government forces, disappeared and were assumed to have been murdered, or were imprisoned without due legal process, and frequently tortured. Witnessing and/or experiencing this, many citizens, including Mrs. Z, fled the country, leaving behind all their personal attachments and material possessions. Mrs. Z never discussed to what extent she experienced these types of trauma. She was admitted close to the beginning of this time of national trauma. She must have escaped relatively early. I was not well enough informed about what was happening in her country to take the initiative and ask her about her experiences before she emigrated. Decades ago the effects of trauma were given much less emphasis than today. It is also possible that I was at some level aware of the potential for an immigrant from this country to have experienced trauma, but was not emotionally prepared to hear from Mrs. Z what she may have experienced. In any event, the opportunity for her to have some help in dealing with whatever trauma she may have experienced was lost. It appears very likely to me that her fears of being killed by people she feared, and her experience of being watched and threatened, had some realistic basis in her experiences in her country of origin.

Individuals who have suffered trauma can be treated with a variety of psychological approaches, including cognitive behavior therapy, psychodynamic group psychotherapy, and psychoanalysis or individual psychoanalytic psychotherapy. A psychoanalytic approach involves helping the traumatized individual both experience the terrifying emotions associated with the trauma and recall repressed memories of the trauma in a bearable way with the support of the analyst. Not everyone who experiences the same type of trauma is similarly traumatized. A psychoanalytic approach also takes into account experiences in an individual's life before the trauma occurred that may make her more vulnerable to experiencing a potentially traumatic event as traumatic, or, on the other hand, more resilient and resistant to the effects of trauma. Advantages of a psychoanalytic approach include the benefits of the treatment being intense and long-term, which offers a greater opportunity for a meaningful relationship to be established between therapist and patient, and the more adequate provision of enough time to enable patient and therapist to experience what, up to the time of treatment, may have been thoughts and feelings that were unbearable for the patient alone. As well, factors not directly related to the trauma that rendered the patient vulnerable to being more severely traumatized are addressed, which is not the case in psychological treatments that are not psychoanalytically informed and do not address the patient's unconscious inner life and the influence of the individual's relationships with early caregivers.

In general, stable, supportive, and loving family relationships, characterized by parents whose relationship with each other is generally positive, are able to empathize with their child, and to maintain an ongoing awareness of and responsiveness to their child's emotional state, tend to foster the development of a positive and resilient image of the self and positive unconscious images of others in the child. Developing positive aspects of one's internal world like this is protective regarding the effects of trauma. As well, what is considered to be traumatic is not merely the traumatic event, but the traumatized individual's lacking the psychological support she needs to psychologically process the impact of the trauma on her. This may be most evident in children who have been molested, where the parents' reaction (presuming it was not a parent who was the perpetrator) is crucial to how the child responds to the trauma. If the parents are pre-occupied with their own feelings about the abuse, at the expense of being responsive to their child's needs to talk about it, for example, or, worse, if they feel guilty and need to project their guilt by blaming the child for being molested, the child is much more likely to experience the molestation as seriously traumatic. If parents respond to the child's experience of trauma with the adequate and consistent provision of love, understanding, and support that generally characterizes their relationship with their child, open to hearing about the child's traumatic experience and comforting her, the child has a much better chance of not being so traumatized. In the case of a national trauma, such as occurred in Mrs. Z's country of origin, the presence of supportive individuals close to Mrs. Z, in addition to whatever internal supportive mental structures had already been instituted in her early years through adequate parental care, would have been protective. To the extent that Mrs. Z's psychotic symptoms represented a reaction to trauma, I would hypothesize that both early protective factors and protective factors at the time of the trauma were limited. With the understanding of the effects of trauma currently available, I would have tried to help Mrs. Z begin to talk about her experiences of trauma during her hospitalization, and continue psychoanalytic psychotherapy with her after discharge.

REFERENCES

Bauer MS, Whybrow PC (1986). The effect of changing thyroid function on cyclic affective illness in a human subject. *American Journal of Psychiatry* 143(5):633–636.

Bion WR (1957). Differentiation of the psychotic from the non-psychotic personalities. International *Journal of Psychoanalysis* 38:266–275.

Bion WR (1967). *Second Thoughts: Selected Papers on Psychoanalysis.* London: Karnac.

Cowdry RW, Wehr TA, Zis AP, Goodwin FK (1983). Thyroid abnormalities associated with rapid-cycling bipolar illness. *Archives of General Psychiatry* 40(4):414–420.

Flagg GW, Clemens TL, Michael EA (1956). The relation of emotional factors to recurrence of thyrotoxicosis. *Canadian Medical Association Journal* 15:993.

Folks DG (1984). Organic affective disorder and underlying thyrotoxicosis. *Psychosomatics* 25(3):243–244.

Garrett MD (1985). Use of ECT in a depressed hypothyroid patient. *Journal of Clinical Psychiatry* 46(2):64–66.

Giannandrea PF (1987). The depressed hyperthyroid patient. *General Hospital Psychiatry* 9(1):72–74.

Hall RCW (1983). Psychiatric effects of thyroid hormone disturbance. *Psychosomatics* 24(I):7–18.

Hermann HT, Quarton GC (1965). Psychological changes and psychogenesis in thyroid hormone disorders. *Journal of Clinical Endocrinology* 25:237.

Joffe RT, Kutcher S, MacDonald C (1988). Thyroid function and bipolar affective disorder. *Psychiatry Research* 25(2):117121.

Katerndahl DA, Vande Creek L (1983). Hyperthyroidism and panic attacks. *Psychosomatics* 24(5):491–496.

Kathol RG, Delahunt JW (1986). The relationship of anxiety and depression to symptoms of hyperthyroidism using operational criteria. *General Hospital Psychiatry* 8:23–28.

Kathol RG, Turner R, Delahunt J (1986). Depression and anxiety associated with hyperthyroidism: Response to antithyroid therapy. *Psychosomatics* 27(7):501–505.

Lassen E, Ewald H (1985). Acute organic psychosis caused by thyrotoxicosis and vitamin B12 deficiency: Case report. *Journal of Clinical Psychiatry* 46(3):106–107.

Loosen PTS, Tipermas A (1983). Thyroid hormones in manic-depressive disorders (letter). *American Journal of Psychiatry* 140(4):511–512.

McGaffee J, Lippmann S, Barnes MA (1983). Psychiatric presentations of hyperthyroidism. *American Family Physician* 27(2):257–260.

Paykel ES (1966). Abnormal personality and thyrotoxicosis: A follow up study. *Journal of Psychosomatic Research* 10:143.

Rodin G, Voshart K (1986). Depression in the medically ill: An overview. *American Journal of Psychiatry* 143(6):696–705.

Rolla AR, el-Hajj GA, Goldstein HH (1986). Untreated thyrotoxicosis as a manifestation of anorexia nervosa. *American Journal of Medicine* 81(I):163–165.

Rosenfeld H (1965). *Psychotic States.* London: Karnac.

Saks E (2014). *The Center Cannot Hold: My Journey Through Madness.* Westport, CT: Hyperion.

Searles HF (1965). *Collected Papers on Schizophrenia and Related Subjects.* New York: International Universities Press.

Segal H (1957). Notes on symbol formation. *International Journal of Psychoanalysis* 38:391–397.

Trzepacz PT, McCue M, Klein I, Levey GS, Greenhouse J (1988). A psychiatric and neuropsychological study of patients with untreated Graves' disease. *General Hospital Psychiatry* 10:49–55.

Wallerstein RS, Holzman PS, Voth HM, Uhr N. (1965). Thyroid hot spots: A psychophysiological study. *Psychosomatic Medicine* 27:508.

Whybrow PC, Prange AJ, Treadway C (1969). Mental changes accompanying thyroid gland dysfunction. *Archives of General Psychiatry* 20:48.

Yeragani VK, Rainey JM, Pohl R, Ortiz A, Weinberg P, Gershon S (1987). Thyroid hormone levels in panic disorder. *Canadian Journal of Psychiatry* 32(6):467–469.

CHAPTER 13

"MY PATIENT IS HYSTERICAL":
ADRENAL CARCINOMA AND HYPERTENSION
PRESENTING WITH CATATONIC STUPOR

This chapter describes a woman referred for psychiatric consultation for "catatonia" who had an adrenal tumor and hypertension. Catatonic schizophrenia is described as occurring in two forms, inhibited or stuporous catatonia, and excited catatonia. Stuporous catatonia involves an absence or pronounced decrease of spontaneous movements and activity, mutism, negativism, stereotypies, echopraxia, and automatic obedience. Excited catatonia involves extreme psychomotor agitation, with continuous talking or shouting, incoherent verbal productions, and often destructive and violent behavior.

Catatonic symptoms provide the clinician with a diagnostic challenge because of the multiplicity of psychiatric, neurological, and medical presentations. Catatonic symptoms may occur in psychiatric conditions, including bipolar disorder, major depression, conversion disorder, and dissociative disorder. Catatonia has been observed in many neurological disorders, including lesions in the basal ganglia, limbic system, temporal lobes, third ventricle, thalamus, and frontal lobe, and in diffuse encephalomalacia, closed head injury, *petit mal* status, postictal phase of epilepsy, Wernicke's encephalopathy, tuberous sclerosis, general paresis, narcolepsy, encephalitis lethargica, and cerebral-macular degeneration.

Braunwald (1989) describes stupor in hypertensive crisis, but does not mention other catatonic signs. Abnormal psychomotor behavior including stupor is a feature of delirium (Lipowski, 1985). Cushing's syndrome may present with psychiatric symptoms, including apathy verging on stupor (Lishman, 1987). A diagnostic hazard lies in patients who develop psychotic features early, when the endocrine disorder may go unnoticed. Metabolic conditions associated with catatonia include diabetic ketoacidosis, hypercalcemia from parathyroid adenoma, pellagra, acute intermittent porphyria, homocystinuria, membranous glomerulonephritis, and hepatic encephalopathy. Catatonia has also been described in toxicity associated with organic fluorides, illuminating gas, mescaline, phencyclidine, amphetamines, ethyl alcohol, aspirin, adrenocorticotropic hormone, fluphenazine enanthate, and in patients receiving high-potency antipsychotic agents (Gelenberg, 1976). Stoudemire (1982) does not mention hypertension or excessive serum cortisol levels as etiological factors of the catatonic syndrome. Case reports associate catatonia and other psychiatric symptoms that are initially felt to represent primary psychiatric conditions with organic disorders (Harris & Menza, 1989; Kirubakaran et al., 1987; Steinberg, 1994; Steinberg & Mackenzie, 1989; Weinberger, 1994). The importance of identifying patients in whom a medical condition presents with psychiatric symptoms is clear. Every patient with a mood or psychotic disturbance requires careful physical screening to rule out treatable medical disease (Martin, 1995). Slater (1965) warns against presuming that symptoms of polysymptomatic patients are non-organic, and indicates that evidence for psychogenesis is not infrequent in patients with organic disorders. However, neither does the presence of a medical condition associated with psychiatric symptoms rule out primary psychiatric disturbance.

CASE HISTORY

Mrs. F, a 59-year-old widow engaged to be remarried, was found by her children to be incoherent and immobile. She was admitted with blood pressure of 230/130 mmHg, and demonstrated unresponsiveness, waxy flexibility, and stereotyped behavior, smacking her lips and alternatively patting her stomach with the palm and dorsum of her hand. She initially was unable to provide a history, would not allow her eyes to be opened, and grimaced and withdrew in response to pain. There were no other significant findings on physical examination. Electrolyte values were within normal limits, apart from an initial slightly low serum sodium level. Five months before admission, Mrs. F was treated for hypertension of 150/90 mmHg with hydrochlorthiazide 100 mg and amiloride 10 mg. Prazosin 2 mg was added one month before admission, and hydralazine 200 mg was prescribed three days before admission.

Mrs. F's previous medical history was unremarkable. Psychiatric consultation was requested as the attending physician believed her symptoms to be due to a primary psychiatric disorder. He felt that hypertension was not the etiology of Mrs. F's other symptoms. Brain computed tomography (CT) scan was normal, which he believed ruled out cerebral edema. The attending physician believed Mrs. F to be exhibiting "hysterical unresponsiveness." The neurology consultant believed that Mrs. F's diagnosis was hysteria, with catatonic schizophrenia as the differential diagnosis.

Mrs. F's son and her fiancé told the psychiatric consultant she had experienced many recent stresses. She had been concerned about allergies, believed she had cancer, and was worried about her heart. She had been diagnosed to have serious hypertension, and was warned about the danger of a stroke. This upset her, as a friend had recently suffered a serious stroke and became hemiplegic. Mrs. F also was preoccupied with the anniversaries of her parents' and husband's deaths. She had nursed her husband during his final illness, which was long and difficult, as was her mother's final illness with cancer. Another source of stress was the return of her youngest daughter, Z, with whom she always had a difficult relationship. Z was admitted to a psychiatric unit three years previously for a suicide attempt, and subsequently refused contact with the family. Z frequently made unjustifiable accusations and unreasonable demands of Mrs. F. Mrs. F's fiancé indicated that none of the other children knew that Mrs. F had made a loan to Z that was not likely to be repaid. Mrs. F was anxious about the other children's reaction to this. Mrs. F herself had no previous psychiatric history. No other family psychiatric history was available.

On psychiatric examination Mrs. F appeared oblivious to her environment. She was able to follow one command, "Squeeze my hand," which she did rhythmically. She nodded twice, but ignored the rest of the interviewer's questions. She moved constantly in bed. Voluntary muscle power appeared to be preserved in all her limbs. Mrs. F was mute, kept her eyes tightly closed, and expressed neither affect nor thought. Her sensorium could not be fully evaluated. She appeared to understand at least part of what was said to her. Her insight appeared very poor. As hypertension was thought unlikely to be the cause of this catatonic state, a provisional diagnosis of brief reactive psychosis was considered, although delirium presenting as the catatonic syndrome seemed a more likely diagnosis, with hypertensive encephalopathy and hydralazine toxicity being the most probable causes.

The psychiatric consultant suggested that Mrs. F be treated symptomatically with haloperidol, beginning with 2 mg three times a day, and that she have constant nursing observation while the medical investigation continued. She responded dramatically, becoming completely lucid four hours after haloperidol was first given, exhibiting none of her previous catatonic symptoms. She was fully conscious and orientated, and expressed concern about Z's poor investments and her own health. There was no abnormality of thought process or content. Her immediate and recent memory and ability to concentrate were intact. Mrs. F remained alert, well oriented, and cognitively intact, with amnesia for the period when she was "catatonic," although she remembered believing at the time that she was being cremated with her husband. Her psychiatric symptoms remitted with the haloperidol before her hypertension decreased. The blood pressure was gradually controlled to 160/100 mmHg.

Ten days after admission, Mrs. F had an episode of anxiety, persecutory ideation, and confusion following a transient increase in blood pressure. Her memory and orientation remained intact. Three weeks after admission, Mrs. F described her "catatonic" episodes, indicating that she was aware of her surroundings and could hear, but could not talk or move. Shortly thereafter, she was found much the same as when admitted, unresponsive and demonstrating waxy flexibility. There were no features suggestive of neuroleptic malignant syndrome. Later that week, she exhibited flattened affect, but was able to communicate coherently, although not to move voluntarily. Her blood pressure was 210/130 mmHg. She had further brief episodes of immobility during that week, but was able to respond verbally during them. Mrs. F described a prodrome to her immobile state: she felt that her thoughts were slowing down, and was aware that she was becoming unresponsive.

Mrs. F had been treated with up to 10 mg haloperidol per day; by three weeks after admission, it did not appear to affect her symptoms, and the dosage was reduced. Medical investigation revealed elevated plasma cortisol level and a right suprarenal mass lesion by CT scan and magnetic resonance imaging (MRI). Mrs. F underwent right adrenalectomy and splenectomy. A cortisol-producing adrenal carcinoma was found. She was subsequently discharged from hospital, having experienced no further catatonic episodes postoperatively. She refused psychiatric follow-up on discharge. She was readmitted three months later for postoperative investigation of adrenal function. Liver metastases and high serum cortisol levels were found. Mrs. F was observed by her family to have had mild catatonic symptoms twice following discharge, but exhibited no psychiatric symptoms during the second admission. She was admitted four months later with metastatic adrenal cancer, and died in hospital two months later of renal failure, metastases, and an abdominal hemorrhage. An episode of confusion was noted during this admission, but there was no recurrence of catatonic symptoms.

DISCUSSION

A high index of suspicion of organic mental disorder is necessary in medically ill patients with psychiatric symptoms, even when there is symptomatic evidence of psychiatric disturbance accompanied by many psychosocial stressors. The psychiatrist must function in his role as a physician, even – perhaps especially – when medical specialists are making psychiatric diagnoses. Concurrent medical and psychiatric investigation is necessary when differentiating medical from psychiatric disturbance is difficult. This obviates unnecessary medical investigations and the withholding of indicated psychiatric treatment when a psychiatric condition can be positively identified, as well as avoiding a psychiatric diagnosis being made by exclusion, with the consequent danger that a psychiatric symptom of a medical condition may not be adequately investigated. Mrs. F's catatonic symptoms appear to have been a manifestation of hypertensive encephalopathy, elevated serum cortisol levels, or both. Apart from the initial symptomatic recovery following haloperidol treatment, the catatonic symptoms recurred during episodes of uncontrolled hypertension. However, many patients with similar degrees of hypertension have normal mental states. With the exception of the hydrochlorthiazide–amiloride combination, which has been associated with stupor, none of Mrs. F's medications are associated with catatonic symptoms. As Mrs. F was started on the combination five months prior to admission, it seems unlikely that her stupor was attributable to medications. An undetected central nervous system tumor may have been a contributing factor to her symptoms. As well, the psychiatric presentation might have represented a functional psychiatric disorder, with the diagnosis of adrenal tumor being incidental.

Another possibility is that Mrs. F, with a family history of depressive disorder, presented with signs of psychotic depression when subjected to physiological stress. Catatonia, like delirium, may be considered to have a multifactorial etiology. Here hypertension and Cushing's disease were biological factors, and Mrs. F's many recent stresses were psychological factors. The many psychosocial stresses to which Mrs. F was exposed may have affected the onset or severity of her stupor, along the same lines that have been suggested regarding psychological factors affecting the course of a delirium (Chapman et al., 1958). In this case the psychoanalytically informed psychiatrist needed to subordinate his psychoanalytic understanding of the patient to his psychiatric assessment of his patient's condition.

CONCLUSIONS

Excessive serum cortisol levels and adrenal carcinoma must be considered in the differential diagnosis of the catatonic syndrome. Appropriate clinical and laboratory evaluation must be undertaken to rule out medical illness in patients with psychiatric diagnoses, especially in patients with psychotic or affective symptoms (Harris & Menza, 1989; Steinberg, 1994). Special care must be taken with patients presenting with acute psychiatric symptoms, with a previous history of normal emotional functioning, and those in whom psychological symptoms may obscure signs of medical illness. *A history of psychological stresses, no matter how severe and complex, does not warrant concluding that symptoms that might represent either psychiatric disturbance or medical disease are psychogenic and represent a psychiatric disorder; appropriate medical investigation to rule out medical disease must be undertaken.*

REFERENCES

Braunwald E (1989). Heart disease. In: Kaplan NM (ed.), *Systemic Hypertension: Mechanisms and Diagnosis*. Philadelphia, PA: Saunders.

Chapman LF, Thettford WN, et al. (1958). Highest integrated functions in man during stress. In: Solomon HC et al. (eds.) *The Brain and Human Behaviour. Proceedings of the Association for Research in Nervous and Mental Disorders*, Vol. 36. Baltimore, MD: Williams and Wilkins, 491–534.

Gelenberg AI (1976). The catatonic syndrome. *Lancet* i:1339–1341.

Harris D, Menza MA (1989). Benzodiazepines and catatonia: A case report. *Canadian Journal of Psychiatry* 34:725–727.

Kirubakaran V, Sen S, Wilkinson CB (1987). Catatonic stupor, unusual manifestation of temporal lobe epilepsy. *Psychiatric Journal of the University of Ottawa* 12:244–246.

Lipowski W (1985). Delirium updated. In: *Psychosomatic Medicine and Liaison Psychiatry*, Vol. 28. New York: Plenum, 1–287.

Lishman WA (1987). *Organic Psychiatry: The Psychological Consequences of Cerebral Disorder*, 2nd edition. Cambridge, MA: Blackwell Science, 437–438.

Martin MJ (1995). Psychiatry and medicine. In: Kaplan HI, Sadock BJ (eds.), *Comprehensive Textbook of Psychiatry*, 6th edition. Baltimore, MD: Williams and Wilkins.

Slater E (1965). Diagnosis of "hysteria". *British Medical Journal* 1395–1399.

Steinberg PI (1994). A case of paranoid disorder associated with hyperthyroidism. *Canadian Journal of Psychiatry* 39:153–156.

Steinberg P, Mackenzie R (1989). A patient with insulinoma presenting for psychiatric assessment. *Canadian Journal of Psychiatry* 34:58–59.

Stoudemire A (1982). The differential diagnosis of catatonic states. *Psychosomatics* 23:245–252.

Weinberger DR (1994). Brain disease and psychiatric illness: When should a psychiatrist order a CT scan? *American Journal of Psychiatry* 141:1521–1527.

PART III

LEARNING FROM INPATIENT AND DAY HOSPITAL PSYCHIATRY

Some may question what the place of psychoanalysis could be on a psychiatric inpatient ward. However, up to the end of the 1970s many inpatient psychiatrists had psychoanalytic training, applying it usefully in inpatient work. Shur (1994) describes how patients and psychiatrists in institutions enact the primitive internal worlds of the patients (and sometimes of the psychiatrists!). Psychoanalytic understanding of these enactments enhances, and sometimes makes possible, adequate functioning on psychiatric inpatient units. The classic work on the internal functioning of psychiatric institutions is *The Mental Hospital* (Stanton & Schwartz, 1954). Psychoanalytically informed partial hospitalization programs can offer effective treatment to many very disturbed patients (Piper et al., 1996).

Chapter 14 originated when one psychiatrist from each Canadian medical school was selected to present a case for publication in the *Canadian Journal of Psychiatry*. The patient's presenting complaint was inability to decide on a name for her child. I use this case to demonstrate how a psychoanalytic understanding of a patient enhances formulation of the patient's problems, and offers a rational approach to the psychotherapeutic aspects of management. In a theoretical digression, the contemporary relevance of the Oedipus complex is described, and how difficulties related to this may be accompanied by a disturbance of thinking.

In Chapter 15, psychoanalytic theory is applied in understanding and managing a psychiatric inpatient, not to suggest that she might benefit from psychoanalytic psychotherapy, but rather that incorporation of a psychoanalytic understanding of her leads to a more effective management approach, especially regarding dealing with staff reactions to disturbing patients. Psychodynamic formulation of a patient, considering attachment and affect regulation, self-image and internal object relations, and transference and countertransference implications, demonstrates how psychoanalytic principles can be applied in non-psychoanalytic settings. Consideration of the patient's personality and recognition of the patient's having a comorbid personality disorder appear important in her management, and have practical implications regarding staff members' understanding of the patient and the consequent identification and handling of difficulties in patient–staff relations. Specific management approaches based on a psychoanalytic understanding of the patient are described.

Chapter 16 describes two patients treated in a psychodynamic group psychotherapy-oriented day treatment program, to which one had been referred from the inpatient unit. One patient's treatment was considered successful; the other's was not. Factors influencing the outcome of these "difficult" patients included considerations of countertransference, the use of a combination of confrontation and support, the therapists' personal difficulties, and what one can conclude about serious deficiencies in our patients' early environment. A digression on the development of the human mind is included. Factors that are prognostically favorable and unfavorable regarding a psychoanalytically informed treatment are described.

REFERENCES

Piper WE, Rosie JS, Joyce AS, Azim HFA (1996). *Time-limited Day Treatment for Personality Disorders: Integration of Research and Practice in a Group Program.* Washington, DC: American Psychological Association.

Shur R (1994). *Countertransference Enactment: How Institutions and Therapists Actualize Internal Worlds.* Northvale, NJ: Jason Aronson.

Stanton AH, Schwartz MS (1954). *The Mental Hospital: A Study of Institutional Participation in Psychiatric Illness and Treatment.* New York: Basic Books.

CHAPTER 14

THE MOTHER WHO COULDN'T NAME HER CHILD: PROBLEMS OF ATTACHMENT, IDENTITY, AND THE CAPACITY TO THINK

I interviewed this patient once and had her admitted to hospital but was not involved in her management. My comments show my learning to think along psychoanalytic lines, compared with my understanding of her when I met her. The unsatisfactory outcome of treatment doesn't detract from what one can learn from it. A theoretical digression about origins and manifestations in therapy of disturbances in thinking is included.

HISTORY OF PRESENT ILLNESS

Mrs. X, a 31-year-old married housewife, was referred for emergency psychiatric consultation because of depressed mood for 11 months since the birth of her second child. She also was unable to decide on a name for this child, who was unplanned. She renamed her daughter five times without finding a name that "fit," feeling unable to feel attached to her until she had found the "right" name. She did not feel she was calling her daughter by name when using these "wrong" names. Mrs. X chose the first name, Joie, after an acquaintance who was described "a joy." This name was chosen two weeks after the child was born. *(This first choice of name now seems to me to represent a concrete approach to naming a child. It seems to refer to Mrs. X's wish that she would experience joy in being a mother and having this child. Perhaps her needing to name the child "Joy" suggests ambivalence about whether she felt joy at being a mother again. Making her wish to feel joy concrete, in a name, appears to represent a more primitive side of Mrs. X's personality. It also suggests that Mrs. X would have difficulty in forming an attachment to her child, which was evident when I met her.)*

Mrs. X felt that the next choice, her husband's, Penelope, was too long a name. She chose another name, Freda, although a cousin whom she disliked had the same name, because it sounded "loving" and "goes with my first daughter's name." Mrs. X recalled a similar difficulty in deciding on the name of the latter, although she denied experiencing overt psychiatric symptomatology during or after the first pregnancy. *This leaves the impression that Mrs. X was ambivalent about being a mother at the time of her first pregnancy too.* She named her older daughter after a cousin, Y, with whom she sympathized. Y's mother required Y to tend to her three younger siblings, despite Y only being 12 years old herself. As well, Y was her own mother's confidante, as Y's father was emotionally unavailable. Mrs. X felt that Y was exploited by her mother. Y as well was neglected by her grandparents, which reminded Mrs. X of her own unsupportive in-laws. *This sounds as if Mrs. X identified strongly with Y in expressing feeling unsupported by her in-laws. However, in-laws are often a convenient target on to whom to displace feelings about one's family of origin that people find consciously unacceptable. For many people it is more comfortable to dislike a mother-in-law, for example, than one's own mother. This is a basis for the many jokes and stories about mothers-in-law. All this suggests that Mrs. X likely felt significantly unsupported in childhood by some members of her family of origin and/or by her husband.*

Since her second delivery, Mrs. X suffered from impaired concentration, initial and terminal insomnia, and decreased energy and appetite, and had gained 15 pounds. She had transient suicidal ideation over several months, but no specific plans. She denied a family history of psychiatric illness. As a child, Mrs. X hated her own given name, which her mother had chosen. This name, she felt, was unusual and often was mispronounced. She also felt her younger daughter would resent her if she didn't choose the right name. *This suggests that Mrs. X had considerable resentment of her mother as a child, which appears to have continued into adult life, expressed by her fantasy that her daughter would resent her. This likely represents a displacement on to her daughter of her own feelings towards her mother. It seems likely that Mrs. X resented her mother as a child for more than just her first name. She seems to have suggested that her mother was not thinking of her in giving her her name, which was unusual and hard to pronounce. This might also reflect difficulties Mrs. X had in establishing an identity of her own, represented by hating her name.*

Mrs. X consciously was pleased to be pregnant, but felt her husband wasn't interested enough. She complained she generally didn't get his full attention when she wanted it, and felt he neglected their older daughter. She also felt unappreciated by his parents, who she believed praised him excessively at her expense, and complained that her own mother behaved similarly. *Mrs. X might have had some legitimate complaints about her in-laws. Nevertheless, these complaints also might represent a displacement of feelings about her parents on to her in-laws. This impression is supported by her complaining that her mother had the same attitude as her in-laws.* Mrs. X found herself downtown several times without remembering why she was there, similar to a problem that prompted neurological consultation years ago. On admission she had been treated for two weeks with clomipramine 150 mg qhs, with little effect.

MEDICAL HISTORY

At the age of 15, Mrs. X was treated successfully for enuresis with urethral dilatation. *My knowledge of urology is very limited. Perhaps Mrs. X suffered from some structural deformity of the urethra that caused enuresis, and was cured by the dilatation, although an online search did not suggest that this was an etiology of enuresis. Another possibility is that the enuresis had an emotional basis to it. If so, today this probably would be subsumed under a diagnosis of somatic symptom disorder. If we could meet the 15-year-old Mrs. X and her family and elicit an adequate history, her enuresis might become understandable from a psychoanalytic point of view on the basis of one of a number of perspectives. Enuresis might represent an unconscious conflict, the expression of an unarticulated, possibly unbearable, feeling, or an unmet psychological need. Enuresis has been interpreted as a hostile act, an expression of fear, and an attempt to deny anxiety, guilt, or depression brought about by hate (Winnicott, 1937). Some authors suggest that enuresis is related to suboptimal parenting, poor child-rearing practices, and disruption of maternal care. I believe some of the above might better be described as a poor fit between mother and infant. Stein (1998) describes a case in which the child's desire for intimacy, following failed mother–infant bonding due to maternal depression, was obtained through enuretic symptoms and interpersonal conflict. He notes that this quest for intimacy through replication of early pleasurable somatic sensations and the utilization of conflict for attention seeking can develop into a cycle involving delinquency, crime, and sexual perversion later in life. He concluded that in such cases, a psychodynamic understanding informing treatment is most likely to succeed (Stein, 1998).*

Mrs. X consulted a neurologist at the age of 15 because of dysarthria and memory problems, inability to understand the teachers or to concentrate on homework, and disorientation when getting off a bus. No neurological problems were found. Depression was diagnosed, but not further investigated or treated. *This description of multiple symptoms not explained by a medical condition suggests that, as a teenager, Mrs. X likely was suffering from an unconscious conflict, unmet psychological needs, or unbearable emotions, or a combination of these, that could not be articulated, and were expressed by a variety of symptoms that often represent neurological conditions. They may have been symptoms of a conversion disorder. The description of an inability to concentrate and disorientation leave the impression that Mrs. X may have experienced some dissociative symptoms. A dissociative state is one involving disturbances or alterations in the normally integrated functions of identity, memory, and consciousness (Yager & Gitlin, 1995). These symptoms might have represented a dissociative disorder. They suggest a regression to a relatively primitive level of mental functioning, prior to a stage characterized by verbalization. With the benefit of hindsight, it would have been wise, especially as Mrs. X was diagnosed with depression, to have her assessed by a psychoanalytically informed clinician, so an appropriate form of psychotherapy could be recommended. It seems likely that Mrs. X's needs were not met by her parents and medical caregivers at the time.*

At 25, Mrs. X again consulted a neurologist for pain behind the eye, stuttering, trouble naming objects, and transient episodes of loss of vision. Multiple sclerosis was ruled out, and neuro-ophthalmological consultation resulted in a diagnosis of "anxiety." *This was a second occasion when referral to a mental health professional with psychodynamic or psychoanalytic training was indicated, but not pursued. Mrs. X again seemed to have symptoms suggestive of a conversion disorder. The suffering that she could not put into words seemed to be expressed in somatic symptoms. Mrs. X's relationship with her physicians appeared to be characterized by a lack of understanding of her needs, which were consequently not met. This seems to recapitulate what appears to have been Mrs. X's experience of her early caregivers. It also reinforces the impression that Mrs. X continued to experience conflicts, unmet needs, and/or painful emotions that she could not articulate in words, which were expressed in medical symptoms. Conversion symptoms are thought to symbolize an unconscious conflict or inexpressible thoughts, feelings, or impulses. Mrs. X's stuttering and transient blindness leave the impression of someone who is having difficulty saying something or cannot bear to see something.*

DEVELOPMENTAL HISTORY

Mrs. X was the second of four children, with an older brother and a younger brother and sister. She described her mother in superficially positive terms, but indicated she could not really communicate with anyone in the family. Her parents constantly fought. Her father was constantly critical of Mrs. X and verbally abusive to Mrs. X and her mother. She felt like her mother's favorite, in that her mother turned to her for consolation regarding her unhappy marriage. She felt she somehow had to make up for her mother's suffering, especially as she believed her birth tied mother to father. *This description suggests that Mrs. X, as a child, felt she had to take care of her mother, reversing the expected roles, and placing excessive emotional demands on her, which she could not be expected to meet. This would help explain her difficulty in articulating her problems, as there apparently was no one to hear them; her mother was described as being preoccupied with her own suffering, and consequently unavailable to receive painful feelings that Mrs. X was experiencing.*

Mrs. X remembered her mother as listless and withdrawn after the birth of both younger siblings; it is possible that her mother had postpartum depression. Mrs. X remembered trying to cook for her mother when she came home from hospital, and was disappointed because she did not appear to appreciate Mrs. X's efforts. As Mrs. X grew older, she increasingly performed household chores, hoping to please her mother, but never succeeding. Mrs. X recalled feeling that if she became close to her father, her mother would be hurt and feel betrayed. She felt she had to take sides, and her mother needed her more than her father. *This leaves the impression that, as a child, Mrs. X had already learned that she had to subordinate her own emotional needs to those of her mother. Children do not do this out of altruism; they hope that if they can provide the parent with enough of what she needs, then the parent will reciprocate and provide the child with what she needs. The child cannot take this care as given, and tries to earn it.*

Ms. X felt that her father envied her close relationship with her mother. *This leaves the impression that her father was somewhat immature and preoccupied with his own difficulties in a manner that probably interfered with his being able to be concerned with the emotional welfare of his children. One possible explanation is that Mrs. X's father never adequately was able to pass through the early oedipal period. That is, he never experienced the entry of his own father into the emotional world in which he as an infant and his mother inhabited in a way that left him feeling enriched by the appearance of a third person, who could introduce him to the world outside the infant–mother dyad. Rather, he may have experienced his father as intruding on him and his mother in an unwanted way. Consequently, he would be inclined to unconsciously hope for a very close, rather infantile relationship with his wife, and resent the intrusion of his own children. On this basis, Mrs. X would likely end up feeling unwanted, at least by her father, from a very young age. All this could have an impact on the development of both Mrs. X's and her father's capacity to think. (I will elaborate on this in the theoretical digression below.)*

One could also infer that Mrs. X might form a rather infantile relationship with her husband, creating an attachment to him as if he were her mother, and unconsciously not welcome the intrusion of her own children. I say unconsciously because such thoughts would be difficult to tolerate consciously, especially if she had felt unwelcome herself as a child. Her difficulty in naming her daughter could be interpreted as a form of postpartum psychiatric disturbance, related to ambivalence about being a mother, independent of her depression.

A Theoretical Digression

The term "Oedipus complex" originally described the experience a preschool/kindergarten-age child has in wishing to possess the opposite-sex parent while feeling a rivalry for the same-sex parent. The extreme version of this is a wish to have sexual relations with the opposite-sex parent, whatever that seems to represent to any individual child, and to kill the same-sex parent, his/her rival. Subsequently, Melanie Klein (1928) thought the Oedipus complex began in the first year of life. The baby, whose world initially essentially consists of her mother, gradually becomes aware of the presence of a third party, her father. This involves the father introducing the child to a world outside the mother–child dyad, and the child becoming aware that mother and father have a relationship that excludes her. This enables the child to begin thinking of what is going on in other people's minds when observing the parental couple, to which she does not belong. That is, the introduction of the father, in this early version of the complex, contributes to a development in the young child's thinking. A successful passage through the Oedipus complex was considered to involve the child accepting that the parents have a relationship from which the child is excluded. From this follows an increasing awareness of and interest in the minds of other people, among other developments in the capacity to think. This involves some capacity to mourn, as well as an awareness that other people are separate from oneself, with different feelings, ideas, impulses, and aspirations. So this is an important contribution to children's processes of separation and individuation, that is, to realizing that they are separate from their mother, and eventually from everyone else, with unique characteristics of their own, including their own capacity to think and their own mental contents that no one else is privy to. Finally, progression through the Oedipus complex involves identifying with the same-sex parent, intending to find a partner of the opposite sex of one's own. Of course, the contemporary focus on fluidity of sexualities and the greater acceptance of non-heterosexual relationships complicates this description.

The term "thinking," as I am using it, is comprehensive of all mental contents, including ideas, fantasies, feelings, wishes, fears, impulses, and daydreams. A person may be inhibited from thinking about specific mental contents, for example, sexual or aggressive impulses. Even normal ambition or an intention towards constructive activity may seem too aggressive to some people. Age-appropriate sexual fantasies of adolescence (and adulthood) similarly may be forbidden. The process of thinking itself may be inhibited, so that a patient may, in a striking way, appear to not be thinking about things that one would expect him to devote significant attention to, for example, his financial well-being, healthcare needs, or difficulties in relationships. Alternatively, a patient's thinking may be limited in its logical or rational qualities. For example, a patient may entertain at different times polar-opposite attitudes with no conscious awareness that what he thinks or feels at one point is totally inconsistent with what he thinks or feels at another point. This involves a splitting of the mind in which two parts of the mind are kept separate, without communication between them. Obviously, this can lead to significant difficulties in one's relationship with the world. With disturbances in the form or content of thinking, reality testing may suffer, either transiently, when an individual is under stress, or more regularly, when such a form of thinking is characteristic of the individual. Some patients may entertain beliefs or convictions that appear delusional, although they may otherwise appear to be rational. Mild forms of these kinds of disturbances of thinking are practically universal, especially when one is under stress. Disturbances in thinking become a difficulty if they are more severe and become the characteristic way a person functions.

Feldman (1989) describes how the development of the child's relationships with each parent and with the parental couple affects her capacity to think. Unconscious internal images of the child's parents form in her mind. In psychodynamic psychotherapy and psychoanalysis, the therapist/analyst is experienced, more or less, as these internal figures. That is, the internal images are projected on to the patient's experience of the therapist. (This actually occurs in all therapeutic relationships, including physician–patient relationships, and, moreover, in all relationships, more or less, but the opportunity to explore this is greatest in psychoanalysis and psychoanalytic psychotherapy.) To express this another way, the quality of the patient's transference is influenced by unconscious internal images of the patient's parents. The more severe the patient's disturbance, the more the qualities of the internal images are projected, and consequently the less the patient's experience of the therapist may represent who the therapist actually is. That is not to say, of course, that a patient is not capable of accurately perceiving some aspect of the therapist's personality, undistorted by her internal images of her parents. In fact, the most severely disturbed patients are often the most sensitive to some realistic aspects of the therapist's personality. An understanding of the nature of and relationships between a patient's internal images ("internal objects") helps a therapist recognize what a patient experienced as a child, which she may re-enact with the therapist.

So we are describing the child's internal world, inhabited by figures derived from early experiences, mostly with her parenting figures. The qualities and functions of these experiences are influenced by projections and distortions. That is, the child's internal objects, her unconscious internal images of others, are derived from early experiences with caretakers, but influenced by her way of dealing with painful emotions like anxiety with unconscious mental mechanisms of defense. In the child's (unconscious) fantasy, these internal figures relate to one another in complex ways, in which the patient's experience of the figures of her childhood remains alive in her mind. This influences her current relationships, including the way she experiences and responds to her analyst, therapist, or physician. In psychoanalysis, both members of the analytic couple find themselves pulled in more than one direction regarding their desires for the other. Each option involves a compromise, and may require a blurring or avoidance of aspects of reality that arouse too much pain or guilt. For example, a female patient may fall in love with her male therapist, in spite of believing that he is married. Her love for her therapist and her awareness of his marital status may end up split in her mind, so that in one part of her mind, she may love and want him, oblivious to the part of her mind that knows he is unavailable. This example clearly is derived from the Oedipus complex, with the therapist being experienced as father.

A session of psychotherapy (or a meeting between a patient and physician) may involve the patient unconsciously and non-verbally influencing the therapist (or physician) such that she exerts subtle pressure on him to act in particular ways based on her early experiences, possibly not represented in words because it may be from a time before she had words to use or before her mind had developed to employ words in thinking. The therapist or physician might experience pressure to perform an action that feels uncharacteristic and professionally inappropriate. Thus, underneath the unremarkable professional interaction, whether psycho-therapeutic or medical, there may lie a more primitive experience of love or hate based on the patient's early experience, that the therapist or physician may be pressured to re-enact. This is one description of transference. The experience of the therapist or physician in this situation can be called countertransference. For example, a patient may indicate how desperate and bereft she is, to the point where her therapist or physician feels an impulse to make himself more available than he usually would to a patient, for example, giving the patient his cell phone number to call at any time on the weekend, as opposed to letting the patient call the on-call service number. One might call this an enactment of an infantile relationship in which the patient acts as if she requires the availability of around-the-clock care, as an infant does. One could say that the physician or therapist has experienced a fantasy of taking care of his patient like an infant. To what extent this is some-thing the patient induced, and to what extent it is based also on the therapist/physician's emotional needs (to be needed, for example) should be explored. For example, if a therapist/physician has a similar longing to be cared for like an infant, he might be very sensitive to the patient's unconscious tacit invitation, identifying with the patient, and be tempted to comply. Of course, this type of enactment never works out well, because the patient's expectations, being temporarily gratified, only continue. Eventually, any therapist/physician will become frustrated and withdraw this around-the-clock care, with a predictably untoward reaction on the part of the patient. It is clear in this kind of case that the therapist/physician has contributed to the poor outcome, which represents yet another experience in which the patient sought care that initially seemed to be offered, but subsequently was withdrawn. This fruitless attempt to gratify a patient's longings for love, which is followed by the therapist/physician's withdrawal, can precipitate suicidal feelings.

A different approach would involve the therapist (or physician) indicating in a gentle way that the patient sounds as if she wants him to be available 24/7, and explore with the patient what that would mean to her, and what she thinks might happen. (That is, begin exploring the patient's wishes, rather than trying to gratify them.) At some point, the therapist/physician would need to outline the limits of how much care the patient can expect. The more tempted the therapist/physician is to stretch or break the boundaries, the more he must be vigilant in thinking about his motivations for doing so. I have heard of therapists taking patients home for the weekend, or even for longer periods of time. There is no shame in having this fantasy or feeling like doing this, but it is clear that enacting it would be destructive. If the therapist/physician has difficulty maintaining his professional boundaries, this is something for him to think about, at his leisure; that is different than enacting a boundary crossing or violation with a patient that benefits neither the patient nor the therapist/physician.

In psychoanalysis and psychoanalytic psychotherapy, the patient's material and the dynamics of the transference situation, for example, the patient's fantasies about her relationship with the therapist, including longings, which she tacitly invites the therapist to fulfill, can lead to understanding the patient's early experience. This can allow the therapist to construct a view of the nature of the patient's early interactions with her parents, and how this may affect how the patient experiences current relationships.

Individuals who negotiate the Oedipus complex in a relatively healthy way have an internal model of parental intercourse that is, on balance, a creative activity. This seems to be directly connected with the development of the individual's capacity to allow thoughts and ideas to interact in a kind of healthy inter-course in his mind. On the other hand, the fantasy that any connection forms a bizarre or predominantly destructive couple seems to result in damaged, perverse, or severely inhibited forms of thinking. In this way, the child's early relationships with his parents, and their relationships with each other, influence his forms of and capacity for thinking.

BACK TO OUR PATIENT

Mrs. X never had a close relationship with her siblings. She resented her younger sister's academic and social successes. She felt her sister did as she pleased, neglecting their mother, yet looking down on Mrs. X for being so close to their mother. *The lack of closeness with her siblings reinforces the impression about Mrs. X's difficulty with three-person relationships.* Mrs. X married at the age of 20 after a one-year courtship. She claimed to have a very satisfactory marriage. She described her husband as friendly and kind, although increasingly absent since their first child was born, due to his work as a middle-level executive, which involved him being out of town several days at a time. She found the increased demands of the children a burden in his absences. *This is especially understandable, to the extent that Mrs. X experienced her husband as her mother and herself as a young child. She would feel especially abandoned by him, and find the demands of children especially difficult because she felt she wasn't being cared for herself. This seems to recapitulate Mrs. X's early experience with her own mother.*

Mrs. X worried about how obedient her older daughter was, wondering why she never showed any defiance, which Mrs. X believed would be appropriate sometimes. She was concerned that her daughter was too much like she was at that age, in contrast to Mrs. X's younger sister. *Perhaps Mrs. X's older daughter unconsciously experienced Mrs. X as needing care, including not being opposed, and conformed to this, hoping that by taking care of her fragile mother, the latter would take better care of her. Children are very sensitive, able to pick up cues from their parents from infancy. The first period when children unmistakably assume personal agency is the "terrible twos," when they learn to say "No!" Mrs. X's daughter's compliance might have originated then or earlier. Some babies learn not to cry, to avoid disturbing their mothers. A second child may experience her older sibling as taking care of their mother, and feel freer to be herself.*

MENTAL STATUS AND PHYSICAL EXAMINATION

On examination, Mrs. X appeared alternately depressed and mildly agitated, or calm and comfortable. Her affect was labile. There was no abnormality of content of thought beyond her preoccupation with her need to find the baby's "right" name. No disorder of thought process was observed except thought blocking after admission. Mrs. X denied other obsessive-compulsive symptoms. There was no evidence of perceptual abnormality. She had mild vague suicidal ideation. Her sensorium was intact. Judgment appeared unimpaired, although she appeared to have little insight, and felt that if only she could find the right name, all would be well. Physical and neurological examination were normal.

DIFFERENTIAL DIAGNOSIS

Mrs. X was admitted to the psychiatric unit directly from her outpatient consultation appointment because of the degree of upset, the chronicity of her symptoms, the question of suicide risk, and the need for the support of a hospital environment. Provisional diagnosis was major depression. Differential diagnosis included dysthymic disorder, adjustment disorder with depressed mood, and obsessive-compulsive disorder.

INITIAL PSYCHODYNAMIC FORMULATION

(My subsequent ideas on formulation are contained in the developmental history section above.) Mrs. X's symptoms reflected a difficulty with identity, both her own and her younger daughter's. *(The child whose mother couldn't name her may well have her own problems with identity.)* This appeared related to frustrations in her attachments with her husband, sister, and parents. Choosing names that suggest joy and love could be interpreted as a defense against contrary feelings possibly aroused by the child's birth. *(This represents the defense of reaction formation.)* It also may represent Mrs. X's attempt to feel more positively about her daughter than she believed her parents felt about her. Mrs. X's resentment of her sister and her identification with her older daughter, whom she felt had been emotionally deprived by her husband, seems to be a recapitulation of her own experience of deficient attention from both parents. Finding a name that "goes together" with her older daughter's name suggests a defense against conscious awareness of resentment towards her own sister. Part of Mrs. X's difficulty with her second daughter might have involved the identification with her first daughter: the baby may represent the envied younger sister. Changing the baby's name thus could be interpreted as an attempt to make the baby more lovable to Mrs. X, as she once tried to make herself lovable to her mother. Mrs. X's identification with her cousin seemed based on unconscious feelings of being neglected and taken advantage of by her mother, and later neglected by her husband and in-laws.

Mrs. X seems to have idealized her mother; however, the latter was described as siding with her in-laws, sympathizing with Mr. X, and not supporting Mrs. X, who gave little evidence that she had a close relationship with her mother beyond trying to compensate for her father's unfriendly attitude. Even Mrs. X's developing a relationship with her own father seemed to be too much of a threat to her mother, who appeared to need Mrs. X to obey her implicitly, do her housework for her, and provide her with solace. Mrs. X grew up preoccupied with her mother's needs, at the expense of her own individual development. This supports the idea that Mrs. X might have had difficulties with self–object differentiation, *distinguishing herself from other people and viewing herself as a separate individual,* which could predispose her to further regression. One could speculate that her mother may have had a poorly developed sense of identity herself, accepting her role as exploited housewife, and not recognizing Mrs. X's needs as separate from her own.

TREATMENT PLAN AND COURSE IN HOSPITAL

Mrs. X's lack of insight regarding interpersonal problems, the severity of the symptoms, and the possibility of an underlying more regressed condition, led to the conclusion that pharmacotherapy would be the mainstay of treatment, with psychotherapy limited to support. *(I do not agree with that conclusion, and would have placed more of a focus on psychotherapeutic treatment starting in hospital if I were managing her care. They say hindsight is 20/20.)* Mrs. X was initially treated with clomipramine 200 mg daily. On the fourth day of admission she was observed to stop talking in the middle of sentences, and appeared not to be initially aware of this, eventually admitting that she could not remember what she was thinking. Because of this and her increasing agitation, haloperidol 5 mg and benztropine 2 mg daily were added. The thought blocking disappeared with the haloperidol. As well, her thinking became more coherent and her mood more stable. *(This leaves the impression that Mrs. X might have been experiencing the beginning of psychotic symptoms, which were relieved by haloperidol. One cannot know whether this represented the natural course of her illness, or whether her admission to hospital might have exacerbated her condition. She might have been reacting to a sense that hospital staff had decided not to approach her therapeutically from a stance of attempting to understand her.)*

Mrs. X's agitation diminished. The haloperidol was changed to trifluoperazine 15 mg because of side effects. As Mrs. X's depressive mood and preoccupations did not improve despite therapeutic serum levels of clomipramine, she was changed to maprotiline 150 mg after five weeks. In hospital Mrs. X experienced several panic attacks, for which no precipitants were identified. She was subsequently treated after nine weeks with amitriptyline up to 200 mg daily, to which was added lithium carbonate up to 1200 mg a day along with trifluoperazine 10 mg a day. Mrs. X remained preoccupied with finding the baby's right name, alternating between feeling depressed and feeling better, always denying that she had a serious problem. It is tempting to suggest that, parallel to Mrs. X's preoccupation with her child's name, the staff appeared preoccupied with finding the right medication for her, as if that would solve her problems. *It now seems unfortunate that, with a lengthy hospitalization, especially on a unit ostensibly specializing in a psychoanalytically informed approach, more attention was not given to understanding Mrs. X's difficulties psychodynamically. This might have led to psychoanalytically informed supportive psychotherapeutic efforts supplementing the medication. A better outcome might have resulted, obviating the need for a lengthy hospitalization.*

Mrs. X was not able to identify specific problems in life beyond that of naming the baby. After ten weeks in hospital, with fluctuating but persistent depressive symptoms, medications were discontinued and she had five electroconvulsive therapy (ECT) treatments, which did not improve her symptoms. An electroencephalogram (EEG) performed after ECT was abnormal, with paroxysmal high-voltage activity and bursts of sharp wave activity, suggesting the possibility of idiopathic epilepsy. Nuclear magnetic resonance (NMR) scan of the brain was normal. Mrs. X was subsequently treated with phenelzine 60 mg, lithium carbonate 900 mg, and alprazolam 1.25 mg. This regimen was later supplemented with L-tryptophan 1500 mg and trifluoperazine 10 mg. Mrs. X continued to experience marked mood fluctuations, depressed mood, agitation, and suicidal ideation, preoccupied with choosing the right name. She was subsequently treated with trimipramine 100 mg, lithium 1200 mg, clonazepam 1 mg, and flupenthixol 1 mg. At the time of writing the original article, Mrs. X had been in hospital seven months, with some improvement, but still having labile mood, hoping to be discharged from hospital soon. I did not receive information about her ultimate disposition.

Now I believe that psychoanalytic therapy is strongly indicated for a patient like Mrs. X, especially given her poor response to medication and ECT. The provision of adequate containment is important. Several appointments per week would be optimal, with considerable sensitivity on the therapist's part. Mrs. X is not unlike many patients who consult psychoanalysts and psychoanalytic psychotherapists, with a reasonable prognosis for significant improvement. Were Mrs. X to be seen with her husband in couple's therapy, this should not be undertaken by Mrs. X's individual therapist. The marriage deserves its own therapist, which would avoid "contaminating" Mrs. X's transference to her therapist, compromising her individual therapy. There is the danger that Mrs. X.'s therapist, seeing the couple in therapy, might favor or be perceived to favor Mrs. X. Alternatively, Mrs. X might resent the therapist for not favoring her, or for having to share her. In my opinion, it is contraindicated for a therapist who is treating an individual to also treat the patient with his partner in couple's therapy. However, occasionally it becomes necessary for a psychotherapy patient's partner to meet with the patient and his therapist if the partner's support in the patient's therapy is necessary, or to obviate the partner's opposing or sabotaging the therapy.

This chapter attempts to illustrate how a psychoanalytic understanding of a patient enhances understanding of the patient's problems and offers a rational approach to the psychotherapeutic aspects of management. (See Chapter 15.)

REFERENCES

Feldman M (1989). Chapter Three: The Oedipus complex: Manifestations in the inner world and the therapeutic situation. In: Britton R, Feldman M, O'Shaugnessy E (eds.), *The Oedipus Complex Today: Clinical Implications*. London: Karnac Books, 103–128.

Klein M (1928). Early stages of the Oedipus conflict. *International Journal of Psycho-analysis* 9:167–180.

Stein SM (1998). Enuresis, early attachment and intimacy. *British Journal of Psychotherapy* 15(2):167–176.

Winnicott DW (1937). Enuresis. *International Journal of Psycho-Analysis* 18:58–59.

Yager J, Gitlin MJ (1995). Clinical manifestations of psychiatric disorders. In: Kaplan HI, Sadock BJ (eds.), *Comprehensive Textbook of Psychiatry*, 6th edition. Baltimore, MD: Williams and Wilkins, 637–670.

CHAPTER 15

FREUD ON THE WARD: INTEGRATION OF PSYCHOANALYTIC CONCEPTS INTO THE FORMULATION AND MANAGEMENT OF HOSPITALIZED PSYCHIATRIC PATIENTS

Here I describe a psychiatric inpatient who would not benefit from psychoanalytic psychotherapy. Nevertheless, psychoanalytically understanding her leads to a more effective management approach, especially regarding dealing with staff reactions to disturbing patients (Shur, 1994). This approach hearkens back to a heritage from the mid-1900s that the present preoccupation with financial efficiency (or profit), pressure for early discharge, and treating symptoms rather than condition or, even better, the patient (Ghaemi, 2008), has abandoned. Consideration of the patient's personality disturbance has practical implications regarding staff members' understanding of her and consequent identification and handling of transference and countertransference manifestations. "Enactments" are the acting out in the patient's relationship with her therapist (or with others, for example, with other patients on an inpatient unit) of a difficulty she has in her relationships with someone else. This parallels a disturbance in the patient's internal world (of images of herself and others), which, being unconscious, she cannot discuss with her therapist. This is enacted in an interaction with another individual, usually with untoward results. For example, a patient experienced a parent as excessively critical and consequently developed a critical attitude towards herself, a sensitivity to criticism from others (feeling that she is being criticized even when this is not intended), and a tendency to criticize others. She may either feel criticized on the ward by another patient who did not mean to criticize her, which may result in interpersonal conflict between them, or may be critical of another patient in a manner that leaves the other patient feeling attacked, with a similar potential for conflict. *These outcomes are the result of the patient (1) projecting a critical parental image on to the other person, while the patient identifies with her internal criticized child self-image and feels criticized; or (2) projecting a criticized child self-image on to the other individual, who feels criticized, while identifying with the internal critical parental image.* Problems that are likely to occur as enactments on the inpatient unit can be anticipated or identified early, and a consistent staff approach prepared when a psychoanalytic understanding of patients is undertaken. A psychoanalytically informed inpatient management approach can help anticipate challenging interpersonal experiences between patients and staff. The development of psychoanalytic thought renders it applicable not only regarding the varieties of patients who can benefit from psychoanalysis or psychoanalytic psychotherapy *per se,* but also regarding the clinical venues in which psychoanalytic concepts usefully can be applied (e.g., Piper et al., 1996).

An important goal in the inpatient treatment of challenging inpatients is that of staff members maintaining their professional stance in the face of sometimes considerable provocation, continuing to provide an acceptable standard of care to these patients and the other patients, and maintaining a therapeutic ward atmosphere. That is, staff members as effective healthcare professionals must survive their management of these patients. Therapeutic goals must be realistic, not only considering the severity of the patients' disturbance, but also considering the treatment medium, that is, an inpatient psychiatric unit.

This chapter is based on a single consultation between an inpatient psychiatrist and a psychiatrist who is a psychoanalyst. The clinical material represents a composite of many patients. This is intended to stimulate the integration of psychoanalytic thinking into the inpatient treatment of psychiatric patients.

CLINICAL EXAMPLE

Mrs. W is a 47-year-old unemployed married woman with two adolescent children who lives in a rural community. Her husband works seasonally. She presented to the local hospital accompanied by her husband after she had ingested a small quantity of gasoline. Earlier that day they had argued and she felt he had belittled her. Mrs. W had accumulated credit card debts without her husband's knowledge. When a collection agency called, he became angry, confronting her regarding overspending. Mrs. W subsequently ingested the gasoline and immediately informed her husband, who brought her to hospital. There also was conflict between Mrs. W and her children, who "don't listen and disagree," unlike when they were younger. Mrs. W acknowledged "giving up" and retreating when faced with interpersonal conflict. Her husband noted that, over the past year, she had become increasingly more withdrawn, contributing little to the running of the household.

Mrs. W has chronic low-back pain and takes prescribed opiates for "help with all my pain." She has a history of alcohol and cannabis abuse, but has not used them recently. She recently developed an internet relationship with a man she pitied, and purchased household items for him. The relationship abruptly ended when he went offline. Mrs. W's involvement with a local support service recently was interrupted by her case worker's illness. Mrs. W frequently visits her family physician, often presenting with a multitude of ailments, and has exhausted his supportive capacities. She has been treated with numerous antidepressants without benefit. Her medical history is essentially unremarkable.

Mrs. W, the eldest of three children, was raised in a large city. Her father worked at a number of unskilled jobs, but mostly was unemployed. Both parents were heavy drinkers. Mrs. W described her early life as "chaotic." Her father was overbearing, threatening, and sometimes physically violent with Mrs. W and her siblings. Early attempts of the children to raise concerns were generally stifled, if not met with overt mistreatment. Mrs. W recalled often retreating to her room whenever upset. Her mother was emotionally absent, consumed by the demands of doing her best to manage the household within limited means. At times her mother was absent for prolonged periods on drinking binges. Mrs. W recalled assuming significant household and childcare responsibilities as a child. She left home at 17, and had a pattern of involvements with men who mistreated and neglected her. Her husband is often absent because of his work. She described him as verbally abusive. Mrs. W typically responds to differences between herself and others by withdrawing and remaining voiceless. During times of conflict, she usually resorts to self-injury; this has escalated over the previous year. Mrs. W's relationships are limited; the little contact she has with others is generally superficial.

Mrs. W was admitted involuntarily to the inpatient psychiatry unit for assessment. The psychiatric team consists of a psychiatrist, a primary nurse responsible for coordinating the nursing care plan, a social worker, an addictions counselor, and a family physician who provides general medical care. The assigned nurse provides nursing care when the primary nurse is absent, so the patient may have several nurses involved in her care during the course of a week.

Individual psychoanalytically based supportive interventions are provided daily by the psychiatrist. Structured group programming, including life skills training, open interpersonal training skills groups, addictions groups, and psychoeducational disorder-specific groups, is offered.

The different attitudes toward Mrs. W expressed by staff members created a schism between those who tried to meet her every need and those who tended to ignore her. Much effort was expended by the treating psychiatrist in managing the conflict among the staff members to create a consistent management approach and help staff understand their reactions. Mrs. W made multiple daily demands for more lorazepam, which further polarized staff members between doting and depriving attitudes. Efforts by some staff members to engage Mrs. W in active treatment were met with cross words by others who felt that excessive demands were made of her. Mrs. W's OxyContin was reduced and discontinued when her husband disclosed she was hoarding and bingeing on the drug. This led to further devaluation of Mrs. W by some of the team. The staff members who found themselves doting on Mrs. W felt exhausted, defeated, and resentful by the end of the day. They felt their efforts were met with ever-increasing demands of time and effort. Other staff members described in confidence their fantasies of "breaking out the therapeutic wooden stick." These fantasies were accompanied by considerable guilt over such negative thoughts.

DISCUSSION

Psychiatric formulation is an essential part of psychiatric management planning. The biological aspect of psychiatric formulation is relatively straightforward, and largely consists of considering what genetic and constitutional factors may contribute to the patient's current condition, and what the patient's current medical status might contribute to his psychiatric symptomatology. The psychosocial aspect of psychiatric formulation is based on psychodynamic formulation. This attempts to explain, with the information available, how the patient got to be where he is on presentation. While diagnosis deals with organizing symptoms into recognizable syndromes and conditions, psychodynamic formulation attempts to utilize information in the individual's psychosocial history in an attempt to explain the basis for his adaptation that led him to his current condition. This includes his personality; current and chronic psychiatric symptoms; self-image and internal object relations (unconscious images of himself and others); ego functions (including his characteristic unconscious mental mechanisms of defense, capacity to think, regulation of emotion, impulse control, and quality of relationships with others); and superego functioning (including conscience and moral standards for himself, and the ego ideal, his partly conscious ideal version of himself). The patient's psychological reactions to illness and management are also subsumed under psychodynamic formulation. (See Chapter 8.) Psychodynamic formulation is based on psychoanalytic theories of development and personality (Steinberg, 1998a, 1998b).

Attachment and Affect Regulation

Mrs. W's history of alcohol and marijuana abuse and opiate hoarding and bingeing suggests that she has difficulty in regulating her affect: "help with all my pain." She appears to rely on substances and to withdraw and be uncommunicative in interpersonal conflicts, rather than seeking support in relationships and trying to address difficulties in relationships directly. This suggests that her positive attachment to her parents, especially her mother, was limited with respect to their early responsiveness to her internal states, helping her as an infant to learn to recognize, experience, and tolerate her feelings. Her establishing an internet relationship suggests that she wanted some attachment beyond what she felt she had with her husband, but was more comfortable with one that was controllable and remote. Sending her internet friend household items might suggest the wish to establish a happier home with him. In sending gifts, she likely was expressing a wish that her parents and probably her husband and children be more generous with her. Her internet friend's disappearance suggests that he exploited her and was not attached to her. This may represent a pattern in her attachments, early and current. This relationship also reinforces the impression of Mrs. W's capacity for deception, in that she never told her husband about this man and her spending money on him.

Mrs. W's case worker's illness appears to have represented a disruption of an important attachment. It likely predisposed Mrs. W to requiring admission, making her more vulnerable to other disappointments in attachments. It may have actually precipitated the need for admission. Mrs. W's reliance on her family physician, draining his capacities, gives a hint of her capacity to demand and to expect care beyond what is reasonable for an adult, which has transference implications for the ward staff: *one would expect her to have a similar demanding attitude towards them, which seems to have been demonstrated.*

Self-Image and Internal Object Relations

Mrs. W ran up debts without her husband's knowledge until a collection agency intervened. She presented herself as depressed and helpless, but exhibited a capacity for personal agency and covert action. These qualities are potential assets that could be enlisted into constructive activity. Mrs. W did not appear as helpless as her presentation suggested. One can foster personal agency in patients like Mrs. W, rather than accepting her passive, helpless stance. She did not treat her husband like a partner, and behaved in a financially irresponsible manner. It was unclear how much this was a response to feeling that her husband did not treat her as an equal partner. One would need to engage her as an active partner in the treatment team, providing her with options, asking her opinion, and indicating the team's need for her input and cooperation, as opposed to allowing Mrs. W to experience herself as the passive recipient of whatever the treatment team decides.

Mrs. W described her father as overbearing, threatening, and violent. One would expect her to have an internal object (the unconscious image of the other) that is persecutory and critical, with an unconscious self-image of a crushed, frightened, and helpless child. This impression is reinforced by Mrs. W's description of early attempts to raise concerns as stifled or leading to mistreatment. This would interfere with Mrs. W's development as a secure individual who functions effectively. A likely transference implication is that Mrs. W would fear the staff members, and be unlikely actively to raise her concerns, especially concerns regarding her relationships with them. She also would tend to experience them as attacking and critical, and might tend to provoke this type of reaction from them. *Klein (1946/1975) described projective identification, in which an individual projects the internal image of another, usually based on early experience, onto a current relationship. Ogden (1979) highlights how individuals can unconsciously provoke people, onto whom they may project these unconscious internal images of others, to behave in a manner corresponding to the internal images, re-creating the interpersonal disturbance internalized in their mind during early relationship experiences.*

Mrs. W described her mother as emotionally absent. One would expect an unavailable, neglectful internal object. Mrs. W took on significant responsibility in the household when her mother was on prolonged drinking binges. This might be seen as a strength in that Mrs. W developed a precocious capacity to function. However, especially in the context of abuse and neglect, this adaptation fosters resentment in the child, who unconsciously longs for the care she never had, and results in an adaptation of pseudo-maturity, leaving the child vulnerable as an adult to regressing to the role of a helpless, demanding child, especially when disappointed in adult attachments. Because Mrs. W's father was mostly unemployed, her basic material needs likely were met only to a limited extent. Her parents' heavy drinking in a situation of limited financial resources is not suggestive of a mature concern for the children's needs, and also suggests that the parents had their own difficulties with affect regulation.

Mrs. W's early life was described as chaotic, likely not an atmosphere in which a stable, positive sense of self and a secure feeling about close attachments would be easy to develop. Mrs. W might re-create this chaos on the inpatient unit, splitting the staff into wished-for loving caregivers (good part-objects, *that is, a view of some staff members that is unrealistically idealized*), and feared neglectful persecutors (bad part-objects, *that is, a view of other staff members that is unrealistically devalued*), who contend with each other. *(The term "part-object" implies that an individual's unconscious view of others is split between idealized all-good and devalued all-bad parts, rather than having a "whole" image of others that is realistically ambivalent, including both positive and negative feelings.)* That is, Mrs. W may project her chaotic internal world, internalized from her experience with early attachment figures, *consisting of longed-for fantasized idealized parental images and devalued, hateful parental images, on to the ward environment, splitting the nurses into two warring camps, reminiscent of her parents' relationship.* Jacobson's (1964) pioneering work in early object relations and Kernberg's (1984) description of the activation of primitive object relations *(idealized and devalued unconscious images of the self and other)* in the hospital setting are applicable to this situation.

Mrs. W left home when young and was involved with neglectful men who mistreated her. That is, she found men who were good targets onto whom she could project her negative internal objects and recapitulate her unhappy early relational experiences. For her, positive experiences in a relationship might be experienced as threatening, a reminder by contrast of her early trauma and disappointment. As well, if Mrs. W did not choose men who treated her as her parents did, she would have to assume more responsibility for what happened to her. Her husband, absent because of work and verbally abusive, seemed to fit her general pattern of attachments.

Transference and Countertransference Implications

Mrs. W's deception of her husband has transference implications. *That is, one can predict from this relationship how she might be inclined to interact in her relationships with others, including caregivers.* She may not be any more direct in her dealings with the treatment team than she has been with her husband, including regarding the expression of her internal states. Mrs. W's ingesting gasoline and informing her husband of this action forced him into the role of agent who had to act in order to save her. This seems like an indirect expression of her anger, with obvious transference implications, *for example, regarding how she may indirectly express anger to the staff.* Mrs. W's expression of frustration with the treatment team may be equally indirect, self-destructive, and provocative. Her self-poisoning suggests that she has a destructive, punitive internal object. With the gasoline ingestion, she appears to project her experience of herself on to her husband, threatening him with danger to his wife's life, and exposing him to an avoidable painful situation. This may have been Mrs. W's way of forcing his hand to provide her with care. It likely evoked mixed feelings in her husband, including concern, anger, fear, frustration, and perhaps a wish that Mrs. W might die.

Mrs. W's feeling that her adolescent children do not listen to her or agree with her suggests she had difficulty in separating from her children, and accepting and enjoying their normative development independent of her. This may have contributed to Mrs. W's depressive mood. It reinforces the impression that she had a disturbance of attachment with her own parents (Wallin, 2007), with resulting internal objects that did not feel reliable. Mrs. W's reaction to her children's normatively separating from her likely exacerbated tensions between her and them. The self-poisoning also may reflect anger at her children, and be an attempt to manipulate them with the message, "I can't live without you." This also has transference implications: Mrs. W may behave in a passive-aggressive or manipulative manner in her relationship with the treatment team. That is, she may express herself and pursue her goals in an indirect and covert fashion. One treatment goal would be to foster Mrs. W's direct verbal expression of her internal states, including her affects, thoughts, wishes, impulses, and fantasies. One countertransference implication *(how one might predict the staff to react to Mrs. W)* is that staff members are likely to become frustrated and angry with her indirect way of expressing herself and her refusal to express herself. The staff would need to contain their reactions. Their anger can be understood as an affect that Mrs. W is still unable to contain within herself, and therefore places into the staff, as she appears to do in her relationships with her husband and children. This can be understood as a concordant countertransference (Racker, 1968), with the staff ending up feeling like other people in Mrs. W's life. Alternatively, in a complementary countertransference, the staff might experience a projection of Mrs. W's internal objects onto them, and end up reacting to Mrs. W as her parents did, preoccupied with their own concerns, as opposed to being concerned with her needs. *That is, Mrs. W, in projecting either a self-image or an internal object onto the staff, may elicit behavior from the staff respectively in two alternative ways: she may identify with her parents, treating the staff as she experienced her parents treating her, inducing in the staff feelings she had as a child; or she may induce the staff to treat her as she experienced her parents treating her, and re-experience how she felt as a child.*

Mrs. W's reaction to her children not listening to her or agreeing with her, as they did when they were younger, suggests she has an unrealistic view of parent–child relationships and human development, likely based on her own early experience. Treatment could involve education about normal development, the importance of separation, and the understandable anxieties it generates. Mrs. W's reaction leaves the impression that her parents likely did not foster her development as an independent individual, but expected continued compliance. She likely did not separate psychologically from her parents in a satisfactory manner. She also does not seem to have learned that uncomfortable affects such as anxiety can be borne. One might conclude that Mrs. W would have difficulty forming positive attachments to staff, and would be threatened, once she does feel attached to them, by any expectation that she function more independently, for example, when going out on a pass, making preparations for discharge, or needing to express an opinion or feelings contrary to those of the staff.

Mrs. W appears to have a strong unconscious wish for parental care, to be provided for like a child or infant, and to never have to function as an interdependent adult. The staff need to accept Mrs. W's wish without positively reinforcing it by doing for her what she is able to do for herself. Some staff may identify with Mrs. W and "spoil" her, feeling sympathetic toward her longings for care. Other staff may react against her unspoken demands, and have a rejecting or even punitive attitude toward her. We all, to some extent, experience the dependent longings that appear evident in Mrs. W. The staff members' countertransference experience depends in part on the extent to which they are consciously aware of these longings and accept them in themselves, as opposed to needing to project them onto Mrs. W, and either indulge her (and themselves by proxy) in them, or attack her for what they cannot accept in themselves. *To the extent that we cannot accept feelings or wishes, such as longing for care, in ourselves, we have difficulty accepting them in our patients. Accepting such unmet longings involves tolerating not having them, mourning what we never had in our early lives, and what we may never have throughout our life. Such mourning is more tolerable if we have had and continue to have some satisfying relationships with others as well as with ourselves. The capacity to mourn is a developmental achievement that many people have difficulty attaining.*

An alternative approach to the above-mentioned reactions is to foster constructive adult functioning in Mrs. W in a firm, patient manner, offering her options of responsible behavior or, better, eliciting such ideas from her. To the extent that the staff dote on Mrs. W, this reflects Mrs. W's successful projection of a fantasized, loving, all-caring parental image, that is, a good part-object, on to the staff. To the extent that the staff reject and attack Mrs. W, this reflects Mrs. W's projection of neglectful, punitive parental images, that is, a bad part-object. Staff members have a contribution to the extent that they accept these projections. They need to be open to recognizing enactments with Mrs. W early, and extract themselves from them (Jacobs, 1986). *An enactment with staff who are idealized, that is, perceived as all-positive, might be gratifying to both patient and staff member, but is not sustainable. When the idealized staff member eventually inevitably disappoints the patient, the experience of the idealized part-object can be rapidly replaced by the patient experiencing the staff member as a devalued all-negative part-object. This explains the rapid change in some patients' attitudes towards their medical caregivers, from unrealistically positive to unrealistically negative.* Mrs. W's tendency to give up and retreat when faced with interpersonal conflict suggests that it might be difficult to engage her in meaningful discussion on the ward, whether individually or in groups. One can use the information elicited in Mrs. W's history to predict her relationships on the ward, so staff will feel less helpless in their anger (which Mrs. W feels), and not view her lack of cooperation as bad behavior to be changed or punished, but rather as an opportunity to engage her in working on these problems, which brought her to the hospital. *The advantage of a psychoanalytic approach is that these interpersonal problems cropping up in her therapeutic relationships provide an opportunity to address the problems therapeutically.*

Mrs. W characteristically responded to differences between herself and others with withdrawal, remaining voiceless. Her self-injuring behavior appears to be an identification with her father, in which she assumes both the roles of her physically abusive father and her abused self. One would expect Mrs. W to assume one of these roles in her relationships with the staff and to project the other role, possibly alternating the choice of roles with different staff members (Racker, 1968). *That is, she may enact with a staff member the destructive relationship with her father, assuming either the role of her father or her child self, and experiencing the staff member in the other role.* Mrs. W's restricted types of relationships and superficial contact with others reflect her early impoverishment in relationships. Meaningful interaction on the ward with this patient, beyond the limited and stereotyped roles she brings to relationships, would be an important achievement.

Some staff members were described as doting on Mrs. W. With them, she apparently succeeded in projecting an all-good part-object. This situation is unlikely to last; the doting staff likely will eventually resent Mrs. W's unspoken but considerable demands. The staff were described as being left exhausted, defeated, and resentful; their efforts were met with increased demands. The fantasies of other staff members of breaking out the "therapeutic wooden stick" suggest that Mrs. W projected a bad devalued part-object on to these staff, who appeared to wish to attack and punish her. The staff who doted on her the most, once they become disillusioned with her, are the most vulnerable targets for this projection. Staff members felt guilty about their negative thoughts about Mrs. W. These reactions are inevitable, and indicate how others experience Mrs. W. A staff relations group (O'Kelly & Azim, 1993) is necessary for staff members to have a venue to express their feelings about patients in a safe, supportive environment, and to come to a consensus about a realistic therapeutic approach. It is essential to identify splits *(between staff perceived as all-good and those perceived as all-bad)* when they occur among staff members, and to repair them. Without ongoing dialogue, staff members risk interacting with Mrs. W either by coddling her or by attacking her, finding themselves at odds with each other. One must not accept the projection of either all-good or all-bad part-objects, but instead provide for Mrs. W, through more authentic relationships with the staff, an example of adult cooperation, of mutuality in relationships (Aron, 1996), and of reflection on how problems, including problems in her relationships with staff, can be approached. *I think it would be more realistic to suggest that one can try to avoid such projections but cannot always succeed. It is essential to recognize as early as possible when one is enacting such a projection from a patient, and engage other members of the staff in discussing this, so the enactment can be reversed, and a more therapeutic interaction can be instituted.*

Most clinicians who had assessed Mrs. W diagnosed depression. This does not consider the contribution of her personality. The current diagnostic label that might best describe Mrs. W is self-defeating personality disorder; the older term, masochistic personality disorder (Lingiardi & McWilliams, 2017) better describes her, although it is now considered politically incorrect by some. Mrs. W appeared to accept that, for her, attachment inevitably involved suffering. She behaved in a manner that fulfilled this unconscious expectation, and ensured that others would suffer with her. The treatment team's job is to disengage from relating with Mrs. W in this fashion, showing her different ways of interacting in their relationships with her. That is, the enactment needs to be identified and then discussed, first among staff, and then with Mrs. W, rather than continue to be acted out with her. *Unfortunately, this type of work with this type of patient may only be possible in an inpatient unit stay of some weeks, or an intensive partial hospitalization program lasting several months, and so currently is available (when it exists) in most jurisdictions only in private hospitals for those who can pay. Nevertheless, applying the principles listed below will help avoid many destructive interactions on the ward, and foster growth among patients (and staff). These principles also can be applied in the psychiatric management of outpatients by psychiatrists and family physicians, whether or not these patients receive formal psychotherapy.*

Management

Integration of psychoanalytic principles in the management of psychiatric inpatients can be useful in the following ways:

1. Staff members reflecting on their experience with patients, including their uncomfortable countertransference affects and impulses, are more likely to see the latter as something to be understood, including being seen as potential communications from the patient, and to discuss them with other staff members. They are thus less likely to respond with destructive behavioral reactions, "countertransference acting out."

2. Staff members recognizing potential assets in the patient's personality, even if they currently are not employed constructively, and identifying them to the patient. Work can be done in helping the patient to exploit them more adaptively.

3. Staff members engaging the patient as an active partner in the treatment team.

4. Staff members recognizing how conflict among themselves may represent a projection of the internal world of the patient.
5. Staff members recognizing the patient's disturbed pattern of attachments to predict and be prepared to manage similar difficulties when they arise in the patient's relationships with them.
6. Staff members fostering verbal expression of the patient's internal states in a constructive manner.
7. Staff members, when appropriate, educating patients about normal development, specific to the patient's psychological difficulties, for example, difficulty with separation.
8. Staff members recognizing and accepting the patient's unconscious wishes without either gratifying these wishes or judging the patient for them, but rather fostering constructive adult functioning and providing a venue for discussing these unconscious wishes as they are manifest in relationships with staff (transference).
9. Staff members anticipating enactments or recognizing them at an early stage, so they can extract themselves from them and create a venue for discussing what hitherto was expressed only in action.

To summarize the approach to patients like Mrs. W, treatment should involve fostering personal agency in her, rather than accepting her passive, helpless stance. This approach should be pursued in the transference *(the relationship with staff members)* by engaging her as an active partner in the treatment team, fostering direct verbal expression of her internal states, including her affects, thoughts, wishes, impulses, and fantasies. Staff will need to contain their frustration and anger with Mrs. W's indirect way of expressing herself and her refusal to express herself. They should foster constructive adult functioning in Mrs. W in a firm, patient manner, offering her options of responsible behavior or, better, eliciting such ideas from her, rather than "spoiling" her, or reacting with a rejecting or punitive attitude. Establishing meaningful interactions on the ward with Mrs. W beyond the stereotyped roles she brings to relationships is essential. The staff need to disengage from relating to Mrs. W in the sadomasochistic fashion to which she is accustomed, and show her a different way of interacting in their relationships with her.

CONCLUSIONS

Consideration of the patient's personality and the recognition of the patient's having personality disturbance and interpersonal difficulties, in addition to depressive symptoms, are important in the management of depressed inpatients. *This applies, of course, to all patients, whatever their symptomatic condition.* Psychodynamic formulation of the patient (McWilliams, 1999) can enhance staff members' understanding of the patient and the consequent identification and handling of transference and countertransference difficulties. Enactments more readily can be anticipated or identified early. Recognition of the patient's personality disturbance may result in changing the inpatient management approach from one of medications as the first-line treatment accompanied by a purely supportive approach to a plan giving adequate consideration to the patient's relationship and personality difficulties. One does not expect to effect personality change during an admission, but one may begin to help patients reflect on their contributions to relationship difficulties and on their internal states in a new way. *This may be the best opportunity a patient has to be introduced in an intensive way to a psychotherapeutic approach that involves the patient reflecting, in a non-persecutory way, on herself and her contribution to difficulties in her relationships and other aspects of her life*. By utilizing psychoanalytically informed supportive interventions that address observable aspects of the real relationship between staff and patient, a new experience may be created that leads to further understanding if the patient undertakes formal psychotherapeutic treatment after discharge. This may foster some hospitalized patients in becoming amenable to a psychoanalytically informed treatment, such as individual or group psychodynamic psychotherapy, or a psychodynamically oriented partial hospitalization program (Piper et al., 1996; Steinberg et al., 2004).

REFERENCES

Aron L (1996). *A Meeting of Minds: Mutuality in Psychoanalysis*. Hilllsdale, NJ: Analytic Press.

Ghaemi N (2008). Towards a Hippocratic psychopharmacology. *Canadian Journal of Psychiatry* 53: 189–196.

Jacobs T (1986). On countertransference enactments. *Journal of the American Psychoanalytic Association* 34: 289–307.

Jacobson E (1964). *The Self and the Object World*. Madison, CT: International Universities Press.

Kernberg OF (1984). *Severe Personality Disorders*. New Haven, CT: Yale University Press.

Klein M (1946/1975). Notes on some schizoid mechanisms. In: *Envy and Gratitude and Other Works 1946–1963*. London: Hogarth Press and the Institute of Psychoanalysis, 1–24.

Lingiardi V, McWilliams N (2017). *Psychodynamic Diagnostic Manual*, 2nd edition. New York: Guilford Press.

McWilliams N (1999). *Psychoanalytic Case Formulation*. New York: Guilford Press.

Ogden TH (1979). On projective identification. *International Journal of Psycho-Analysis* 60:357–373.

O'Kelly JG, Azim HFA (1993). Staff–staff relations group. *International Journal of Group Psychotherapy* 43, 469–483.

Piper WE, Rosie JS, Joyce AS, Azim HFA (1996). *Time-limited Day Treatment for Personality Disorders: Integration of Research and Practice in a Group Program*. Washington, DC: American Psychological Association.

Racker H (1968). *Transference and Countertransference*. Madison, WI: International Universities Press.

Shur R (1994). *Countertransference Enactment: How Institutions and Therapists Actualize Primitive Internal Worlds*. Northvale, NJ: Jason Aronson.

Steinberg PI (1998a). Attachment and object relations in formulation and psychotherapy. *Annals of the Royal College of Physicians and Surgeons of Canada* 31(1):19–22.

Steinberg PI (1998b). Supportive therapeutic relationship with an HIV-AIDS patient. *Annals of the Royal College of Physicians and Surgeons of Canada* 31(1):23–26.

Steinberg PI, Rosie J, Joyce AS, O'Kelly JG, Piper WE, Lyon D, Bahrey F, Duggal S (2004). The Psychodynamic Psychiatry Service of University Alberta Hospital: A thirty year history. *International Journal of Group Psychotherapy* 54(4):521–538.

Wallin DJ (2007). *Attachment in Psychotherapy*. New York: Guilford Press.

CHAPTER 16

PSYCHOANALYTIC APPROACHES INTEGRATED INTO DAY TREATMENT AND INPATIENT SETTINGS[3]

This chapter describes two patients treated in a partial hospitalization program informed by psychoanalytic principles. One treatment was deemed as successful, and the other unsuccessful. I outline factors influencing the clinical outcome of these "difficult" patients. These are composite cases with information derived from the history of several patients.

A "SUCCESSFUL" TREATMENT IN AN INPATIENT UNIT AND A PARTIAL HOSPITALIZATION PROGRAM

This patient, with a quite severe personality disorder, participated in the psychodynamic group psychotherapy-oriented day treatment program (DTP) of the University of Alberta Hospital Department of Psychiatry. (See Piper et al., 1996, for a detailed description of DTP and outcome research validating its work.)

Mr. M, a 41-year-old unemployed man who abused drugs and lived with a common-law partner, presented to a hospital emergency department saying he was going to shoot himself. He faced both long-term problems and current stressors. His drug abuse and financial debt were escalating. He lost his driver's license after driving while intoxicated. His partner was threatening to leave him. He appeared agitated and depressed. Mr. M had received counseling for his problems several times, but never maintained an ongoing therapeutic relationship, and currently was without a counselor. He was involuntarily admitted to a psychiatric unit for observation and evaluation.

On inpatient units, patients generally are not treated with psychodynamic psychotherapy. However, as with partial hospitalization programs, psychoanalytic concepts serve as a useful foundation of inpatient treatment by providing understanding and direction for individual patients and the patient group as a whole. (See Chapter 15.) During the first few days, Mr. M was very demanding in his attempt to obtain medication for his symptoms. Once he made threatening gestures. He also deliberately knocked over pills from the medication cart, for which he was placed in seclusion. He constantly made special requests and tested the resolve of the staff. He was noted by staff to be particularly vulgar, argumentative, and hostile toward female patients. Female staff reported that he seemed to invade their personal space. He seemed oblivious to their withdrawing and indicating their discomfort with his standing so close to them. Despite his aggravating behaviors, he succeeded in winning the compassion of some staff members, who viewed him as wounded and hurt. The ability to split staff into one group who maintain a favorable attitude towards him, and another group with an unfavorable attitude in their evaluation of his actions, is common among such patients. (See Chapter 15.)

---

3   The original portion of this chapter is reprinted with permission from *Psychodynamic Psychotherapy for Personality Disorders: A Clinical Handbook*, (Copyright©2010). American Psychiatric Association. All Rights Reserved.

Part of what makes such a patient "difficult" is the emotional reactions he induces in staff, their counter-transference. One way of understanding the situation of splitting the staff is that Mr. M's behaving in a disturbing or even hateful way involves projecting a hateful aspect of himself, which he cannot bear conscious awareness of, into the staff. Some staff accept this projection and experience their hatred consciously, directing it at him. The hateful aspect of Mr. M might represent early experiences of being treated in a hateful way. One cannot determine to what extent such a patient's parents, for example, were objectively hateful, and to what extent the patient's sensitivities to his parents' treatment of him, or other intervening factors, for example, a mother's postpartum depression, or severe poverty, making it impossible adequately to nourish him, may also have intervened. In any event, one can interpret the outcome being that Mr. M recapitulates his early experience of being treated hatefully in inducing similar treatment, or at least, feelings, in some of the staff. The staff who maintain a favorable attitude towards him likely identify with him in some way. One explanation for this reaction is that Mr. M projects a longed-for, perhaps idealized unconscious image of a parent into them. Staff members who have at some point in their lives behaved or felt like behaving the way Mr. M did on the ward might be more accepting of this type of projection, although on the same basis they could reject it, not accepting it in themselves. The outcome of such a staff split involves dissension among the staff, described in Chapter 15.

The inpatient unit ran a supportive psychodynamically informed psychotherapy group. The day after Mr. M was placed in seclusion, he was informed in the group by the leader that both patients and staff were concerned about him, and his behavior of the day before could not be tolerated. Some patients reinforced these comments; some added that they were afraid of him. Mr. M momentarily seemed affected by this feedback, but soon dismissed the patients' comments, except those of Mrs. Q, who was 20 years older than he. She described how she had not been the mother that her son, who was also a drug abuser, needed. With tears in her eyes, she told Mr. M she didn't want to see him on skid row, eventually dying of an overdose, as her son had. This moved Mr. M. This group seemed to mark a turning point in his hospital stay. He appeared to have experienced Mrs. Q as a concerned maternal figure, likely based on her seeming to experience him as the son she had lost, hoping not to lose him again.

Mr. M spent 13 days in hospital. On discharge, he was in better general health, not having used drugs for two weeks. He accepted his psychiatrist's referral to DTP, appearing skeptical about its potential benefit. His psychiatrist believed that without intensive treatment he inevitably would revert to self-destructive patterns of behavior. His discharge diagnosis was mixed personality disorder with narcissistic, borderline, and antisocial traits.

Mr. M was told his admission to DTP was contingent on not drinking alcohol, using illicit drugs, or behaving in a threatening or violent manner. Violations of these conditions would result in his discharge. He agreed, but had a casual attitude towards them. Having the entire DTP staff involved in the admission process helps staff cope with patients' behavior problems and deal with their countertransference reactions. *It also makes splitting of the staff more difficult.*

During the first week, after an outburst of temper in a group, Mr. M was prescribed quetiapine to help him control his temper. (See Chapter 5.) During his third week, Mr. M arrived late one morning, unshaven, appearing disheveled, and with a bruise and cut on his face. He had been drinking and fighting the night before. Staff asked him what had triggered the fight. He told the staff to mind their own business. Mr. P, a 28-year-old man in his 16th week of the program, confronted Mr. M, reminding others that he too had a history of drinking and fighting, and knew he could avoid these behaviors. He said he had learned in DTP what triggered such behaviors and how to control them. Part of the solution for him was learning that he needed to confront the person he was angry with directly and discuss things in a calmer way. Mr. P added that patients were discharged from DTP for similar behavior violations. Mr. M asked if he would be discharged. After consultation with staff, Mr. M was informed that he could stay if he recognized the seriousness and destructiveness of his behavior and was committed to stopping it. He agreed.

What seemed to be supportive to Mr. M was a combination of confrontation by a patient who had been in his shoes, and being given a chance to continue his psychotherapeutic work in DTP. That is, a confrontation involving someone whose opinion was hard to dismiss, combined with remaining welcome to continue to work therapeutically in DTP with firm limitations on acting out, seemed to be effective. In DTP patients often will listen more readily to other patients, especially those with similar problems, than to staff, whom patients often see as not understanding the difficulties they face.

During a small-group session, Mr. M was asked what had precipitated his drinking and fighting. He deflected the question again by claiming he didn't know. Ms. S, a 25-year-old patient, reminded him that in the small-group session preceding this episode, several patients had confronted him about his lack of concern for others. She pointed out how his attitude put people off, and disclosed how as an adolescent she had assumed a similar attitude of not caring about her mother that obviated her having the kind of relationship with her mother she had longed for. She joked about the similarity between them, being tough guys with soft insides. Mr. M was surprised to hear he was regarded as uncaring, adding that he appreciated the patients' concern for him. *Again, one observes a patient responding to a fellow patient who said that she had been in his shoes.*

An important feature of DTP is the weekly staff relations group (SRG) (O'Kelly & Azim, 1993). It provides staff with an opportunity to examine feelings and other reactions to difficult patients such as Mr. M. Sometimes staff feel guilty about their negative reactions, viewing them as a sign of unprofessional behavior. As noted above, patients with personality disorders often succeed in splitting staff regarding their reactions to the patients, making it difficult to arrive at a consensus about therapeutic approaches to such patients. Some staff members had negative countertransference reactions toward Mr. M, who assumed little responsibility for his substance use. Other staff seemed more sympathetic. One staff member, Mr. T, allowed Mr. M to dominate several group discussions. Another staff member, who was sympathetic to Mr. T, gently suggested in SRG that Mr. T himself had a rather dominant personality, perhaps making it difficult for him to recognize the negative effects of Mr. M's behavior. This confrontation took place over several SRG sessions before being constructively resolved. Mr. T agreed he was giving Mr. M "too much slack," and aligned himself more with the approach taken by other staff. Another staff member, Mr. U, found himself intimidated by Mr. M, to the point that he almost dreaded coming to work. In SRG he linked this predicament to his situation as a child with an intimidating and bullying brother. Mr. U received support from other staff members, who encouraged him to continue discussing his difficulties with Mr. M in SRG, which he found very helpful.

It is clear from this example that therapists bring their own conflicts, unmet needs, and other difficulties to work with them, just like everyone else. The benefit of SRG is that staff members receive support from each other in becoming aware enough of the difficulties they are facing with patients, and what their particular sensitivities and vulnerabilities are that make them prone to these difficulties. This enables them to work more constructively with patients and other staff. This kind of feedback can lead to personal growth on the therapists' part. SRG is not a psychotherapy group, but can result in personal growth of staff members. This does not replace therapists having a personal psychotherapy or psychoanalysis, which generally enables therapists to be more effective therapists than they would be without therapy. Only in psychoanalytic training are candidates required to have their own lengthy therapy, that is, psychoanalysis. In other psychotherapy training programs, this is up to the student therapist, apart from some psychodynamic psychotherapy group training programs, which require some experience as a group therapy patient.

Mr. M completed the 18-week DTP. He appeared to have benefited considerably, particularly regarding his relationships with others. Toward the end of treatment, he actually was supporting staff in confronting patients, describing his own experiences in DTP. The staff believed that the combination of support and confrontation offered by both staff and patients on an intensive basis enabled Mr. M. to respond well to DTP. Mr. M ended with cordial relationships with most staff and patients. The last month of his treatment involved no temper outbursts, with him actively involving himself constructively in groups.

After DTP, Mr. M attended the weekly follow-up psychotherapy group for patients who complete DTP and wish to continue treatment. Staff believed the follow-up group would enhance the psychotherapeutic work he had begun in DTP. They believed his ability to benefit from a weekly group was only made possible by his experience in DTP. Had he attended such a group rather than DTP, it is doubtful he could have benefited, and probably would have dropped out.

DTP patients occasionally are admitted to the psychiatric inpatient unit on an emergency basis, usually when staff have a significant concern about suicide risk, but also if psychotic symptoms persist or worsen, or if a patient appears dangerous to others (Steinberg & Duggal 2004; Steinberg et al., 2008).

AN "UNSUCCESSFUL" TREATMENT IN DTP

In this case, concerns about suicide precipitated hospitalization. Mrs. R, a 57-year-old divorcee, was raised in a rural village, the youngest of seven siblings. Her mother was neglectful and sometimes physically abusive. She did not work outside the house, regularly abused alcohol, and did not maintain sanitary standards in the house, or provide regular meals. Mrs. R's older siblings often prepared dinner when coming home from school, if their mother was drunk or moody. Mrs. R largely was raised by her eldest brother, who was ten years older. He was friendly and at times supportive, but understandably preoccupied with his own concerns. Her father, a manual laborer, worked many hours of overtime, apparently to avoid his wife. He was friendly but often unavailable, not protecting Mrs. R from her mother. Mrs. R learned early that she could get some attention from her oldest brother and her father by behaving flirtatiously with them. She often "told on" her older siblings to her eldest brother, informing him of their misbehavior. *This is a description of a child whose upbringing likely involved very significant deficiencies in terms of her emotional, and even her basic physical, needs. She likely could not have internalized satisfactorily an image of a caring other person inside of her to help her develop an ability to care for herself. As well, this family provided a discouraging model on which to base expectations of future relationships, which is accomplished unconsciously. I believe Mrs. R's eldest brother's friendly and supportive attitude was a mitigating factor without which she might have ended up much worse off. However there does not seem to have been an adult available consistently to think of Mrs. R's experience as an infant and child, and help her bear it and put it into words that the child eventually could understand in a way that would help the child develop her mind, starting with learning to speak.*

I wish to expand briefly on the theory of the development of the human mind expounded by Wilfred Bion, who suggests that, for infants, experiences like physical pain are terrifying. If one thinks of it, much of what an infant contends with is physical and emotional regulation, without which he will feel increasing discomfort, for example, having wet diapers, being hungry, needing to sleep but not able by himself to fall asleep, and needing intimate contact with a mothering figure. Infants are completely helpless regarding meeting these needs. In fortunate circumstances, what Winnicott calls a "good enough mother" (Caldwell & Joyce, 2011), really a reliably available adult of either sex, not only meets the infant's concrete needs, but also communicates to the infant some understanding of how he is feeling. This often is accomplished by speaking dramatically to the infant in a high-pitched voice, putting words to the infant's discomfort or situation. Little by little, the infant associates the sight, smell, voice, tactile feel, and other sensory features denoting the mother's (let us say) presence, and he calms when he experiences his mother coming to care for him, even before he sees her. The mother's capacity to experience what the infant is experiencing, the mother's reverie, and to express it back to the infant transformed, mitigating the infant's feeling of terror, for example, gradually is internalized by the infant, who becomes able to experience the emotions that his mother has named for him as emotions. This is a first step towards being able to think about one's own mind. It requires a parent or parents who have the child in mind and are able to express the child's experience in a way that the child understands.

As the child grows older and begins to understand words, he can internalize his parents' interested attitude towards his mind, and gradually develop a similar interested attitude towards it. That is, not only does the infant internalize the mother's "metabolized" version of his experience, but also the process of thinking about his experience. In less fortunate cases, when due to any number of possibilities, such as a mother who is depressed or has some other psychiatric disturbance, is too busy with work responsibilities or too many children to pay enough attention to the child, or simply never had the attention she needed when she was young, the infant of parents who do not have him in mind and do not respond in the way described above will be less likely to develop much capacity to think about how he is feeling, that is, to reflect on his own experience.

Mrs. R presented herself rather dramatically, often attracting the attention of men. She soon became friendly with Mr. W, flirting with him. He responded with many chivalrous behaviors and became enamored with her, wishing to spend time alone with her. Mrs. R experienced difficulty engaging in DTP. Patients were irritated with her attention seeking with men while neglecting women. Staff found her emotionally superficial. *Rather than becoming involved in DTP, in which she could learn more about herself, Mrs. R focused on eliciting the gratifying attentions of the man she chose as her partner in DTP. This is acting out, expressing in behavior a problem that would be more productively discussed. (The problem not discussed was Mrs. R's motivation for restricting her relationships to flirting with or ignoring people.)*

During her fourth week, Mrs. R was confronted by other patients because of inconsistencies in her description of relationships in DTP. She was accused of spreading malicious gossip. The group leader attempted to modulate the intensity of the confrontation, but was hampered by his own negative countertransference toward her. Mrs. R denied the allegations and fled to another room. Mr. W intervened, expressing to staff his concern about her suicidal comments. He took Mrs. R's side, criticizing staff who allegedly had allowed events to escalate. As is routine, the psychiatrist and several staff members met with Mrs. R to assess suicide risk.

Although the staff believed that her claim to suicidal intent was unconvincing, the psychiatrist had her evaluated by the emergency psychiatry consultation team. She was admitted to the psychiatric unit overnight, Her admission coincided with her discharge from DTP. In retrospect, the staff believed that she was never committed to the psychotherapeutic work of DTP, and wished to be discharged. Her manner of discharge left some of the patients who had confronted her feeling responsible for her discharge. Her discharge diagnosis was histrionic personality disorder with dependent traits.

As this case illustrates, inpatient treatment is usually prompted by a crisis of some sort. The main objective is to provide support and observation in an effort to stabilize the patient until outpatient care can be arranged or resumed. Although group treatment usually is a regular part of the ward regimen, it may represent only a small part of it. It is not likely to be aimed at modifying long-standing personality traits. In North America, the length of stay in hospitals or residential centers has decreased significantly in response to escalating costs. Thus, in many cases, inpatient treatment is very brief. Exceptions include prison systems that include a strong rehabilitative objective for inmates who have antisocial personality disorders or traits. Kibel (2003) describes a psychodynamic approach to working with patients in residential treatment groups. If inpatient settings and day treatment settings share a common theoretical foundation, work within each setting and movement of patients from one setting to the other are facilitated.

CONCLUSION

Predicting patient suitability for day treatment is important. It is effective for patients with personality disorder, including borderline personality disorder. Research suggests that patients with a history of "mature" relationships, and who are older and are married are more likely to remain in day treatment. *(In my experience, people with mature relationships are unlikely to be referred to DTPs, which largely treat patients with significant personality disturbance whose relationships are far from mature.)* Patients in day treatment with previous psychiatric hospitalization improve more on interpersonal functioning than those without. Clinical experience suggests that patients with antisocial traits, psychotic symptoms, organic dysfunction, recent substance abuse, and criminal behavior do not do well in DTPs (Piper and Steinberg, 2010). None of this is surprising, but it does not help explain the reasons for the different outcomes of Mr. M and Mrs. R.

Mr. M's positive and constructive response to his interaction with Mrs. Q, his fellow inpatient, changed the hospital staff's view of him from an unpromising patient to someone who might benefit from DTP. His history and behavior to them were discouraging regarding him being amenable to any form of psychotherapy. His responsiveness to Mrs. Q was an important prognostic sign, and was followed with similar responsiveness to Mr. P and Ms. S. Nothing in Mr. M's history suggested that he might be so responsive. One difference between the histories of Mr. M and Mrs. R is that little was elicited of Mr. M's early life, so perhaps he had some positive relationship experiences with early caregivers that might have enabled him to respond positively to his co-patients. Mrs. R's history of early relationships was discouraging. The abuse and neglect described would not predispose her to respond positively to the interventions of others.

I include in the Appendix of the first introductory chapter lists of positive and negative prognostic factors for selecting patients for psychoanalytic psychotherapy. This may be helpful in deciding which patients physicians might refer for psychoanalytic psychotherapy. If the family physician is not sure about whether or not to refer a patient for psychoanalytic psychotherapy, it is useful to be acquainted with some psychiatrists and other therapists who perform psychoanalytic psychotherapy themselves and "run a patient by" them, or have one see the patient in consultation to determine if the patient is appropriate for this type of therapy. The average family doctor does not have the time to make herself an expert in this type of assessment, although she can benefit by learning from the opinions she receives from these consultants.

REFERENCES

Caldwell C, Joyce A (eds.) (2011). *Reading Winnicott.* London: Routledge.

Kibel HD (2003). Interpretive work in milieu griups. *International Journal of Group Psychotherapy* 53:303–329.

O'Kelly JG, Azim HFA (1993). Staff–staff relations group. *International Journal of Group Psychotherapy* 43:469–483.

Piper WE, Steinberg PI (2010). Psychodynamic approaches in day treatment and inpatient settings. In: *Psychodynamic Psychotherapy for Personality Disorders: A Clinical Handbook.* Washington, DC: American Psychiatric Publishing.

Piper WE, Rosie JS, Joyce AS, Azim HFA (1996). *Time-limited Day Treatment for Personality Disorders: Integration of Research and Practice in a Group Program.* Washington, DC: American Psychological Association.

Steinberg PI, Duggal S (2004). Threats of violence in group-oriented day treatment. International Journal of Group Psychotherapy 54(1):5–22.

Steinberg PI, Duggal S, Ogrodniczuk J (2008). Threats of violence to third parties in group psychotherapy. Bulletin of the Menninger Clinic 72(1):1–18.

PART IV

NON-CLINICAL TOPICS

Outside of psychoanalytic and academic circles, the extent to which psychoanalytic ideas have been applied over the last 120 years in many non-clinical areas, including literature, art, music, sociology, and anthropology, generally is not appreciated. This section provides a taste of psychoanalytic concepts applied in three non-clinical areas relevant to medicine, and in particular to medical studies.

In Chapter 17, I show how both examiners and candidates in oral certification examinations can increase their understanding of examination anxiety by applying object relations theory. Unconscious images of self and others that examiners and candidates may project onto each other can affect the examination outcome. The examiner must observe himself, the candidate, and the other examiner, lest a transference affecting the examination's progress occur, to avoid an enactment that may interfere with the examination. Unconscious processes may prejudice the examiner's attitude towards a candidate, thus jeopardizing the examination's fairness and validity. I describe how a candidate's anxiety may interfere with his optimal functioning and affect the outcome of the examination, and how this might be managed.

In Chapter 18, I describe what physicians might do for themselves to prevent their lives becoming so painful that they consider suicide. I discuss unconscious motivations for physicians to overinvolve themselves in their work at the expense of relationships and recreational activities. Physicians are advised to limit their ambitions, and to lead a life balanced among love, work, and play, as opposed to placing too heavy a burden on work to provide satisfaction and meaning in life.

In Chapter 19, I observe that male physicians who sexually abuse adult female patients do so as a result of character disturbance, severe psychiatric disorder, or when they are emotionally vulnerable; these are not mutually exclusive categories. The several options needed to deal with this abuse are discussed. It needs to be determined whether abusive physicians can be rehabilitated, and what kind of education provides the most effective prevention.

CHAPTER 17

ATTACK OF NERVES:
ORAL EXAMINATION ANXIETY IN PHYSICIANS

This chapter examines anxiety in oral certification examinations from an object relations point of view. This theory is useful in attempting to maintain appropriate boundaries in oral examinations to foster a fair, valid assessment of the candidate's competence. Neither candidate nor examiners can "be themselves" entirely, but must function within limits conducive to assessment of the candidate's competency (Ferron, undated). Freud described therapeutic neutrality: the therapist must limit his responses to the patient so they are realistic, appropriate, centered on the needs of the patient, and largely conscious (Langs, 1974). Examiners must similarly adhere to "neutral" behaviors, neither being unduly familiar, encouraging, or personal, nor taking a critical, adversarial, or unnecessarily authoritarian stance. The examiner cannot best judge the candidate's competence in any of these polarized modes of relating. Otherwise, it is more likely that the examiner will elicit an untoward personal reaction that may obscure the candidate's level of competence, making the evaluation process more difficult or even impossible, if this is the habitual stance of the examiner towards examination candidates, or towards anyone in a position of lesser status or power.

Freud (1900/1953) interpreted examination dreams in terms of other challenges that an individual faces with anxiety, noting that one generally only dreams of examinations in which one already has been successful. Several authors (Bauer, 1978; Blum, 1926; Flugel, 1939; Schmideberg, 1933) connect examination dreams with castration anxiety. Thorner (1954) compares examination anxiety, depersonalization, and hypochondria in patients who have an unconscious sense of internal persecution. He concludes that anxiety connected with academic examinations represents a fear that one's evil tendencies or worthlessness will be uncovered and exposed, with consequent ruin.

Other authors describe a variety of issues related to examination anxiety, including a strong need to establish a sense of mastery (Stengel, 1936) and changes taking place in a series of examination dreams paralleling the patient's increasing freedom and spontaneity (Kafka, 1979).

This paper approaches examination anxiety from an object relational viewpoint, emphasizing the influence of individuals' real experiences, including unmet emotional needs and interpersonal conflicts (as opposed to fantasy), on the unconscious internal images one has of oneself and others (that is, self-image and internal objects).

There is evidence of significant psychopathology, including high rates of substance abuse and suicide, among physicians (Michalon & Iracema, 1998; North & Ryall, 1997). In the case of psychiatric examination candidates, it is also relevant to consider evidence of unconscious motivations for practicing psychotherapy, which are related to unresolved unconscious conflicts and unmet needs (Sussman, 1992). This also applies to some extent to physicians in general, as I will discuss. This evidence is consistent with the suggestion that some candidates in board certification examinations are likely to struggle with negative unconscious images of themselves and others that may affect their functioning in the stressful venue of the oral examination.

ORAL EXAMS, TRANSFERENCE, AND INTERNAL OBJECT RELATIONS

Oral certification examinations, like psychiatric assessment interviews and ongoing psycho-therapeutic interviews, are situations with considerable potential for eliciting transference reactions from the participants (Greenson, 1967). The examination candidate, depending on her earlier experiences (especially with caretakers and other authorities), may react in a more extreme manner than appears warranted by the examination situation. The reality is daunting enough in that the oral examination is the last hurdle before the candidate qualifies to practice, and she may not be eligible for a license to practice medicine until this examin-ation has been passed. In addition, when the candidate appears to experience anxiety on the basis of previous unresolved experiences with authorities or parental figures, careful man-agement by the examiner is necessary to optimally assess the competence of the candidate. The question is, to what extent does the re-experiencing of painful early experiences and associated feelings influence one's behavior and functioning in the oral examination situ-ation? In my opinion, "neurotic difficulties" (Maleson et al., 1980) leading to anxiety in oral examinations are based significantly on transferences between candidate and examiners that occur during the examination. These transferences can be examined from the viewpoint of projected self- and object-images and the resultant re-experiencing of early unmet needs, painful affects, and unresolved conflicts.

Physicians who are oral examination candidates may experience anxiety based on factors they have in common that motivated them to become physicians. The need to help others, the fantasy of being able to cure or discover cures for disease, the longing for admiration, and the willingness to assume considerable responsibility and to sacrifice much of what others rou-tinely enjoy are commonly seen in physicians. While many of these qualities are superficially admirable, and while society relies on individuals who possess these qualities, the unconscious motivation for them often includes narcissistic personality features related to the physician's early experience of his mothering figure being unable to provide adequately for her own or her child's needs. *The term "narcissistic" in this context refers to the child's learning to relegate his subjective experience of himself to a secondary position while focusing on his mother's subjective experience, in an attempt to "heal" his mother. This adaptation involves a disturbance in the child's experience of himself as an autonomous individual, potentially interfering with his sense of himself as separate from others, that is, his experience of him-self, including his feelings, wishes, fears, independent thinking, aspirations, and personal agency. The result is an individual to some extent divorced from his subjective experience of himself, who has not developed aspects of the self he needs to pursue satisfying and meaningful experiences in different aspects of life.*

The gifted child (the future physician) responds by attempting to help her mother by devoting herself to her mother's needs at the expense of developing an adequate awareness of her own needs, of learning how to fulfill them, and of pursuing her own interests (Miller, 1981). The grandiosity of this child in believing that she can fulfill her mother's needs (hoping that her mother then will have more to offer her) may be the best adaptation she could find in childhood, but extracts a heavy toll as the child grows older and continues to focus on the envir-onment for gratification, rather than developing a growing awareness of herself. *This grandiosity can be understood as a grandiose defense against the sense of helplessness that a child might naturally experience when her needs were unmet and she undertook to take care of her mother.* When the individual is a phys-ician candidate in an oral examination setting, grandiosity and omnipotence are qualities that may jeopardize chances of success. To some extent, examination anxiety may be considered a "normal" phenomenon, that, if not overwhelming, may actually be adaptive, helping the candidate both prepare for the examination and focus on it during the examination. Additionally, this anxiety can help to curtail the grandiosity described above. A candidate is more likely to pass an oral examination if she is properly prepared, and does not behave in an arrogant manner.

Object relations theory provides an approach to understanding different candidate–examiner relational constellations (Steinberg, 1998). Unconscious images of self and others begin developing very early in life and continue to be influenced by our experiences throughout life. These unconscious images are more strongly influenced by early interpersonal experiences, especially with parenting figures. The child's self-image is based largely on an internalization of her parents' attitude towards her. To the extent that parents have a generally positive attitude towards their child, she will be inclined to develop a positive attitude towards herself. The converse is true of the unfortunate child whose parents have a generally negative attitude towards her. Excessive frustration, disappointment, neglect, and abuse in early relationships lead to negative internal images of self and others.

We tend to project our self-images and internal objects (our images of ourselves and the other) on to other people. A sign of relative psychological health is that these projections are not so strong that they interfere significantly with our realistic evaluations of others on the basis of our experience with them. Persons functioning at lower levels of psychological development have a predilection to project good or bad part-objects on to others, with a correspondingly unrealistic idealization or devaluation of them. *Excessive projection, which might be either characteristic of an individual functioning at a lower (or more primitive) level of development, or might occur when a person regresses under stress, results in an unrealistic perception of the other person, too strongly based on the contents of the projection (of the self-image or internal object) rather than on realistic perceptions based on one's experience of the other person. By "part-objects," I am referring to one-dimensional, black-and-white, unrealistic images of self and others, for example, an idealized or denigrated view of oneself or the other, rather than a more nuanced ambivalent view, which encompasses both positive and negative attributes. Part-objects, polarized views of self and others, are thought to originate in very early mental life, before positive and negative aspects of the self and other can be integrated in the young child's mind. The implication is that, at a very early age, infants do not experience parents as containing both positive and negative attributes. Rather, the infant experiences her parent as good if they are engaged at the time in a gratifying experience, and bad if they are engaged in an ungratifying experience. At this point of the infant's development, she does not experience the "good" parent and the "bad" parent as the same individual. Infants and children in whom the parent–child fit is too problematic, or whose early experiences were too frustrating, may never get beyond this split experience of others, which remains outside of conscious awareness.* People generally functioning at lower levels of psychological development tend to experience others as all good or all bad, as opposed to tolerating positive and negative feelings concurrently about someone else. Individuals under significant stress may regress and function at a more primitive developmental level than is their norm. An oral certification examination is clearly such a stress.

The extent to which a candidate projects self- and object-images onto the examiners, and the extent to which these images are polarized, depends on several factors, including the candidate's general level of psychological development, how stressful he finds the examination experience, and the extent to which he is subject to unrelated concurrent stresses. A candidate who had generally supportive parents will tend to project a relatively benevolent object image onto the examiners, and will respond to the examination as an opportunity to show his competence as a consultant. A candidate who grew up in an atmosphere where separation and individuation were not supported by his parents, and where dependence was reinforced, may project an internal object onto the examiners characterized by a tendency to intrude and encroach. He may have more difficulty in establishing himself as an expert with his own opinion in the examination, and look for opportunities to defer to the expertise of the examiners. He also may relate to them in a dependent fashion, unconsciously inviting a benign care-giving attitude on their part. These are not likely to be constructive adaptations in the examination situation.

The candidate who as a child was treated with harshness and punitiveness, and experienced his parents as hostile and unaccepting, will be inclined to project a corresponding severe internalized object onto the examiners, and tend to react adversely, either with exaggerated fear or hostility. *One might describe this as a paranoid reaction.* This may interfere with his ability to cope with the examination situation, either by significantly increasing the candidate's anxiety or by fostering an adversarial stance, resulting in his becoming provocative of, or rebellious towards, the examiners, with an increased risk of an untoward result. A candidate may behave grandiosely, attempting to project a threatened, helpless, vulnerable self-image onto the examiners. This projection is unlikely to be accepted by the examiners, who may respond by becoming prejudiced against the candidate, especially if the projection corresponds accurately to a similar unconscious self-image in them that results in their feeling threatened.

When the candidate appears to be having such a "personal" reaction, the job of the examiners, as individuals in positions of greater power and experience, is to support the candidate in functioning at his optimal level of competence. They must avoid the tacit invitation to become benignly patriarchal, intrusively overactive, or punitive. That is, they must try to identify the internalized self- or object-image the candidate is projecting on to them, and not be pressured into assuming that role, analogous to a psychoanalyst identifying the patient's projective identification and "metabolizing it," as opposed to merely reacting to the feelings and impulses the patient elicits in the therapist (Gabbard & Wilkinson, 1994). *In other words, the examiners have to be aware of how the candidate may be influencing the way they are feeling, and not act on this in a destructive way, but reflect on it, and use their feelings to influence the way they support the candidate, helping him to focus on the objective of the meeting, which is to evaluate his professional competence.*

Difficulties may ensue when the examiners' and candidate's mutual projections "fit." An interaction may occur, for example, in which the candidate projects a hostile, critical parental image on to the examiner, and the examiner in turn identifies with his own critical internalized parents and projects a frightened, helpless self-image on to the candidate. In these circumstances, an enactment may occur, an untoward "personal" reaction on the part of both candidate and examiner that is played out in reality (Plakun, 1998). *In an enactment, unconscious factors motivate the behavior of individuals towards each other, such that an unconscious internal relationship scenario in each party to the interaction, which usually is based on real early experiences, often with caregivers, is recapitulated between the two parties in the present, often to the detriment of one or both of them.* This may jeopardize the examination's fairness and validity. It would be important for the other examiner (when there are two) to be aware of the potential for this, to intervene in a tactful way during the examination if necessary, and to bring this up in the post-examination discussion with the examination board if she feels the interaction affected the outcome of the examination.

Examiners also are vulnerable to transference reactions. Although they have much less at stake than candidates, they may have personal reactions to examination or candidates. An examiner who projects an aspect of herself onto a candidate may behave according to what she would have wanted from her own parents, and treat the candidate in a particularly benevolent, kindly, and supportive manner. On the other hand, an examiner may project a vulnerable, humiliated self-image onto a candidate, identifying with the parent as aggressor, and tend to treat the candidate in an inappropriately aggressive fashion, browbeating or deriding him, possibly eliciting fear and humiliation in him – reactivating the situation of how the examiner once felt with her parents.

In the case of an examiner with grandiose tendencies, grandiosity may defend against feelings of anxiety, low self-esteem, and helplessness in a manner that interferes with the examiner's capacity to assess the candidate. This situation would turn the examination into a defense on the examiner's part against an awareness of her threatened self-image by projecting it onto the candidate. Alternatively, an examiner (rarely) may experience herself as a frightened child, and project a more controlling object-image representing her parents onto the candidate, allowing the candidate to dominate the examination. An anxious candidate may elicit any of the above reactions, depending partly on the examiner's tendencies. These reactions of candidates and examiners correspond to different types of countertransference in psychoanalysis, including complementary and concordant countertransferences described by Racker (1968). The potential for difficulty in the interaction between the examiners, which might affect the examination outcome, is considered below. In addition, transferences that may occur between candidate and patient during the oral examination are not discussed here, but may influence the reciprocal reactions between candidate and examiner, analogous to the parallel process of psychotherapy supervision (Ekstein & Wallerstein, 1972).

The work of Bion and his followers offers a different perspective. One might consider the candidate whose anxiety before or during the examination is severe enough to impair his functioning possibly being overwhelmed by proto-emotions, precursors of emotions that cannot be distinguished from each other, and cannot be thought of or experienced consciously, or from physical sensations. In these circumstances, a candidate either has regressed to a level, or characteristically functions at a level, where his emotions cannot be articulated verbally, and are experienced in a more primitive manner in which physical sensations and emotions are not distinguished. This could become an unbearable experience for the candidate, who would require someone to help him contain these somato-psychic types of early experience. Before the examination, this might be a mentor, family member, teacher, or supervisor. The containing person could help the candidate articulate his anxieties, giving words to them, a process that, with the emotional support being provided, may reduce the candidate's anxiety to more manageable proportions. If not, the candidate might benefit from being referred to a psychotherapist or psychoanalyst for psychotherapy before the examination. Brief forms of psychoanalytic psychotherapy have been developed when time is limited, for whatever reason (Levenson, 2017). From a technical point of view, psychoanalysis, psychodynamic psychotherapy, or even sensitive support by a non-therapist may help the candidate to convert his proto-emotions into thoughts accompanied by feelings, or, at least, provide a temporary infusion of thoughts accompanied by feelings from the other person. This process is what is thought to underlie the mother's experience of reverie in containing an infant's unbearable feelings. This process is gradually internalized by the infant, and eventually develops into the infant's capacity for thought, that is, thinking thoughts accompanied by feelings. A similar process occurs in psychoanalysis and psychoanalytic psychotherapy.

DISCUSSION

Candidates have the right to expect fair and impartial behavior on the part of their examiners; hopefully, this generally occurs. If a candidate feels an examiner deviates from his expected role, the candidate needs to manage her anxiety and adhere to the role of junior consultant, giving her medical opinion to senior colleagues. If she is aware of possible motivations for the examiner's behavior, she can help to manage her own anxiety. The candidate may also monitor her emotional reactions to the examiner's behavior in attempting to avoid an untoward behavioral reaction. For example, depending on the personality of the candidate, she may react to an overly aggressive examiner either by becoming unduly aggressive or submissive, or by not giving her opinion as completely or confidently as she otherwise would. A candidate might react to a seductively friendly examiner by being lulled into a state of unwarranted relaxation and not function optimally, given the realistic expectations of the examination situation. Alternatively, a candidate might be taken aback, given the state of mind induced in her by an unexpectedly pointed series of questions. The candidate needs to observe her reactions to the examination as they occur. Her awareness of her own personality tendencies will facilitate an appropriate response to the examiners, as opposed to projecting a self- or object-image onto them in a wholesale manner, perhaps acting on these projections in potentially self-destructive ways.

Candidates also may struggle with their own emotional reactions to the examination situation, independent of the examiner's behavior. Most candidates likely repeatedly rehearse the examination and its hoped-for and feared outcomes in their minds. To some extent, this is normal, healthy anticipatory thinking. At some point, however, depending on its frequency, duration, and the related affective intensity, it may become a preoccupation or obsessional ruminations. If the candidate feels too apprehensive about the examination, or is considerably more anxious than reality warrants, some self-analysis at least is called for. The candidate may ask herself what her motivation may be for the excessive anxiety along the lines already described. Candidates for oral examinations in psychiatry should be in a better position to do this, given what their training should include. As suggested above, the overanxious candidate may consider a brief form of psychoanalytic therapy to help deal with her anxiety by understanding its unconscious basis, if it is excessive, especially if she fears it might affect the examination outcome. Alternative symptomatic treatments for control of symptoms of anxiety include cognitive behavioral therapy and medication. I believe, especially in cases of candidates for psychiatric certification examinations, that if the candidate expects to need a symptomatic treatment for anxiety, it would be advantageous to consider exploring the unconscious basis of her anxiety. The advantage of a psychoanalytic form of treatment is that it often provides the individual not only with symptomatic relief, but also helps her to find more adaptive solutions to problems in life that are not directly related to the problem that motivated her to seek treatment, that is, anxiety regarding the examination. It also is clear that the psychiatrist who has some familiarity with her unconscious conflicts and relational difficulties is in a much better position to assess and manage patients with similar conflicts and difficulties than she would be without such an awareness (Gabbard, 1996).

Similar relational configurations based on corresponding transferences and/or projective identifications also may occur between the examiners. These may be based on differences in theoretical or technical approaches, seniority, or other factors to which the individual examiners are sensitive. Such reactions may have an impact on the outcome of the examination. For example, one examiner may feel that the other is favoring the candidate, and will try to balance this by treating the candidate in an unduly challenging manner. A caricature of an examination occurs when the examiners debate the very issues about which they should be questioning the candidate. These considerations may also be applicable in relationships between psychiatric educators and residents. As people in positions of power and authority in relation to residents, educators likely experience the same kinds of transferences that candidates are prone to bring to oral examinations. Educators who are invested in their residents succeeding in the examinations may help residents identify unconscious transferential factors in situations of evaluation, and may address these specifically as they relate to the resident's preparation for the oral examinations.

Personal reactions on the part of candidates and examiners in oral board certification examinations cannot be eliminated. Undesirable behaviors of examiners can be limited by adherence to established guidelines (Ferron, 1998). The examiners are responsible for identifying signs of untoward "personal" reactions in the candidates or themselves, and should respond appropriately. The application of object relations concepts can assist the examiners in these considerations. The examiner's willingness and ability to be introspective and observant, to notice how he, his fellow examiner, and the candidate are behaving and appear to feel during the examination, will help him manage the examination in a manner that optimizes its fairness and validity.

CONCLUSIONS

By applying object relations theory, both examiners and candidates can increase understanding of anxiety in oral certification examinations in order to enhance the fairness and validity of the examinations. Unconscious images of self and others that examiners and candidates may project on to each other can affect the examination. The examiner must observe himself, the candidate, and the other examiner, lest a transference affecting the process of the examination occur, and to avoid an enactment that might interfere with the examination. The result of these observations should appropriately support the candidate in functioning at an optimal level of competence. Unconscious processes may prejudice the examiner's attitude towards a candidate, thus jeopardizing the examination's fairness and validity. The candidate's anxiety, based on projections onto the examiners, may interfere with her optimal functioning and affect the outcome. If a candidate's anticipatory anxiety is excessive, she needs to decide if it needs to be managed on a symptomatic or psychotherapeutic basis. Candidates and examiners both need to monitor their feelings during the examination in order to optimize the latter's fairness and validity. All these issues may also be considered in the relationship between psychiatric educators and trainees.

REFERENCES

Bauer SF (1978). Nothing to worry about: A clinical note on examination anxiety. *Psychoanalytic Quarterly* 47: 606–613.
Blum E (1926). The psychology of study and examinations. *International Journal of Psychoanalysis* VII:457–469.

Ekstein R, Wallerstein RS (1972). *The Teaching and Learning of Psychotherapy*, 2nd edition. New York: International Universities Press.

Ferron D (1998). Guidelines for conduct of oral examination. *Annals of the Royal College of Physicians and Surgeons of Canada* 31(1):28–30.

Ferron D (undated). The concept of acceptable competency and the certification examinations of the Royal College. The McLaughlin Centre for Evaluation, Royal College of Physicians and Surgeons of Canada.

Flugel J (1939). The examination as initiation right and anxiety situation. *International Journal of Psychoanalysis* XX:275–286.

Freud S (1900/1953). *The Interpretation of Dreams. Standard Edition of the Complete Psychological Works of Sigmund Freud*, Vol. IV. London: Hogarth Press, 273–276.

Gabbard GO (1996). Lessons to be learned from the study of sexual boundary violations. *American Journal of Psychotherapy* 50(3):311–322.

Gabbard GO, Wilkinson SM (1994). *Management of Countertransference with Borderline Patients*. Washington, DC: American Psychiatric Press.

Greenson R (1967). *The Technique and Practice of Psychoanalysis*. New York: International Universities Press.

Kafka E (1979). On examination dreams. *Psychoanalytic Quarterly* 48:426–447.

Langs R (1974). *The Technique of Psychoanalytic Psychotherapy*, Vol. II. New York: Jason Aronson.

Levenson H (2017). *Brief Dynamic Therapy*, 2nd edition. Washington, DC: American Psychological Association.

Maleson F, Fink P, Field H (1980). Board certification anxiety. *American Journal of Psychiatry* 137(7):837–840.

Michalon M, Iracema L (1998). Physicians as patients – substance use and psychiatric illnesses among medical trainees and practitioners: A professional predicament. *Annals of the Royal College of Physicians and Surgeons of Canada* 31:379–383.

Miller A (1981). *Prisoners of Childhood: The Drama of the Gifted Child and the Search for the True Self*. New York: Basic Books.

North CS, Ryall JE (1997). Psychiatric illness in female physicians. *Postgraduate Medicine* 101:5, 233–236, 239–240, 242.

Plakun EM (1998). Enactment and the treatment of abuse survivors. *Harvard Review of Psychiatry* 16:318–325.

Racker H (1968). *Transference and Countertransference*. Madison, CT: International Universities Press.

Schmideberg M (1933). Ein Pruefungsneurose. *Zeitschrift fuer Psychoanalyse paediatrische* XIX:198–202.

Steinberg PI (1998). Attachment and object relations in formulation and psychotherapy. *Annals of the Royal College of Physicians and Surgeons of Canada* 31(1):19–22.

Stengel E (1936). Pruefungsangst und Pruefungsneurose. *Zeitschrift fuer Psychoanalyse Paediatrische* X:300–320.

Sussman MB (1992). *A Curious Calling: Unconscious Motivations for Practising Psychotherapy*. Northvale, NJ: Jason Aronson.

Thorner HA (1954). Three defenses against inner persecution. In: Klein M (ed.), *New Directions in Psychoanalysis*. London: Tavistock.

CHAPTER 18

HEALERS CARING FOR THEMSELVES AND EACH OTHER: PREVENTING SUICIDE IN MEDICAL STUDENTS, RESIDENTS, AND OURSELVES

Statistics about physician suicide have been alarming for decades. I recall that 40 years ago it was described as being 30 times greater than that in the general population, with psychiatrists and ophthalmologists, along with dentists, having the highest rates. This is higher than contemporary figures. Because of their greater knowledge of and better access to lethal means, physicians have a higher suicide completion rate than the general public. The most reliable estimates of successful completion of suicide range from 1.4 to 2.3 times the rate achieved in the general population. Although female physicians attempt suicide far less often than their counterparts in the general population, their completion rate equals that of male physicians, thus exceeding that of the general population, 2.5–4 times the rate by some estimates. Underreporting of suicide as cause of death by sympathetic colleagues certifying death may skew these statistics; consequently, the real incidence of physician suicide may be higher than prevailing estimates. Sussman (1995) found suicide rate among psychiatric residents to be 4 in 100,000, much higher than for any other medical specialty. Kleespies et al. (2011) describe large surveys indicating that psychologists are at risk for depression, anxiety, substance abuse, and suicidality. They find that healthcare professionals, including physicians, dentists, and nurses, are at elevated risk for suicide. They conclude that further research is needed to confirm if there is a heightened risk of suicide for psychologists.

Physicians, residents, and medical students who die by suicide often have untreated or undertreated depression or other psychiatric conditions. The culture of medical training is very demanding, and can be critical and shaming of anyone who does not conform to expectations. Limits have been set in many residency programs regarding on-call frequency, but there is pressure to ignore them, especially in surgical specialties, which are well known for long hours.

Psychoanalysis began as the study of unconscious motivation of repressed (because unacceptable to conscious awareness) sexual or aggressive impulses that became symbolized by a conversion symptom. It has expanded to explore unconscious motivations of many aspects of life. Unconscious motivations to become a physician include fear of illness (that often is related to illness in the physician's family of origin), with a consequent unconscious wish to heal one's parent, similar to wishes that often motivate one to become a psychotherapist or psychoanalyst, and a denial of mortality, which can assume the form of an omnipotent/manic defense against the awareness of the inevitability of aging, illness, and death. An omnipotent/manic defense consists of a denial of normal human limitations, combined with feeling that one can accomplish anything — feeling like Superman. This defense is difficult to sustain for any length of time in people who still maintain some contact with reality. When it collapses, it often is followed by what it is intended to defend against: feelings of depression, despair, hopelessness, and powerlessness. This gives some indication of some physicians' potential vulnerability to depression and suicidal feelings.

Often learning about medicine involves employing defenses against fear of illness, including intellectualization (focusing on intellectual aspects of a problem at the expense of the emotional aspects) and isolation of affect (separating the affect from the feared thought content). One could describe becoming a physician to frequently involve a counter-phobic defense against the fear of illness. That is, the feared situation is not avoided, but is confronted head-on in an attempt to master it. The unconscious fantasy is,

"I will be a physician and take care of sick people, avoiding illness myself." Another way of describing this is that the unconscious fear of illness is projected onto the patient. (All physicians remember "medical students' disease," in which the student fears she has the symptoms of a succession of the diseases she studies. This represents the return of the repressed – in this case, the repressed fear of illness.)

Many individuals are motivated to be effective and compassionate physicians who render their communities considerable service on the basis of these defenses. However, the accompanying danger is that, to the extent that the physician is unconsciously preoccupied with defending against awareness of her fear of illness, this may affect her treatment of her patients such that she has difficulty distinguishing between their needs and her unconscious needs. This may result, in some cases, in a cavalier attitude towards illness, reassuring patients who realistically cannot be reassured by reassurance, and who will feel their concerns are unheard. An extreme example of this would be if the physician needed to deny the possibility of illness to the extent that indicated investigations or treatment were withheld. Another possibility is that the physician might be overly scrupulous in investigating and treating his patient's condition, resulting in unnecessary tests, procedures, and treatments that might be both wasteful and expose the patient to needless risk.

I wish to make a connection between a child's need to cure her parent, which involves an excessive burden on the young future physician, with the excessive kinds of demands that some people make of themselves that can get them in trouble in situations like oral examinations, described in Chapter 17. One can understand both cases as representing an excessively demanding figure in the patient's internal world that I have described as a persecutory internal object. This may be based, at least in part, on demands the child's parents made on her beyond what she could meet, which Miller (1981) describes. These could include curing a parent's emotional disturbance, becoming the success a parent longs for, or providing a parent with what the parent's partner isn't providing emotionally. These early experiences often have their parallel in the adult life of physicians, not setting limits on what they think they can accomplish, including working excessively long hours, allowing themselves to be emotionally overburdened by demanding patients who don't respect the physician's boundaries, and generally trying to do the impossible – omnipotence again! Working under the burden of such a demanding internal master can make physicians more vulnerable to despair and accompanying suicidal feelings.

This chapter is based on a presentation given to medical and dental students after a classmate committed suicide. I was asked to advise the students how to prevent this by outlining signs that might suggest a colleague who may be suicidal should be assisted in seeking appropriate treatment. (What follows applies to students, residents, and practicing physicians; I will use the term "physicians" to refer to all.) I provided a modicum of the information requested, and then focused on what physicians might do for themselves to prevent their lives from becoming so painful that suicide would seem an option. I discuss unconscious motivations for physicians to overinvolve themselves in their work at the expense of relationships and recreational activities. Physicians are advised to limit their ambitions and to lead a life balanced among love, work, and play, as opposed to placing too heavy a burden on work to provide satisfaction and meaning in life. A secondary benefit of this approach is that the physician then will be in a better position to notice someone else's distress and be able to offer help.

When a colleague may be suicidal, something must be done about it. This situation is analogous to having a patient who is at risk. The most appropriate approach is to ask about this tactfully and directly. It may be an obvious concern when the person tells you that he is depressed or desperate, feels hopeless, or is suicidal. It is important to provide emotional support, and to ensure that he receives timely psychiatric evaluation and treatment. Medical associations sometimes can direct physicians and their families to speedy psychiatric assessment. *A colleague with a major psychiatric disorder, such as an acute major depression or psychotic disorder, may be at high risk, and should have emergency psychiatric assessment. Colleagues whose problems are more long-standing that appear related to their personalities may not require urgent assessment, and often can benefit from long-term psychoanalytic psychotherapy or psychoanalysis, but may not be aware of the availability, or even existence, of these treatments, and would need to be directed to appropriate therapists for assessment. Without treatment, a significant proportion of them may become at risk for suicidal ideation and behavior. The high rates of completed suicide among physicians make active intervention essential.*

At times, the warning signs are less obvious. Then one might ask the individual how she is feeling, gradually enquiring more specifically about suicidal ideation. She may divulge that she has contemplated suicide. If a person is determined to commit suicide, it is difficult or impossible to prevent this, even with the best psychiatric care available. After the event, people may remember a comment that they feel they should have recognized as an indication that the individual was suicidal, or believe that something they failed to pay attention to should have prompted them to take action. Colleagues who are acquaintances and friends of an individual who commits suicide may feel guilty and remorseful as they blame themselves, while feeling sad and angry as they mourn the death of someone they knew and to whom they may have been closely attached. *This may represent a turning against themselves of the anger they feel towards the individual who has committed suicide, for abandoning them in this violent way, and perhaps reminding them of some feelings of despair of their own.*

When a physician believes that a colleague might be suicidal, he should try to explore with the colleague the risk of self-destruction. If the person is determined to commit suicide, she may not divulge it, but may later proceed to commit suicide. Most people, however, when they are feeling suicidal, are ambivalent about it; there is a healthy part of them that wishes to live. This is the part one needs to contact, the part to appeal to, the part who will cooperate in their getting help.

Physicians commit themselves for their professional lives to taking care of people. One problem with which they are confronted continuously is the limits to the care they can provide. To expect to prevent all suicides is as unrealistic as hoping to prevent all mortality from diabetes or cardiovascular disease. People die, whether they are patients, friends, colleagues. or family members, and sometimes they die by their own hands. It is unrealistic to expect that this always can be prevented, even in a colleague or a friend. It is important to consider the psychological side of physicians' needs to care for people in trying to prevent these tragedies from happening.

Miller (1981) writes about the gifted, intelligent child who many medical students were in their youth. There is no family without problems; relevant questions include, how severe are the problems, and what resources are there in the family to cope with them? If a gifted, intelligent child is growing up in a family with significant ongoing problems, and the parents' capacity to deal with the problems is limited, the child may end up volunteering or being enlisted to help. There might be little amiss with this. The child might even have a positive experience thereby, and gain confidence in the experience. On the other hand, the child might gradually assume the role of problem-solver or caregiver, and learn to relegate her needs and wishes to a secondary position to those of the family. This can happen in many ways, for example, by providing emotional support and practical help or, eventually, financial assistance to parents; by assuming parental responsibilities, taking care of siblings, feeding them, and sending them off to school; or by becoming the confidante of one or both parents. This manner of relating, which might be the best adaptation the child can find to the family's problems at the time, may become a pattern that continues in the child's life into adulthood. This may help explain why a medical student may be willing to sacrifice time during adolescence and young adulthood that might otherwise have been devoted to the pleasures of youth, but instead is spent in demanding study and clinical work. Concrete rewards in life accrue to those who choose medicine as a profession, including having an interesting career, being well remunerated, attaining a respectable position in society, and having the opportunity to continue to learn. For some physicians, the concrete rewards that their practice offers are insufficient, and they look to increasing professional accomplishments, recognition, and even power to gratify them, and to justify all the time and energy they have devoted to their studies and clinical work, and, sometimes, the work of caring for their families of origin.

The sacrifice that the gifted child makes is not made without an expectation of an ultimate reward that may never be forthcoming from the parents. The more the gifted child is involved in providing care for the family, the more this affects his personality, and the more he becomes a caregiver and learns how to relate in that manner. At the same time, the more the parents are preoccupied with their own difficulties, and the more the gifted child ends up being preoccupied with their difficulties, the less they have time, energy, and attention to devote to the child's need to develop, and to explore his interests, talents, ambitions, and aspirations. The child might be rewarded for assuming the role of caregiver, at least by receiving some appreciation from his parents, *but might grow up longing for much more attention, affection, and interest than his parents can provide. This sense of unmet emotional needs usually is repressed (blocked out of conscious awareness), but continues to affect the individual thus burdened.* Tendencies that start in childhood usually continue into teenage years and young adult life. The result may be a gifted child who grows up learning how to be a caregiver, *with an unconscious longing to be cared for himself that continues to be unfulfilled. In addition to the longings continuing to be frustrated in adult life, another problem is that physicians may bring these unmet needs into their relationships with their patients, sometimes with results that are not in the patients' best interests. (Chapter 19 deals with the most egregious examples of this.) Substance abuse is another destructive means of soothing oneself in the lack of satisfying interpersonal experiences.*

Unconscious motivations in choosing to be a professional caregiver are well recognized (Bowlby, 1980: 16; Sussman, 1992). The gifted child may experience gratification related to a sense of competence for the care she provides. This gratification, however, is accompanied by a sense of neglect of the child's needs, because she is focusing too much on the family's needs. One solution that some gifted children use in coming to terms with their feelings about this price is to excel in other activities, including hobbies, academic pursuits, or sports. This may provide some gratification in itself, as the child achieves at a high level in the same way as she originally did in helping the family. There may also be praise from teachers and coaches, which enhances the accomplishment's attractiveness, and may provide the child in these relationships with something that has been missing at home. The danger is that the child's ambition, the lust for achievement to feel good about herself, and to use it as a medium by which to relate to other people, may become overdeveloped, at the expense of developing a capacity for involvement in a variety of interpersonal relationships, and a capacity for enjoying non-competitive recreational and vocational activities for their own sake. If a child's relationship needs are neglected as she devotes herself to helping her parents in the hope that they eventually will have more to offer, she may eventually turn to other achievements besides helping her parents to give herself a sense of importance, mastery, and self-esteem. This is especially likely if the parents reinforce this tendency by expressing gratification at these accomplishments.

A sense of achievement and ambition combined with a hope for public admiration may, in some individuals, become a substitute for close relationships, intimate communication, and personally rewarding activities. The individual then becomes overly oriented towards hard work and distant, if not unrealizable, goals of achievement, away from more immediate and wholesome (at the risk of making a value judgment) sources of gratification, including enjoying close relationships, having fun, and being engaged in activities that are meaningful to the individual. Thus, the person who experienced early neglect may substitute achievements and public acclaim for satisfying relationships, enjoyable activities, and an internal sense of peace and integrity. *Some individuals are quite high-functioning superficially in a given academic, vocational, recreational, or sporting pursuit, but function less well in situations other than their chosen area of excellence, in particular, in interpersonal relationships. These individuals have sacrificed social development, the opportunity for close interpersonal relationships, and a capacity to be interested in constructive social activity, for the limited benefits of public recognition, financial success, and/or power. They may not even value the area in which they excel for its own sake, but rather for what it brings them, and seem unable to invest interest in other people, ideas, or activities.*

The rewards that achievement offers are limited. Sometimes people discover this in a painful way. This can occur after a long and conventionally successful professional, business, or academic career, either when an individual finds that, having devoted excessive time and energy to work, he missed too much else in life, or when he retires and finds that there is little left to live for. This disappointment may also occur during the years of formal education, when he isn't awarded the gold medal for which he worked so assiduously and which he needed to receive so badly. *These individuals often are described as narcissistic. Eventually their obliviousness to other people and the superficiality of their gratification get them into difficulties. Frequently they manage to ride on a wave of success in early adult life, but at some point in middle age, or when they retire and lose the substitutes for wholesome satisfaction that their career provided them, they experience the emptiness of their lives and frequently become depressed. One often sees desperate attempts to forestall the realities of aging, with individuals refusing to leave positions in which they are no longer capable of functioning competently, or attempting to maintain authority over family members who have long outgrown the need or wish for this. One could call this an omnipotent defense against the helplessness of aging, and a refusal to mourn what they have deprived themselves of in life, in an attempt to circumvent despair (Sussman, 1995).*

For all individuals, an important protective factor against suicidal feelings and behavior is the establishment of positive-enough unconscious internal images of self and others, that is, a positive enough self-image and internal objects. This should favor positive relationships between these internal figures, so they can work together in influencing individuals to take care of themselves and enhance the likelihood of positive experiences with other individuals in the world. The establishment and maintenance of a positive self-image and positive internal objects come about, to a considerable extent, by the internalization of qualities of others with whom we have positive relationships, and the internalization of feelings about these relationships, which also favor realistic positive expectations about potential relationships. This of course begins in the first relationships with parental figures, who are most influential (in happy circumstances) in the establishment of a positive self-image and internal objects, and expectations of positive relationships with others. Medical studies and practice (and, no less, psychoanalytic study and practice) offer many opportunities for internalizing positive experiences. These include relationships with fellow students and eventually physicians and analysts at a peer level, as well as relationships with teachers, supervisors, mentors, and professional leaders, such as hospital department chiefs and chairs of academic department, and relationships with subordinates, such as students and residents when one is a consultant. Of course, adult experiences with friends and family on an ongoing basis are similarly internalized and influential, and, last, but not least, our relationships with our patients. All of these types of relationships naturally have the capacity to generate negative interactions as well, some of which can be very hurtful, and may favor the development of a more negative self-image, more negative internal objects, and the unconscious expectation of more negative experiences in relationships with others. Unfortunately, this results not just in an unconscious expectation of negative experience with others, but also a perception of negative experience (that others without the same negative experience of relationships might not perceive), and even possibly a provocation or invitation to negative experience with others, which can involve a self-fulfilling prophecy and a vicious cycle. That is, people whose experiences have been too negative for them to cope with are at greater risk of developing negative self-images and internal objects. This influences them to expect negative experiences with others, to interpret interpersonal experiences more negatively than might be realistic, and even to induce others to engage with them in negative experiences.

One way of thinking about a person who is suicidal is that he is under the influence of a murderous internal object (unconscious image of the other) that may correspond, more or less, to the individual's early experiences with parental figures. Ferenczi (1929) describes children who are unwelcome to their parents when they arrive, for any number of reasons. Their chances for survival are lessened because of this. If they do survive infancy and early childhood, they still may have unconscious self-destructive tendencies, manifest in a variety of ways, including accident-proneness, substance abuse, or a tendency to become suicidal when under stress. They may even be more susceptible to serious illness that may lead to death. Ferenczi notes,

> these children had observed the conscious and unconscious signs of the aversion or impatience of the mother ... their desire to live had been broken by this. In later life relatively slight occasions were then sufficient motivation for a desire to die, even if this was resisted by a strong effort of will ... pessimism, scepticism and mistrust became conspicuous character-traits in these patients, [as well as] ill-disguised longing for (passive) tenderness, repugnance to work, incapacity for prolonged effort, and thus a certain degree of emotional infantilism, naturally not without attempts at forced character-strengthening.
>
> (Ferenczi, 1929: 126–127)

While an individual (who is not chronically suicidal) might become suicidal at any given moment, usually precipitated by some unbearable loss, blow to self-esteem, or other catastrophic experience, it is not as if this is just a transient state that can be overcome and forgotten about. The tendency to become suicidal is greater in some individuals than in others. It is part of one's personality make-up. This can be dealt with in psychoanalytic work, whereas symptomatic treatments may reduce the person's immediate suicidal risk, but not their proclivity to become suicidal under stress. Becoming suicidal might be described as a very concrete and dangerous manifestation of psychic deadness (Ogden, 1995), something which is, more or less, not uncommon.

Rather than focusing on what one can do to prevent colleagues from committing suicide, physicians first can focus on doing their best to reduce their own risk of becoming suicidal, succumbing to depression, resorting to substance abuse, or other self-destructive solutions. This is a preventive approach to the high levels of psychopathology that have been observed in physicians (Michelon & Leroi, 1998). To the main two areas of human endeavor that Freud described, love and work, a third, play, for which there was for most people less emphasis in Freud's era than in ours, can be added. Medical students generally have no difficulty with work, although the danger of their overdoing it is clear. Regarding love, no accomplishment at work or professional recognition can replace the satisfaction and gratification that come from positive attachments with people to whom one is close. Neither can achievement in one's career replace the excitement or pleasure obtainable from a recreational activity that is unrelated to one's chosen work, however valuable this work is. The importance of play, both recreationally and as a necessary part of development and creativity, both in childhood and adult life, has been recognized (Winnicott, 1971). It is important to have a limit to one's ambition. It is not necessarily a disadvantage to be ambitious, but the person who always has to climb one rung higher on the ladder might find that she is never satisfied, or that it is lonely at the top. It is unwise to base one's satisfaction in work solely on conventional success. *A different measure of success, based on an individual's own interests and desires, rather than on what one perceives is valued by society, is the capacity to immerse oneself in what one is passionate about. This is more likely to help develop a sense of personal integrity and inner peace.* One may never satisfy all of one's ambitions. It is more reasonable to have as a goal continuing to learn, to hone one's professional skills, to discover or create something, or to explore an interesting area.

CONCLUSION

The physician who is too dependent on ongoing achievement and professional recognition, and who lacks the ongoing support of non-work-related positive attachments and gratification from interests, will be at increased risk for disappointment, depression, and even suicidal thoughts when the workplace doesn't provide what he demands of it. Based on early relational experiences, he may place too heavy a burden on work to provide gratifications that also should be derived from other areas in life. No amount of conventional success can substitute for the development of the self-respect, purpose, and integrity that can be achieved with a proper balance of work, love, and play. Physicians must care for themselves first. Those who do, who lead a reasonably balanced and thoughtful life and derive satisfaction from several areas of life, won't have all their eggs in one basket. When there is a hole in the basket, and they don't get the gold medal or the promotion, when their research isn't published in the most prestigious journal, or when they must relinquish the basket at retirement, they won't be left with no eggs. Physicians need to take care of themselves and their loved ones. If they do, as a secondary benefit, they will be in a better position to notice when someone else, like a colleague, is having difficulties and to try to help. *Of course, the above thoughts apply to healthcare professionals in general, and, for that matter, to everyone.*

REFERENCES

Bowlby J (1980). *Attachment and Loss Volume 3: Loss.* New York: Penguin.

Ferenczi S (1929). The unwelcome child and his death-instinct. *International Journal of Psychoanalysis* 10:125–129.

Kleespies PM, Van Orden KA, Bongar B, Bridgeman D, Bufka LF, Galper DI, Hillbrand M, Yufit RI (2011). Psychologist suicide: Incidence, impact, and suggestions for prevention, intervention, and postvention. *Professional Psychology-Research and Practice* 42(3):244–251.

Michelon M, Leroi I (1998). Physicians as patients – substance use and psychiatric illnesses among medical trainees and practitioners: A professional predicament. *Annals of the Royal College of Physicians and Surgeons of Canada* 31:379–383.

Miller A (1981). *Prisoners of Childhood: The Drama of the Gifted Child and the Search for the True Self.* New York: Basic Books.

Ogden TH (1995). Analyzing forms of aliveness and deadness of the transference–countertransference. *International Journal of Psychoanalysis* 76:695–709.

Sussman MB (1992). *A Curious Calling: Unconscious Motivation for Practicing Psychotherapy.* Northvale, NJ: Jason Aronson.

Sussman M (ed.) (1995). *A Perilous Calling: The Hazards of Psychotherapy Practice.* New York: Wiley.

Winnicott WD (1971). *Playing and Reality.* New York: Tavistock Publications.

CHAPTER 19

PROFESSIONAL BETRAYAL: SEXUAL ABUSE OF ADULT FEMALE PATIENTS BY MALE PHYSICIANS

INTRODUCTION

This article deals with sexual abuse of adult female patients by male physicians, by far the most commonly identified form of sexual abuse of adult patients. Sexual victimization has been divided into two groups: situations in which one person exerts force over another (rape); and situations in which one person exerts pressure over another person of unequal status. In the latter case, the individual in authority uses sex to take advantage of someone with less power (Burgess, 1981). McPhedran et al. (1991) distinguish between sexual impropriety and sexual abuse for penalty considerations. Sexual impropriety is defined as verbal behavior that is seductive or sexually demeaning to a patient, including inappropriate procedures and comments. Sexual abuse is defined as including physician–patient sexual activity, and any conduct with a patient that is sexual, or may be reasonably interpreted to be sexual, including sexual intercourse, kissing and touching breasts or genitals. The American Medical Association's Council on Ethical and Judicial Affairs has concluded that sexual contact during a physician–patient relationship is unethical, that sexual contact with a former patient may be unethical, that education on ethical issues in sexual misconduct should be included in medical training, and that it is especially important to report offending colleagues (Council on Ethical and Judicial Affairs, American Medical Association, 1991).

Revelations of sexual abuse by individuals such as physicians and priests, whom society has put in a position of trust and authority (Bates & Brodsky, 1989; Gabbard, 1989; Rutter, 1989), make it necessary to examine how and why this abuse occurs, and what can be done to prevent it and deal with it (Gamell et al., 1988; Kardener et al., 1973; Perry, 1976; Strasburger et al., 1990). Much harm is done to female patients by sexually abusive male physicians (Butler & Zelen, 1977; Davidson, 1977; Nadelson, 1989: 229–231; Rutter, 1986: 71–91; Valiquette et al., 1990).

In one anonymous questionnaire, it was found that 5–7.2% of physicians engaged in sexual intercourse with patients (Kardener et al., 1973). In another survey, 7.1% of male and 3.1% of female psychiatrists acknowledged having sexual contact with patients (Gartrell et al., 1986). One estimate suggested that 10% of all physicians sexually abuse their patients (McPhedran et al., 1991). These figures are based on voluntary reports and cannot be considered definitive. Important considerations include treatment for the abused patient (Moscarello, 1990), prevention of abuse, and prevention of recurrence.

PHYSICIAN'S CONTRIBUTION

Male physicians who sexually abuse their female patients have been divided into two groups (Gartrell et al., 1986; Kardener et al., 1973; Rapp, 1987). The first group includes physicians who are vulnerable to sexual involvement with their patients on the basis of a time-limited situation. These physicians often have psychological symptoms such as depression or anxiety related to an interpersonal loss or disappointment, or loss of a gratification that was a substitute for an interpersonal relationship. Examples would be marital separation or discord, or a financial or professional setback. The second group includes physicians who are susceptible because of their character. They have narcissistic and/or antisocial traits, and take advantage of their patients' vulnerability and trust. *(In my opinion, the physician who is sexually abusive on the basis of his character has a severe personality disorder.)* They are opportunistic and unaware of or unconcerned with how the gratification of their impulses will affect others, or how it will affect themselves and their career in the long term. These "characterological" abusers experience little remorse compared with the "situational" abusers. The characterological abusers tend to repeatedly abuse patients, and only stop when the abuse is discovered. They are likely to be less amenable to psychotherapeutic intervention, to have a poorer prognosis, and to be more inclined to repeat their abuse than situational abusers.

Most abusive physicians probably do not fall into absolute situational or characterological categories: it probably is more accurate to place each individual somewhere on a continuum, with situational features at one end and characterological features at the other. As a result, a physician may be characterologically predisposed to abusive behavior, which may be precipitated by increased stresses in his life. A third group of abusive physicians includes those with severe psychiatric disturbance, such as severe depression and psychotic conditions. The distinction between situational and characterological abusers is based on psychiatrists' self-reports; one needs to objectively delineate these groups. This might identify a group of abusers who could be successfully treated. *One physician allegedly could identify which of his patients would comply with a non-verbal invitation to fellatio. This might represent an individual with in the characterological category with narcissistic and/or antisocial personality traits.*

Twemlow and Gabbard (1989) divide abusive therapists into the psychotic, the antisocial, and the love-sick. They think many therapists who fall in love with patients are narcissistic, and become love-sick over a patient when in a life crisis. The therapist and patient each unconsciously believe they can satisfy a need or resolve a conflict in the other. The therapist may project aspects of himself onto the patient, who may respond as though she is his projected self-representation. The tendency for the therapist to fall in love with his projected reflection is linked to a desire for union with a hidden or split-off aspect of himself. The love-sick state can be seen as a regression to a pleasant boundary-less state preceding the development of ego boundaries. *This refers to a chronologically early developmental stage characterized by the experience of being merged with the mother that infants are thought to experience, before learning to distinguish between themselves and others, which capacity gradually develops in the first months of life.*

I am uncomfortable with using terms like "love-sickness," which do not correspond to a diagnostic category, like antisocial personality disorder and narcissistic personality disorder. If love-sickness is not to be considered a diagnostic category, one should attempt to use the present diagnostic classification to describe this clinical picture, rather than invent a new term. Twemlow and Gabbard appear to be suggesting that love-sickness is an experience of narcissistic individuals under stress. This suggests that love-sick individuals represent a subgroup of narcissistic patients who have a strong situational contribution to the abuse.

The male physician who sexually abuses his female patients often cannot find meaningful relationships and satisfying sexual outlets outside his population of patients, some of whom are vulnerable to his invitation or coercion to intimacy. Physicians are financially reimbursed for providing medical care to patients. This care includes consideration of the patient's psychological needs. Physicians who place these needs secondary to their impulses have defaulted in their commitment to provide professional care for their patients. The concept of countertransference includes the unconscious feelings of the physician regarding the patient in any doctor–patient relationship (Slakter, 1986). Physicians must consider their reactions to their patients, and use these reactions constructively, in their patients' best interests. This includes a physician's awareness of having sexual interest in his patient that he needs to contain, rather than act on. Inherent in a physician's sexual involvement with a patient is not only abuse of the patient, but also a self-destructive tendency in the physician (Sreenivasan, 1989), who in abusing his patient damages his professional and personal self-respect, jeopardizes his marriage and family relationships, and risks losing his professional identity and capacity to work, as well as his income.

While the physician is deemed to be at risk for repeating abusive behavior, he should not be practicing clinical medicine. Objective evidence that psychiatric treatment is effective for the rehabilitation of situational abusers would support attempts made to rehabilitate them. Gathering such evidence is complicated by difficulties inherent in the objective study of psychotherapy. *It also is complicated by the difficulty in providing psychotherapy when there is an ulterior motive for the patient to engage in psychotherapy beyond the motivation of symptom improvement or personal growth, such as the concrete benefit of being permitted to return to the practice of medicine.*

Sexual misconduct usually starts with relatively minor boundary violations, leading to a pattern of increasing intrusion, culminating in sexual contact. A slide down the "slippery slope" is more common than an abrupt shift from talking to sexual intercourse (Gutheil & Gabbard, 1993). A common sequence involves the physician and patient addressing each other by first names, having personal conversations intruding on clinical work, some body contact, meetings outside the office, sessions during meals, attendance at social events, culminating in sexual contact (Simon, 1989).

Inherent in the slippery slope is a change in the nature of the physician–patient relationship. The patient consults the physician for professional services from which the latter can derive professional satisfaction. As the relationship changes, both physician and patient seek other forms of satisfaction from it. The physician may be motivated by wishes for a closer relationship than he feels he can have outside his patient population and for sexual gratification, which otherwise may be unavailable to the physician, or he may be able to achieve it only in a relationship with a patient where he has the advantage of power. Similarly, the patient may be searching for emotional gratification that is unavailable to her in other relationships, gratification that goes beyond the satisfaction of being understood and cared for professionally by a physician.

Sexual exploitation of female patients is an extreme violation along a spectrum of boundary violations that are possible in clinical practice. Heightened awareness about the concept of boundary crossings should improve patient care and management of risks by raising doubts about any departure from the usual practice in relating to patients (Gutheil & Gabbard, 1993). Both physicians and patients need to abide by the contract implied in the professional relationship. However, given the physician's expertise and power and the patient's vulnerability, boundary violations, including sexual exploitation, are the physician's responsibility. The professional nature of the physician–patient relationship and the limits that it imposes on both physician and patient must be made explicit in medical school and reinforced in postgraduate and continuing medical education.

Sometimes the self-serving claim is that sexual intimacy with a doctor can be helpful to a patient (Herman et al., 1987; McCanney, 1966; Shepard, 1971). However, there inevitably is a mutually self-destructive quality in the physician–patient relationship when their interactions include sexual relations. There may also be a narcissistic need to have power over the patient, to be accepted sexually, and to be found attractive by the patient. All this implies psychological disturbance in the physician. Unless this disturbance is successfully treated, the abusive physician cannot be returned safely to the practice of clinical medicine.

It has been suggested that male physicians' sexual misconduct with female patients harms at least some of these patients (Rapp, 1987). Most psychiatrists (Herman et al., 1987) assume that any physician–patient sexual contact is harmful to the patient, if for no other reason than that the physician has abdicated his role of provider of care. This usually is only the beginning of the harm to the patient, who may experience the sexual abuse as a repetition of previous mistreatment. *In my opinion, there is no question that male physicians' sexual involvement with female patients is harmful to all of the latter. The physician, by virtue of providing care for the patient and having access to both privileged information about the patient and to the patient's body for examination purposes, is in an in loco parentis position. This is directly comparable to the access parents have to their child's thoughts, feelings, and body for the purpose of caring for the child. There is a parallel between sexual abuse of children by parents and sexual abuse of patients by physicians. The privileged access parents and physicians have to children and patients respectively is in order to care for them. Any use physicians make of this access besides caring for their patients in a manner that is in the patient's best interests likely is a boundary crossing and potentially abusive. The physician does not become sexually involved with a patient on the basis of the patient's best interests; this occurs because of the physician's desires. Patients whose trust has been abused by a caregiver or someone else in authority early in life, be it a parent, other relative, babysitter, teacher, member of the clergy, or sports coach, are more vulnerable to abuse by individuals in authority in adult life, including their physicians. In these cases, the physician's sexual involvement is a re-traumatization of vulnerable individuals who often still are dealing with the effects of the earlier trauma. Apart from anything else, the patient, whose trust has already been violated, will lose trust further in a situation where there was potential for building trust with an authority.*

Because of the emotional intimacy inherent in the practice of psychotherapy and psychoanalysis, standards for maintenance of boundaries with patients are, in general, necessarily stricter for psychotherapists and psychoanalysts than for physicians as a group. Authors differ about whether, from an ethical point of view, a psychotherapist may become sexually involved with a former patient following termination of therapy. Appelbaum and Jorgenson (1991) suggest that impaired decision making, coercion, fraud, and exploitation of a fiduciary relationship must be considered, but conclude that a one-year waiting period after termination of psychotherapy is adequate. Herman et al. (1987) argue that the prohibition against sexual contact between patients and their psychotherapists should be permanent, because "neither transference nor the real inequality in the power relationship ends with the termination of therapy." This also could be applied to the physician–patient relationship. It is a question of to what extent there is a difference regarding the maintenance of professional boundaries between physician–patient relationships and psychotherapist–patient relationships, and whether physicians' former patients are more capable of competently consenting to sexual contact with their physicians (after a reasonable period has elapsed following termination of their professional contact) than psychotherapists' former patients.

I agree that the prohibition on psychotherapist–patient sexual relations should be permanent, if only because the transference, which unconsciously influences the patient's perceptions, feelings, and experiences of the therapist, does not end when the therapy ends, so the patient's unconscious attitude towards her former therapist continues to be imbued with feelings associated with other relationships, and may in addition involve idealization, rendering her vulnerable to being manipulated on that basis. As well, the therapist's ethical standards should include avoiding exploiting the patient in the interest of the therapist's desires; this extends beyond the duration of psychotherapy. I conclude that it is a matter of judgment regarding when a physician–patient relationship ethically may not become a romantic/sexual involvement after a "suitable" time has passed. Each case should be considered on its own merits. The more the physician–patient professional relationship resembles a psychotherapist–patient relationship, for example, regarding the depth of personal confidences the patient has entrusted the physician with, the more a subsequent romantic/sexual relationship with the patient would be inappropriate, even after significant time had elapsed. Of course, when physicians are engaged with some form of psychotherapy or psychological counseling with patients, the same permanent prohibition to a romantic/sexual relationship would apply as does with a psychotherapist. Naturally, the same prohibition applies to psychoanalysts as to any other psychotherapist. I believe that many, if not most, physician–patient relationships largely consist of that of caregiver and one to whom care is given, more or less resembling a parent–child relationship, that make a romantic/sexual relationship inappropriate no matter how long a waiting period has elapsed after the professional relationship has ended; transference is timeless. This may be especially hard on single physicians working in small communities, where most or all of the available potential romantic partners are their patients.

Psychoanalysts have been very active in making valuable contributions to the literature on boundaries and boundary violations. The American Psychoanalytic Association (Dewald & Clark, 2001) authorized an Ethics Case Book for the practice of psychoanalysis. Gabbard and Lester (1995) wrote the authoritative textbook on boundaries and boundary violations in psychoanalysis, which is valid, I believe, for practitioners of all psychotherapeutic modalities. Much in these volumes is applicable to medical practice.

THE PATIENT'S CONTRIBUTION

While considering the patient's unconscious contribution to becoming sexually involved with the physician does not reduce the physician's culpability, optimum patient care makes it necessary to consider the possibility that the patient has contributed to the occurrence of the abuse. *This does not involve blaming the victim, but seeing to what extent, if any, the patient allows herself to become involved with her physician in a way that increases the risk of abuse, rather than decreasing it, which is self-destructive. To the extent that an individual involves herself in a way that increases that risk, this may be understandable in that people who have been abused or whose boundaries have not been respected in childhood are at a higher risk of being abused in adult life.* Physicians in training should be taught about the types of behavior that invite abuse from physicians, and the types of emotional reactions to patients that are warning signs about an unconscious invitation to abuse the patient (Slakter, 1986). The physician can then recognize the danger before it occurs, and can prevent it.

Object relations theory is one approach to understanding an individual's vulnerability to being abused by a physician. It proposes that individuals have unconscious mental images of self and other, mostly developed in the first years of life. These images are based largely on the infant's and young child's real experiences with people around her, and are affected by how children perceive stimuli and experience and are able to think about them. Generally, if one's parents are relatively kind, patient, and effective in taking care of their child, and show interest in their child's mind, including what the child thinks and how the child is feeling, the child will develop a positive sense of herself as someone deserving good care, confident enough to pursue her own interests and wishes, and able to recognize people who are wholesome to interact with, distinguishing between them and less suitable people. She realistically can trust her feelings in making these judgments. This implies that she has reasonably good reality testing in terms of judgments about people. Her unconscious images of others, "internal objects," generally are benign, friendly, and helpful. She would generally be attracted to people in the world demonstrating these qualities. Experiences with other caregivers and people in authority, such as relatives and teachers, also influence the child's self-image and internal objects.

The experience of less fortunate children with their parents may involve neglect, abuse, or a lack of interest in their minds, for example, parents who are preoccupied with their work or are self-centered and don't recognize their children as separate individuals with their own feelings, thoughts, wishes, needs, and aspirations. These children are prone to developing images of themselves as unlovable, unvalued, and unworthy of care. To some extent this self-evaluation is true; these children's potentials have not been nurtured by their parents as have those of children with more involved parents. If some potential in such a child has developed, it may reflect her parents being gratified by this development, but not in a manner leaving her feeling valued for herself, but for what she can achieve. Unconscious images of others (internal objects) in these children are likely to be unloving, uncaring, uninterested, and potentially persecutory. When these children grow up, they are prone to form attachments with individuals demonstrating these qualities. They are less likely to feel deserving of good treatment. If they are treated well, they may be suspicious of it or anxious about it, as it represents a painful contrast with their experience as children. Generally, individuals become attached to people who resemble their internal objects. The more positive their internal objects, the more likely they are to find people to have positive relationships with. The converse applies to individuals with more negative internal objects. A patient with negative internal objects projects those internal objects on to a correspondingly negative person in the world, that is, one resembling the internal objects, who tends to recapitulate with the patient in the present the unsatisfactory type of relationship she had with her early caregivers. This projection may involve expecting mistreatment, accepting mistreatment, or even unconsciously inviting mistreatment.

To the extent that a female patient has been treated poorly in childhood, and has grown up with a poor self-image and a negative internal object, she will likely have both a longing for better treatment in adult relationships, especially with caregivers, who represent her parents, the original caregivers, but also tend to be attracted to individuals corresponding to her negative internal objects. One example of the latter is the sexually abusive physician. Some women with a background of abuse, severe neglect, or significant lack of interest in them on the part of their parents will be vulnerable to such a physician.

Some of these patients can benefit by exploring in psychotherapy the ways they expect, invite, or accept abuse. They might explore the abuse as involving a self-destructive style of relating or fulfilling an unmet attachment need, or as an expression of aggression towards the physician. This exploration would have to be done while making it clear that the patient is not culpable for the abuse. The issue of culpability must be separated from an exploration of patients' unconscious motivations to comply with sexual involvement with physicians. It is not in patients' interests to remain unaware of their motivation to invite or permit abuse if they can benefit from this insight.

When I was a neophyte psychotherapist, a patient informed me after a couple of months that she knew I was like other men, and when I was ready to have sex with her, she would comply. This made me intensely anxious. I felt I had to tell her that we would never be involved in that. Given my experience since then, I believe that now I might respond by asking her, "What then?" Rather than dealing first with the concrete reality that we would never have a sexual relationship, I would invite her to consider what would happen if I accepted her invitation. If a patient overtly invites her physician or therapist to become involved in sexual intimacy, he can then explore and interpret how she contributes to a repetition of self-destructive patterns in other relationships, where she complained that men take advantage of her. If the physician accedes to her invitation, it justifies her transference hatred, that is, her hatred of him, to the extent that it is based on a displacement of feelings associated with other relationships. *In complying with a patient's invitation, a physician disqualifies himself from engaging in just what he undertook with his patient, competent medical care serving the patient's best interests.* The patient then could take her revenge by getting him in trouble with his regulatory body. This example illustrates the exception to the rule. Patients rarely initiate sexual intimacy with their physicians; generally physicians do.

MANAGEMENT OF THE ABUSIVE PHYSICIAN

A balanced approach is needed to protect patients from further abuse by offending physicians, while avoiding an over-punitive reaction to physicians accused of or found guilty of sexual abuse (Shekter, 1991). The patient's needs must be the first priority. Consideration of patient safety must be paramount rehabilitating abusive physicians. One needs to determine if a treatable group of abusive physicians exists, and then distinguish physicians amenable to treatment from those feeling they have done nothing wrong or who can't resist impulses to abuse patients. This involves identifying the mainly "situational" abusers. Physicians whose abuse is associated with major psychiatric illness require ongoing treatment and evaluation of their safety to return to clinical practice.

Options for dealing with physicians found guilty of sexual impropriety or abuse must be available, so that disciplinary bodies have more options than allowing the physicians to resume practice or banning them indefinitely from practice (College of Physicians and Surgeons of Ontario, 1992). Apart from mandated psychiatric treatment with at least temporary revocation of their medical license, possibilities include supervised practice, limited clinical practice, and non-clinical medical employment. The College of Physicians and Surgeons of Ontario has proposed recommendations to deal with three levels of sexual offense, including sexual impropriety (demeaning words and gestures), transgression (sexual touching), and violation (including intercourse). One needs effective self-governing bodies for the medical profession, rather than regulatory bodies revoking medical licenses that may be reinstituted by the courts (Gray, 1991).

PREVENTION THROUGH EDUCATION

The sexual abuse of patients must be addressed in the education of physicians. Gartrell et al. (1988) found 0.9% of psychiatric residents reporting sexual involvement with patients, and concluded that education about sexual exploitation is needed in psychiatric residency programs. Its aim should be primary prevention of the abuse (Burgess, 1981). Blackshaw and Patterson (1992) describe educational activities that should occur in the training of psychiatric residents, including the provision of information about ethical prohibitions early in the residents' training, such as the Canadian Medical Association's code of ethics annotated for psychiatrists (Mellor, 1980). Didactic seminars are necessary to teach about sexual exploitation of patients. Residents should be familiar with the tendency of traumatized patients to re-experience the trauma. Kaplan (1979, 1985) recommends that residents learn about gender-related issues and the impact of traditional gender role behavior on identity, self-esteem, self-image, and the restriction of options for both sexes.

In one Canadian academic department of psychiatry, residents receive one lecture on boundaries overall, which includes sexual boundary violations. Medical students in this faculty receive an orientation in first year with a number of lectures and interactive seminars on ethics, which includes most of the teaching done on sexual abuse. This likely is typical of Canadian medical schools and psychiatric residencies, and does not seem likely to be adequate either regarding quantity or the need in learning for repetition of important principles. Hopefully these lectures are supplemented by repeated discussions of boundaries and boundary violations in clinical teaching at both undergraduate and graduate levels. It seems unlikely that these recommendations, made decades ago, are being carried out.

The best opportunity for teaching psychiatric residents how to manage countertransference feelings occurs during psychoanalytic psychotherapy supervision. While acting on sexual attraction toward patients is forbidden, talking about erotic countertransference is encouraged: it must be clear that this not be met with criticism or negative repercussions (Book, 1987; Pope et al., 1986). Psychotherapy supervisors should raise the topics of therapist–patient sexual attraction and sex role stereotyping when supervisees don't raise them. Blackshaw and Patterson (1992) indicate that those issues apply equally to undergraduate and continuing medical education.

Psychiatric educators should become involved at the undergraduate level, not only because of the psychiatric ramifications of the abuse, but also because of that discipline's ability, based on psychoanalytic concepts, to understand the basis for it and to be involved in its prevention and management. Blackshaw and Patterson's conclusions about the need for formal teaching of medical students on sexual abuse of patients and continuing medical education for practitioners are supported by the Ontario Medical Association (Gray et al., 1991). This likely won't prevent characterological abusers from abusing their patients, but may render individuals at risk of becoming situational abusers more aware of situations involving vulnerability, of available treatment, and of peer support, to avoid abusing their patients and endangering their careers. This would also help other physicians to respond effectively when treating an abused patient, an abusive physician, or a physician who consults them about impulses to sexually abuse his patients who has not committed the abuse.

Medical students must be instructed about options available to them, for example, to refer a patient to a colleague if a physician does not feel that he can deal with his temptation to become sexually involved with a patient. They must be taught about the importance of being aware of a developing sexual interest in their patients and its possible relationship to disappointments or losses in their own relationships or frustration in their sex lives. They must be aware of the availability of psychotherapeutic consultation and individual psychotherapy with a mental health professional, and the availability of consultation with a colleague about the management of a "seductive" patient. Some Canadian provincial medical associations make available to their members counselors and psychotherapists to help physicians and medical students deal with these problems, similar to help available to physicians suffering from substance abuse. Medical students must be aware that it is their responsibility to find a solution enabling them to treat their patients while maintaining the acceptable standard of patient care, as opposed to acting either on impulse or on the patient's invitation. The future physician should be aware that he will have to deal with these issues, and not involve his patients as a solution for his own problems.

Some aspects of medical education on this topic may best be handled in seminars in which students (or practicing physicians) interact with each other, One example might be how to advise a colleague who consults you about his sexual feelings for a patient. Legal questions, such as how to react if you suspect or know that a colleague is sexually abusing a patient, should be discussed. The question of how the physician can seek help when he has already abused a patient should also be addressed. Little information is available on the prevention of sexual abuse (Pope, 1987). Information also should be presented in continuing medical education and postgraduate programs.

Twemlow and Gabbard (1989) indicate that one prophylactic measure against boundary violations is the avoidance of non-sexual dual roles with patients. The therapist–patient relationship should be strictly professional, uncontaminated with socializing outside the therapy hour. They emphasize the need for the psychotherapist to engage in continual intrapsychic monitoring as part of his professional practice, in order to predict and avoid situations where the therapist's wish to receive affirming responses from his patient becomes so great that he becomes at risk of falling in love with her and acting on his sexual wishes with her. *Physicians, especially family physicians, may be acquainted with members of their patient's families or even, especially in small communities, regularly interact socially with their patients. Many would argue that, given these sometimes inevitable types of interactions, the principles of maintaining boundaries inherent in the practice of psychotherapy and psychoanalysis do not apply to physician–patient relationships. In my opinion, this is a relative issue. The closer the physician can come to avoiding dual relationships with his patients, the more intact the professional boundaries will remain, with a reduced risk of sexual boundary violations. This needs to be managed on a case-by-case basis, custom-made for each physician. The physician in a very small town who inevitably interacts with his patients in all sorts of ways, shopping at their stores, socializing with them regularly, and seeing them in the street and at public events, needs to be all the more vigilant regarding maintenance of appropriate professional boundaries. Physicians working in a big city find it easier to avoid interacting with their patients outside of their professional involvement, thus maintaining professional boundaries and lowering the risk of sexual abuse. It is the physician's responsibility to behave in a manner in the best interests of his patients. This sometimes involves sacrifices of some potentially enjoyable social experiences. This is a small price to pay to reduce the risk of boundary violations that not only damage the patient, but also jeopardize the career, income, self-respect, and marriage of the physician involved.*

CONCLUSIONS

Sexual enactments between physicians and patients are destructive largely because the physician, who has undertaken to treat his patient according to what is in her best interests (which sometimes includes helping her better understand and come to her terms with feelings about experiences of exploitation and abuse) instead repeats the exploitation, or simply offers treatment that includes sexual exploitation. This may recapitulate previous abuse, but generally injures patients, eroding their capacity to trust, rather than helping them. Because of how destructive this abuse is, emphasizing prevention of abuse is essential. Additionally, education regarding physician vulnerability to become abusive and the concrete costs to the physician of being a perpetrator must occur in undergraduate and postgraduate medical training. One can't convince a predator not to predate, but education may help depressed, "love-sick," and other vulnerable physicians.

One needs to determine which psychotherapeutic approach is most effective in treating abused patients. *This will depend partly on variables specific to the individual patient. Although specific clinics and symptom-oriented treatments are available for survivors of abuse, physicians are probably less well acquainted with psychoanalytic treatments for abused patients. These treatments address not only symptoms related to the abuse, but the personality of the patient who experienced the abuse. That is important in not only helping a patient to recover from trauma-related symptoms, but also to understand what the trauma has meant to her, and to relate it, when appropriate, to earlier traumatic experiences of trauma and neglect predisposing her to becoming involved in a traumatic situation with her physician (Gartner, 2017).*

One also needs to determine if there is a group of abusive physicians who can be rehabilitated. More ambitious would be to identify potentially abusive physicians early in their training, or, better, during the admission process to medical school. Can one identify potential "characterological" abusers? One must determine what forms of education are most effective in helping prevent physician sexual abuse. One could describe a physician and a patient becoming sexually involved as two troubled people inappropriately seeking solace in a relationship self-destructive to both. The responsibility for avoiding this is the physician's; he is the caregiver and he is in the position of power. Awareness about the danger of sexual abuse of patients should help prevent it and contribute to maintaining a high standard of medical care. *This must become a standard and unquestioned part of medical culture, and, by extension, of our societal culture. It is an especially timely concern, given the MeToo movement. Physicians have an opportunity and a responsibility, especially given our sometimes lamentable contemporary political and social circumstances, to set an example to society regarding preventing abuse, and, when it occurs, dealing with it responsibly.* It is the responsibility of the medical profession to prevent sexual abuse of female patients by male physicians whenever possible, to prevent its recurrence in offending physicians, and to provide treatment for the abused patients in the most effective way possible.

REFERENCES

Appelbaum PS, Jorgenson L (1991). Psychotherapist–patient sexual contact after termination of treatment: An analysis and a proposal. *American Journal of Psychiatry* 148(11):1466–1473.

Bates CM, Brodsky AM (1989). *Sex in the Therapy Hour: A Case of Professional Incest.* New York: Guilford Press.

Blackshaw SL, Patterson PGR (1992). The prevention of sexual exploitation of patients: Educational issues. *Canadian Journal of Psychiatry* 37:350–353.

Book HE (1987). The resident's countertransference: Approaching an avoided topic. *American Journal of Psychotherapy* XLI (4):555–562.

Burgess AW (1981). Physician sexual misconduct and patients' responses. *American Journal of Psychiatry* 138(10):1335–1342.

Butler S, Zelen SL (1977). Sexual intimacies between therapists and patients. *Psychotherapy: Theory, Research and Practice* 14:139–145.

College of Physicians and Surgeons of Ontario (1992). *Members' Dialogue* Dec (11).

Council on Ethical and Judicial Affairs, American Medical Association (1991). Sexual misconduct in the practice of medicine. *Journal of the American Medical Association* 266(19):2741–2745.

Davidson V (1977). Psychiatry's problem with no name: Therapist–patient sex. *American Journal of Psychoanalysis* 37:43–50.

Dewald PA, Clark RW (eds.) (2001). *Ethics Casebook of the American Psychoanalytic Association.* New York: American Psychoanalytic Association.

Gabbard GO (1989). *Sexual Exploitation in Professional Relationships.* Washington, DC: American Psychiatric Press.

Gabbard GO, Lester SP (1995). *Boundaries and Boundary Violations in Psychoanalysis.* Washington, DC: American Psychiatric Publishing.

Gamell N, Herman JL, Olarte S, Feldstein M, Localio R (1988). Management and rehabilitation of sexually exploitive therapists. *Hospital Community Psychiatry* 39(10):1070–1074.

Gartner RB (ed.) (2017). *Trauma and Counter Trauma, Resilience and Counter Resilience: Insights from Psychoanalysts and Trauma Experts.* London: Routledge.

Gartrell N, Herman I, Olarte S, Feldstein M, Localio R (1986). Psychiatrist–patient sexual contact: Results of a national survey. I Prevalence. *American Journal of Psychiatry* 143:1126–1131.

Gartrell N, Herman J, Olarte S, Feldstein M, Localio R (1988). Psychiatric residents' sexual contact with educators and patients: Results of a national survey. *American Journal of Psychiatry* 145(6):690–694.

Gray C (1991). Healers who harm: Ontario college takes aim at physicians who abuse patients. *Canadian Medical Association Journal* 144(10):1298–1300.

Gray J, Graham W, Finlayson R, et al. (1991). OMA responds to task force's preliminary recommendations. *Ontario Medical Review* July 9–13:15.

Gutheil EG, Gabbard GO (1993). The concept of boundaries in clinical practice: Theoretical and risk-management dimensions. *American Journal of Psychiatry* 150(2):188–196.

Herman JL, Gartrell N, Olarte S, et al. (1987). Psychiatrist–patient sexual contact: Results of a national survey. II: Psychiatrists' attitudes. *American Journal of Psychiatry* 134:164–169.

Kaplan AG (1979). Toward an analysis of sex-role related issues in the therapeutic relationship. *Psychiatry* 42(1):112–120.

Kaplan AG (1985). Female or male psychotherapist for women: New formulations. *Psychiatry* 48(2):111–121.

Kardener SB, Fuller M, Mensh IN (1973). A survey of physicians' attitudes and practices regarding erotic and non-erotic contact with patients. *American Journal of Psychiatry* 130:1077–1081.

McCanney JL (1966). Overt transference. *Journal of Sexual Research* 2:227–237.

McPhedran M, Armstrong B, et al. (1991). Preliminary report of the task force of sexual abuse of patients. *College of Physicians and Surgeons of Ontario Journal* May 27.

Mellor C (1980). The Canadian Medical Association code of ethics annotated for psychiatrists. The position of the Canadian Psychiatric Association. *Canadian Journal of Psychiatry* 25(5):432–437.

Moscarello R (1990). Psychological management of victims of sexual assault. *Canadian Journal of Psychiatry* 35(1):25–30.

Nadelson CC (1989). *Sexual Exploitation in Professional Relationships*. Washington, DC: American Psychiatric Press, 229–231.

Perry JA (1976). Physicians' erotic and non-erotic physical involvement with patients. *American Journal of Psychiatry* 33:833–840.

Pope KS (1987). Preventing therapist–patient sexual intimacy: Therapy for the therapist at risk. *Professional Psychology Research and Practice* 18:624–628.

Pope KS, Keith-Spiegal P, Tabachnick BC (1986). Sexual attraction to clients. *American Psychologist* 41(2):147–158.

Rapp MS (1987). Sexual misconduct. *Canadian Medical Association Journal* 137:1934.

Rutter P (1986). *The Wounds of Women, Sex in the Forbidden Zone*. Los Angeles, CA: Jeremy P. Tarcher, 71–91.

Rutter P (1989). *Sex in The Forbidden Zone: When Men in Power – Therapists. Doctors, Clergy and Others – Betray Women's Trust*. New York: Fawcett Crest.

Shekter R (1991). Chilling, dangerous and unpalatable: Health law expert looks at sex abuse document. *Ontario Medicine* Aug 19:2.

Shepard M (1971). *The Love Treatment: Sexual Intimacy Between Patients and Psychotherapists*. New York: Peter Wyden.

Simon RI (1989). Sexual exploitation of patients: How it begins before it happens. *Psychiatric Annual* 19:104–fl.

Slakter E (1986). *Countertransference*. Northvale, NJ: Jason Aronson.

Sreenivasan V (1989). Sexual exploitation of patients: The position of the Canadian Psychiatric Association. *Canadian Journal of Psychiatry* 34:234–235.

Strasburger LB. Jorgenson L, Randles R (1990). Mandatory reporting of sexually exploitive psychotherapists. *Bulletin of the American Academy of Psychiatry and Law* 18(4):379–384.

Twemlow SW, Gabbard GO (1989). The love-sick therapist. In: Gabbard GO (ed.), *Sexual Exploitation in Professional Relationships*. Washington, DC: American Psychiatric Press.

Valiquette M, Sabourin S, Lecomte C (1990). The psychological sequelae of sexual intimacy in patient–therapist relations. Université de Montreal. Presented at 98th annual convention of the American Psychological Association, Boston, August 1990.

ENVOI

Something bothering me about the end of most books is the author never formally saying goodbye. Books that I like best are those in which the author becomes a live person to me, with whom I feel I get acquainted while reading her book. In both fiction and non-fiction, if the author is effective, she has invited me into her mind or into an intimate dialogue on something she is passionate about. After this relationship, that has a predictable ending, I miss the author not offering me a farewell. I know she can't experience my response to what she has written. Of course, I do not know how much of a person I have become to any particular reader, but I will say goodbye to you. The form of farewell that I wish to extend is an attempt at sharing something of what I have learned as a psychiatrist and psychoanalyst. At least it will send you, the reader, on your way, with a notion of what I think is important, in addition to my good wishes for you and your work. I will not repeat what I have already written, but rather offer something to leave an impression with you of what I have been trying to convey.

The Talmud says, if you want to study, first get a friend. I wish to emphasize the importance of having a group or, better, several groups of colleagues with whom to share ideas and grow professionally. This could include a study group, individual friends and colleagues, attending conferences, all both in person and/or through online video. Other venues include ongoing supervision with a respected colleague individually or in a group, meetings with coworkers such as a staff relations group in an outpatient clinic or hospital inpatient unit, and less formal meetings with colleagues or coworkers.

One cannot emphasize enough the importance of listening to our patients, which is not always easy. What they have to say may be hard for anyone to listen to, or especially difficult for particular clinicians, based on our own sensitivities, especially if it concerns a sore spot for us, an unresolved conflict or unmet need, or if we are tired, having a bad day or just at the end of a long day, or preoccupied with our own problems. Simultaneously, one has to listen to oneself and one's reaction to the patient, which can tell you a lot about the patient.

Always consider the possibility that, in addition to whatever medical condition your patient might have, some of his complaints may represent difficulties in his internal psychological world and/or his world of relationships with others, including his relationship with you. I wish to highlight this last point. Your patient may express in a metaphor, or by overtly describing complaints about someone else, how he feels about you. It might not be a complaint, but could just as easily be an expression of appreciation or even love.

Maintaining good professional boundaries is very important. This is easier when one has gratifying relationships and activities outside of work, which are very important to establish and maintain, throughout one's life, given the inevitable multiple losses that are involved in living, especially as one ages, of relationships, gradually reducing capacities for physical activity, mental acuity, and unavoidable inability for various reasons to continue enjoying some activities.

Psychoanalysis and psychoanalytic psychotherapy should affect the life of the patient for the better, although he may feel that he is sadder but wiser. He likely is not sadder, but better able to feel his sadness, hopefully without being as dominated by it. One recalls Freud's indicating that psychoanalysis was able to convert hysterical misery into common unhappiness. Psychoanalysis should be transforming to the individual undertaking it. Inevitably the analyst also to some extent is transformed, and sometimes healed, in every successful analysis. I hope this book helps the reader to see and think of his patients in different ways, and in particular to imagine hidden aspects of his patients that interact with their physicians and their experience of illness, affecting their medical conditions and the management of these conditions. If this book is successful, it should help physicians try to understand their patients in ways they did not understand them before, accept the limitations of what they can do, and interest them further in their work with their patients.

"Doctor on the Couch," a subtitle I considered for this book, could refer, among other things, to the profession of medicine being subjected to psychoanalytic exploration, the motivations for becoming a physician being subject to the psychoanalytic exploration, or a physician undertaking personal psychoanalytic treatment. Miller (1981) and Sussman (1992) write about unconscious motivations for becoming a physician and a psychotherapist, many of which overlap, which may interest some readers. Some individuals' development leaves them with a sensitivity that makes them vulnerable to difficulties when undertaking a medical career. These difficulties may result in psychiatric symptoms and problematic symptoms and behaviors, including depression, suicidal ideation, substance abuse, sexual abuse of patients, compulsive overwork, excessive preoccupation with the welfare of one's patients, marital difficulties, or a grandiose attitude towards what they can accomplish. They engage in their work without recognition of normal human limitations, sometimes becoming overly ambitious and too focused on professional advancement (for example, regarding publishing books and articles), on attaining promotion to academically exalted or administratively powerful positions (at the expense of a balanced life of work, love, and play), or just on making a lot of money. What I have written about regarding patients obviously may apply to physicians as well: emotional disturbance that remains out of an individual's conscious awareness, usually because it concerns conflicts or unmet needs that are unbearable to think about, may manifest as physical symptoms, or as the exacerbation or even precipitation of a recognized medical condition. I hope this book has been an invitation for physicians struggling with their own difficulties to know that psychoanalysis offers an opportunity for them to understand the motivations for their behavior, for how they feel, and what they think, as opposed to continuing to enact unconscious wishes, fears, and other feelings in impulsive and self-destructive behaviors or painful and sometimes dangerous physical symptoms and conditions.

I do not know how much, if at all, my thoughts are original (Ogden, 2003). I have not seen the ideas about medicine in this book collected in written form elsewhere. My ideas are derived from my professional life, including clinical experience, teaching and being taught, supervising and being supervised, reading, and above all, my personal psychoanalysis. I note that all of these activities, including reading, involve contact with another person's mind and the chance to have a relationship with another person (Ogden, 2005, 2009). I suspect that successful writing resembles successful psychoanalysis and psychoanalytic psychotherapy to some extent. The reader allows himself to be moved, transformed, or in some way significantly influenced, if the writer touches him in some personal way that affects him, similar to the effect of these therapies.

Physicians who are interested in incorporating psychoanalytic thought into their clinical practice can do so in a number of ways. Balint groups are a useful way of expanding one's thinking in the company of like-minded individuals. I have tried to indicate what psychoanalytic literature might be most accessible to physicians.

Physicians who are interested in developing skills related to psychoanalysis further may undertake some form of supervision with a psychoanalyst to talk about their cases. This could involve not only psychotherapy supervision, if the physician is performing psychotherapy with her patients, but also discussions about patients in whom the physician believes psychological factors are influencing the course of her patients' illnesses or their compliance with the management of their illnesses. Finally, the time-honored way of understanding the unconscious, which is required of all psychoanalysts in their training, is having personal psychoanalysis. This is a significant expenditure of time and money, and generally is not undertaken unless an individual is experiencing significant suffering and/or difficulties in relationships. Clinicians who undertake a personal analysis, including psychoanalysts, usually find that in addition to the personal benefits of better understanding their unmet needs and unresolved conflicts, a collateral benefit is understanding their patients better too, and being better able to listen to them, resulting in their treatment of patients becoming more effective. (Not coincidentally, considering the above opportunities, the three pillars of psychoanalytic training are didactic teaching, involving considerable reading, supervision of psychoanalytic treatment, and, most importantly, personal psychoanalysis.)

Becoming a psychoanalyst, like most other complex and worthwhile endeavors, is not a goal that one can achieve completely, any more than one can attain perfection as an artist. One continues to become a psychoanalyst throughout one's career. In fact, one becomes a psychoanalyst with every new patient one treats, reinventing psychoanalysis with each patient (Ogden, 2004). One has the chance to continue to grow, develop, and learn on an ongoing basis, with all the attendant opportunities, joy, fascination, difficulties, pain, and dangers. I have dedicated the remainder of my professional life to this.

Often, whether with a patient, a supervisee, or a group of colleagues at a meeting, I hesitate about whether to say what I am thinking. I am used to this by now, and don't think this hesitation is a bad thing, although it is based in my case on the recurring question, "Is this going to be helpful to my patient or supervisee?" or "Will my colleagues think this is worth saying, or is it too obvious, trivial, or unoriginal?" I have become braver with the passing years, and usually say what I was hesitating about, parallel to Bion saying that you, and no one else, are the analyst your patient will be seeing tomorrow. Similarly, what I am thinking at the present time is what I have to offer my patient, supervisee, or the group of colleagues. I am frequently surprised by how positively some colleagues respond to what I have hesitated in saying. I am too experienced not to know that it is impossible to predict what, of all we say to a patient, becomes important to her, and often hear, sometimes years later, that what I almost didn't bother saying, feeling it was trite or marginally relevant, was just what affected my patient the most. Being open to saying what I think does not mean I am advocating "wild analysis." However, I feel that we have to be open to messages from our unconscious, which also may be originating from the unconscious of the people around us, including our patients, and may lead to fruitful lines of thought in either or both of us. Of course, much besides the content of we say affects our patients – not just the attention we pay them, but what they see it costs us to try to pay attention to them, which doesn't always come easily, but with a struggle. This can happen when what they say touches a raw nerve with us (of which they at least unconsciously often are aware) or when we are already having a bad day; it can then be especially hard for us to bear.

One regret I have in writing this book is that, with the space available, I have not been able to convey much detail about the richness of the burgeoning of psychoanalytic thought, especially over the past half-century, which has led to the application of psychoanalysis in an increasing number of clinical and academic areas. I would be remiss in not making explicit the fact that the ideas expressed in this envoi are based on psychoanalytic thought.

In contemplating writing this book, I was surprised at not finding other attempts in the literature to apply psychoanalytic thought to the practice of medicine. Who was I to travel on a journey on which perhaps wiser and more experienced heads had hesitated to embark? I wondered if I were undertaking something ill advised or even impossible, and inexorably destined to fail. I offer this book with the same hope (that I described in talking to patients, supervisees, and colleagues) that readers may find something of value to them in it.

REFERENCES

Miller A (1981). *Prisoners of Childhood.* New York: Basic Books.

Ogden TH (2003). What's true and whose idea was it? *International Journal of Psychoanalysis* 84(3):593–606.

Ogden TH (2004). This art of psychoanalysis: Dreaming undreamt dreams and interrupted cries. *International Journal of Psychoanalysis* 85(4):857–877.

Ogden TH (2005). On psychoanalytic writing. *International Journal of Psychoanalysis* 86(1):15–29.

Ogden TH (2009). Rediscovering psychoanalysis. *Psychoanalytic Perspectives* 6(1):22–31.

Sussman MB (1992). *A Curious Calling: Unconscious Motivations for Practicing Psychotherapy.* New York: Jason Aronson.

GLOSSARY

Alpha-function A mental function that transforms sensuously apprehensible stimuli into elements useful for thinking, dreaming, and laying down for memory. This is a model for how we deal with the apprehension of reality. The analyst receives projections from the patient, metabolizing or digesting them through alpha-function and returning them to the patient in a more bearable form. This is analogous to a mother's central role in helping her infant manage emotional pain. This has been described as the ability of the patient to put unbearably painful feelings into the analyst and leave them there long enough for them to be modified by their sojourn in the analyst's mind.

Conflict, unconscious mental Conflict refers to the unresolved tension between different agencies of the mind. For example, a young man might find a female classmate to be very sexually attractive. One could describe this as an id impulse. However, he may have been raised on a very strict religious basis such that sexual feelings, to say nothing of sexual relations, are totally unacceptable outside of marriage. One could describe this as a superego prohibition when this parental attitude has been internalized by the young man. One solution to this conflict between id and superego is to render the conflict and the sexual feelings unconscious. In this situation, the tension between id and superego continues. The purpose of rendering the conflicts and the unacceptable impulse unconscious, involving the defense of repression, is to reduce anxiety about an aspect of mental contents, in this case, a sexual impulse not acceptable to the individual. If the feelings associated with the conflict are too strong, a psychiatric symptom may result.

Countertransference In the broad sense, countertransference refers to the analyst's total experience of the patient, including the analyst's reveries and fantasies about and emotional reactions to the patient, which can provide information about the patient. In the original, narrow sense, countertransference refers to unresolved psychological disturbance in the analyst stirred up by his exposure to the patient; that is, the analyst's transference to his patient.

Defenses Defenses are unconscious mental mechanisms designed to reduce anxiety and other uncomfortable feelings about unconscious conflict and unmet emotional needs, usually originating in childhood.

Displacement A defense in which thoughts, feelings, impulses, or attitudes concerning one individual are redirected towards another individual. For example, if it is dangerous for a child to express anger at a potentially violent father, the anger may be displaced towards the mother if she characteristically responds in a more understanding and gentle way. Displacement is a central feature of transference, in which thoughts, feelings, impulses, and other mental contents related to important individuals in the patient's life are re-experienced in the relationship with the analyst, or with a physician.

Ego The executive function of the mind that balances the demands of the superego and id, and external reality.

Ego functions These include judgment, relation to reality, capacity to think, relations with important others, regulation of emotion, impulse control, frustration tolerance, motility, and unconscious defenses required to contain painful feelings to bearable levels of intensity.

Enactments Experiences that occur between analyst and patient which, rather than thinking or discussing an experience between the two, are expressed in some form of action. This is potentially destructive if, for example, it involves abusive or exploitive behavior on the part of the analyst, such as sexual relations with a patient. Enactments also can involve a playful way of working through difficult aspects of the patient's relationships or experiences of himself that analyst and patient are not able to talk about in a productive way.

Fit In psychotherapy or psychoanalysis, fit refers to how well analyst and patient are suited to work with each other. This largely depends on the personalities of patient and analyst, in particular how flexible they are. It is the analyst's responsibility to know if the fit of the therapeutic dyad is too poor for them to work together, although sometimes the patient will have this sense.

Id This refers to the repository of instinctual impulses, such as sexuality and the capacity for aggression, as well as a capacity for imagination, playfulness, and creativity.

Internal objects Unconscious internal representations of others in one's mind. They largely are based on one's early experiences with caretakers, especially parents, but do not correspond exactly to the parents' characteristics, depending on how the child perceives the parents, which partly depends on the child's temperament.

Narcissistic Narcissistic personality features popularly refer to excessively self-centered people. However, a wide range of characteristics may be considered narcissistic. Narcissistic individuals often use grandiosity as a defense against low self-esteem. Central affects of narcissistic individuals include shame, envy, and contempt. Idealization and devaluation are often employed to manage painful feelings. Some narcissistic individuals behave with an overt sense of entitlement, devaluing others, and appearing vain and manipulative or charismatic and commanding. Others behave ingratiatingly, seeking people to idealize, are easily wounded, and envy others seen as superior. Narcissistic features are evident in everyone to some extent.

Neurotic This refers to unconscious conflicts between the agencies of the mind, the ego, superego, and id. When conflicts become closer to conscious awareness, one becomes anxious. Unconscious mental mechanisms of defense are utilized to keep conflicts outside of conscious awareness. The term "neurosis" refers to conditions such as anxiety disorder, obsessive-compulsive disorder, and conversion disorder, in which these conflicts are identifiable in the individual. Each neurosis has characteristic anxieties, conflicts, and defenses that are usually found in individuals suffering from that neurosis.

Oedipus complex Originally, the Oedipus complex referred to the combination of loving and hostile wishes that children experience towards parents, classically wishing for the death of the same-sex parent, perceived as the rival, and sexual desire for the opposite-sex parent. Contemporary psychoanalytic thought has expanded this concept to include development of the mind and personality. One's experience of the transition between the original mother–infant dyad to the triadic experience of mother, father, and infant has implications regarding children's introduction to the world outside of the infant's original world of his mother, and being able to recognize that other people have relationships excluding him. This leads to children becoming able to think about their own minds, and to be aware of and be able to think about the minds of others. It also helps to develop a capacity for mourning, as children recognize that their mother has a relationship with someone else, and the parental couple enjoys experiences with each other from which children are excluded. This also may increase the children's envy.

"Primitive"   This can refer to thoughts, feelings, and impulses related to mental functioning of early life, representing feelings of infancy, such as terrifying, violent thoughts, experiences of falling endlessly into an abyss, experiencing oneself as not existing, thinking in illogical or unrealistic ways, experiencing overwhelmingly painful or frightening feelings, or having violent or unwanted sexual impulses.

Projective identification   This is a mental mechanism involving relations between unconscious images of the self and others, having to do with the ridding of the self of unwanted aspects of the self. Originally, unwanted fantasies and images of oneself, another, and/or one's relationship with others were, in fantasy, thought to be deposited into another person. A contemporary understanding of this mechanism involves an interpersonal aspect in which one individual influences another to feel, think, and/or act in a way that the projecting individual cannot tolerate experiencing in himself. Recent history provides an evocative example of projective identification. Once during a meeting of the Supreme Soviet, Khrushchev was enumerating Stalin's errors. Someone in the audience of several thousand called out, "Why didn't you confront Stalin about this at the time?" Khrushchev screamed, "Who said that?" This was followed by dead silence. Khrushchev then replied, "Now you know why." Rather than providing a logical explanation, Khrushchev induced in the audience members the emotions he and others felt at the time of Stalin's violent misuse of power, communicating his terrifying experience directly to them. An individual similarly uses projective identification to induce in another an emotional experience, evacuating the feeling into the other, rather than having to continue to experience it himself (the projective aspect), while still remaining in touch with the experience (the identification aspect).

Projection   This involves the experiencing in someone else of a personal quality, such as a thought, feeling, or impulse, that an individual finds unbearable to recognize in himself. For example, an envious person, rather than experience envy in himself, may feel that someone envies him, and may even accuse her of doing so. In projective identification, by contrast, the envious person might actually incite envy in another person, rather than just believe that she is envious.

Proto-mental emotions   These are the precursors of emotions in infants not yet able to experience emotions *per se*. Infants initially don't distinguish between proto-emotions and sensory experience; somatic and psychological experiences have not been differentiated at this point. Individuals with psychosomatic conditions often are thought to have deficiencies in this differentiation and limitations in the capacity to experience emotions, with consequent transduction of the emotions into somatic symptoms.

Psychodynamic   This refers to a type of psychotherapy based on psychoanalytic concepts with some differences in the therapeutic frame and more limited therapeutic goals. Typically, patients in psychodynamic psychotherapy meet on a weekly or perhaps twice-weekly basis, and usually do not use lie on a couch. The therapist is often more active and perhaps more overtly supportive than in a psychoanalysis. The terms psychoanalytic psychotherapy and psychodynamic psychotherapy usually are used interchangeably. Psychodynamic formulation refers to the use of psychoanalytic principles to understand how a patient has developed, including attempting to explain the basis for the patient's symptoms and personality style.

Psychosis   Psychosis refers to psychiatric conditions in which the capacity for experiencing reality as it is consensually agreed upon (reality testing) is lost. These conditions are frequently characterized by hallucinations and delusions. In psychoanalytic parlance, the term "psychotic" is used in various ways. One can describe psychotic and non-psychotic parts of one's personality. Some defenses, such as projective identification, splitting, projection, and denial, when heavily relied upon, are considered characteristic of psychotic thinking. Anxieties that usually occur in more primitive mental states involve concerns about one disappearing, falling endlessly, ceasing to exist, losing one's identity as an individual, merging into another person, becoming mentally fragmented, or losing one's mind, and are described as psychotic anxieties.

Repetition compulsion This is a tendency to repeat situations one has experienced in the past, despite the fact that they are painful and/or result in disadvantageous outcomes for the individual. The motivation for this is unconscious, and may involve unconscious guilt or hostility. For example, an individual may choose a partner who resembles aspects of his parents with which he consciously would not wish to be associated. A person with domineering parents who demanded compliance might choose a wife with those qualities. Alternatively, such an individual might treat his children in a similar domineering way, in spite of consciously not intending to do so.

Splitting Splitting is considered a primitive defense in which aspects of mental contents, such as one's view of oneself or another person, are unconsciously divided and kept apart. For example, an individual may split his positive feelings about a friend from his negative feelings, and experience only positive or only negative feelings towards the friend, as opposed to the ambivalent experience of being aware of both positive and negative feelings simultaneously. This might result in alternating between idealizing and devaluing the friend, depending on whether the positive or negative feelings are being experienced, such that the friend is experienced in one of two opposite ways, rather than the individual having a more consistent attitude towards the friend.

Superego The superego refers to the internalization of attitudes of early caregivers, parents in particular. This develops into one's conscience and moral standards for oneself, as well as one's unconscious ideal version of oneself, the person one aims to become (the "ego ideal").

Transference The transference originally referred to distortions in the patient's perception of the analyst based on feelings, thoughts, impulses, and attitudes towards other important people in the patient's life that become displaced on to the analyst. In the broader contemporary sense, transference is taken to include all of the patient's experience of the analyst, including her accurate perceptions of him.

Unconscious The unconscious originally referred to a mental space where sexual and aggressive drives are located; a repository for childhood relational schemas (unconscious understanding of current relationships based on early relationships); where mental contents unacceptable to conscious awareness are repressed; and the location of defense mechanisms by which these mental contents are kept out of conscious awareness. A more contemporary view of the unconscious includes it being a source of energy, pleasure, and passion, creating experiences and meaning, a generative system with the capacity for creativity and an evolving sense of aliveness and the capacity to make a passionate commitment to life.

Inpatient and Day Hospital Psychiatry

INDEX

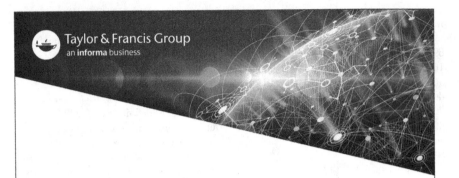

Printed in the United States
By Bookmasters